This volume summarises how recent exciting advances in immunology have cast new light on our understanding of autoimmune endocrine disease. These diseases range from relatively common disorders such as diabetes and thyroid diseases to much rarer conditions. They all, however, provide challenges for the scientist and clinician alike in integrating the immunological basis of the problem with its medical consequences. This volume sets out to distil these scientific advances and highlights their role in clinical disorders.

The new developments in immunology and immunogenetics are clearly explained in the first two chapters as an introduction to understanding the aetiology and pathogenesis of autoimmunity. The remainder of the book details the autoimmune disorders which may affect individual endocrine organs. Each condition is dealt with in the same way, facilitating comparisons between these diseases, and particular emphasis is placed on the lessons learned from animal models of endocrine autoimmunity.

The volume is a completely self-contained account and is suitable for all those with an interest in autoimmune disease, including clinicians, endocrinologists and immunologists.

Autoimmune endocrine disease

CAMBRIDGE REVIEWS IN CLINICAL IMMUNOLOGY

Series editors:

D.B.G. OLIVEIRA
Lister Institute Research Fellow, University of Cambridge, Addenbrooke's Hospital, Cambridge.

D.K. PETERS
Regius Professor of Physic, University of Cambridge, Addenbrooke's Hospital, Cambridge.

A.P. WEETMAN
Professor of Medicine, University of Sheffield Clinical Sciences Centre.

Recent advances in immunology, particularly at the molecular level, have led to a much clearer understanding of the causes and consequences of autoimmunity. The aim of this series is to make these developments accessible to clinicians who feel daunted by such advances and require a clear exposition of the scientific and clinical issues. The various clinical specialities will be covered in separate volumes, which will follow a fixed format: a brief introduction to basic immunology followed by a comprehensive review of recent findings in the autoimmune conditions which, in particular, will compare animal models with their human counterparts. Sufficient clinical detail, especially regarding treatment, will also be included to provide basic scientists with a better understanding of these aspects of autoimmunity. Thus each volume will be self-contained and comprehensible to a wide audience. Taken as a whole the series will provide an overview of all the important autoimmune disorders.

Autoimmune Endocrine Disease   A. P. Weetman

Immunological Aspects of Renal Disease   D. B. G. Oliveira

Autoimmune endocrine disease

ANTHONY P. WEETMAN
Professor of Medicine,
University of Sheffield Clinical Sciences Centre

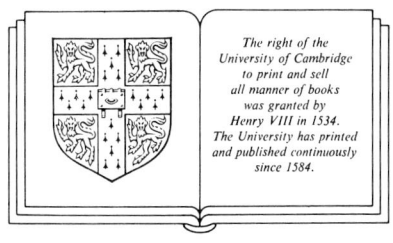

The right of the
University of Cambridge
to print and sell
all manner of books
was granted by
Henry VIII in 1534.
The University has printed
and published continuously
since 1584.

CAMBRIDGE UNIVERSITY PRESS

CAMBRIDGE
NEW YORK PORT CHESTER MELBOURNE
SYDNEY

Published by the Press Syndicate of the University of Cambridge
The Pitt Building, Trumpington Street, Cambridge CB2 1RP
40 West 20th Street, New York, NY 10011–4211, USA
10 Stamford Road, Oakleigh, Victoria 3166, Australia

First published 1991

Printed in Great Britain at the University Press, Cambridge

British Library cataloguing in publication data
Weetman, Anthony P.
  Autoimmune endocrine disease.
  1. Endocrine system. Diseases
  I. Title
  616.4079

Library of Congress cataloguing in publication data
Weetman, Anthony P.
  Autoimmune endocrine disease / Anthony P. Weetman.
    p.   cm. – (Cambridge reviews in clinical immunology)
  Includes bibliographical references.
  Includes index.
  1. Endocrine glands – Diseases – Immunological aspects.
2. Autoimmune diseases. I. Title. II. Series.
  [DNLM: 1. Autoimmmune Diseases – immunology. 2. Endocrine
Diseases – immunology.   WK 100 W398a]
RC649.W44   1991
616.97'8 – dc20   91-10959   CIP

ISBN 0 521 40161 5 hardback

Contents

Foreword

I was particularly pleased when Tony Weetman asked me to write a foreword to his monograph on autoimmune endocrine disease since as well as following his career as an undergraduate we had worked together in Newcastle and Cardiff over a number of years. It is appropriate first to examine his credentials to write this book. He obtained his general medical training in Newcastle and at the Royal Postgraduate Medical School in London and the Welsh National School of Medicine in Cardiff. His immunological interest developed following a first class honours B Med Sci in Newcastle when he trained in immunology with gastroenterology. After obtaining a first class honours MB, BS in Newcastle in 1977 he was awarded a distinction for his MD thesis on 'B Lymphocytes in Autoimmune Thyroid Disease'. He trained in clinical endocrinology with me and with Alan McGregor, Graham Joplin and Steve Bloom, and in clinical and laboratory immunology with Alan McGregor in Cardiff, Tony Fauci at the National Institutes of Health and Keith Peters in London and Cambridge. He was awarded a Wellcome Senior Research Fellowship in Clinical Science in 1985 and gave the 1991 Goulstonian Lecture at the Royal College of Physicians on 'Autoimmune thyroid disease'. He was appointed to the Sir Arthur Hall Chair of Medicine at the Northern General Hospital in Sheffield in 1991 where he succeeded Professor Donald Munro.

With this pedigree it would be difficult to find anyone more appropriate to produce this monograph on Autoimmune Endocrine Disease. It is the first of a series of Cambridge Reviews in Clinical Immunology edited by D. B. G. Oliveira, D. K. Peters and A. P. Weetman. The aim of the series is 'to make the recent advances in immunology, particularly at the molecular level, in the field of autoimmunity, understandable and accessible to the clinician' and also to provide sufficient clinical detail, especially relating to treatment, to provide a useful background to basic scientists. In this volume these objectives have been achieved remarkably well.

The first two chapters deal lucidly with the new developments in immunology and immunogenetics. The rest of the book outlines the impact of autoimmune disease on the different endocrine systems – the thyroid, type 1 diabetes mellitus, the adrenal, the gonads and the pituitary. There is a final chapter on polyendocrine autoimmunity. Each condition is dealt with in the same way with a brief introduction and sections on animal models of the disease, immunogenetics and environmental factors, T cell function, B cell responses, effector mechanisms and finally treatment, so comparison between the diseases is aided.

This volume is a model of clarity applying the lessons of basic immunology to the autoimmune endocrine diseases. I commend it to all of those with an interest in endocrine disease in general and autoimmune disease in particular including clinicians, endocrinologists and immunologists. It is an illustrious introduction to a new and exciting series.

R. Hall CBE, BSc, MD, FRCP
Professor of Medicine Emeritus
University of Wales College of Medicine
Cardiff

Preface

The purpose of this book is to give a comprehensive overview of recent research in autoimmune endocrine disease. These conditions vary from being common to extremely rare, with consequent disparity in the understanding of their aetiology and pathogenesis. Moreover, the results of research are published in a wide variety of journals covering immunology, endocrinology, diabetes and gynaecology. It therefore seemed worthwhile trying to assemble the information about all types of endocrinopathy in one volume. Generally, the features of autoimmune disease affecting each endocrine organ are considered under the same headings, preceded by an analysis of the data from animal models which have been crucial to the expansion of our knowledge.

The book is aimed at physicians involved in treating endocrine disorders, as well as basic researchers who are interested in a broad perspective of these forms of organ-specific autoimmunity. For the former, who may have found immunology and molecular biology cabbalistic, the first two chapters provide a synopsis of the immune response and immunogenetics and address specific issues raised in subsequent sections. The book has deliberately been written single-handed and as succinctly as possible. Obviously this has introduced some bias and loss of perspective, but I hope this is partly compensated for by allowing the development of a concise and homogenous structure which will facilitate comparisons between target organs. I have tried to include new references up to the autumn of 1990 and in general have cited reviews or new references summarising old work where possible.

I am grateful to many people who have shared their views with me and helped to shape those expressed here, particularly Professor Reg Hall, Professor Alan McGregor, Dr Anthony Fauci and Dr David Volkman. The support of Professor Keith Peters, the Medical Research Council and the Wellcome Trust has also been invaluable. More proximally, I am indebted to Mrs Barbara Langlois and Miss Kay Bynon for their expert secretarial skills. Finally, this book would not have been possible without the tolerance and encouragement of my wife and family.

Cambridge   Anthony Weetman

Abbreviations used

ACTH	adrenocorticotrophic hormone
ADCC	antibody-dependent cell-mediated cytotoxicity
APC	antigen presenting cell
Asp	aspartate
BB	Bio Breeding (rat strain)
C	constant region (T cell receptor or immunoglobulin); also a component of complement
CD	cluster of differentiation
CFA	complete Freund's adjuvant
D	diversity region (T cell receptor or immunoglobulin)
EAE	experimental allergic encephalomyelitis
EAT	experimental autoimmune thyroiditis
ELISA	enzyme-linked immunosorbent assay
Fab	fragment of immunoglobulin producing antigen binding (after papain digestion)
Fc	fragment of immunoglobulin which is crystallisable (after papain digestion); determines biological function
$FRTL_5$	Fischer rat thyroid cell line – 5
FSH	follicle stimulating hormone
HLA	human leucocyte antigen (equivalent to H-2 in the mouse)
hsp	heat shock protein
Ia	immune response associated (equivalent to MHC class II)
IFN	interferon
IL	interleukin
ICAb	islet cell cytoplasm antibody
ICAM	intercellular adhesion molecule
ICSAb	islet cell surface antibody
J	junctional region (T cell receptor or immunoglobulin)
LAK	lymphokine-activated killer
LATS	long acting thyroid stimulator
LATS-P	long acting thyroid stimulator-protector
LFA	lymphocyte function-associated antigen
LH	luteinising hormone

Lyt	a system of murine T lymphocyte antigens
MAC	membrane attack complex
MBP	myelin basin protein
MHC	major histocompatibility complex
MIF	migration inhibition factor
Mls	minor lymphocyte-stimulating
NK	natural killer
NOD	non-obese diabetic (mouse strain)
OS	Obese strain (of chicken)
PCR	polymerase chain reaction
RFLP	restriction fragment length polymorphism
SLE	systemic lupus erythematosus
T3	triiodothyronine
T4	thyroxine
TBII	TSH binding-inhibiting immunoglobulin
Tg	thyroglobulin
TNF	tumour necrosis factor
TPO	thyroid peroxidase
TSAb	thyroid-stimulating antibody
TSH	thyroid-stimulating hormone
V	variable region (T cell receptor or immunoglobulin)

–1–
The immune response and autoimmunity

In this chapter, the sequence of events in a normal immune response is detailed, from antigen uptake by accessory cells, through T cell stimulation, to antibody synthesis by B cells. These interactions allow the body to react to a myriad of foreign antigens; ideally this ought to occur without harmful recognition of autoantigens. The means by which such responses are normally prevented are reviewed, together with an appraisal of the potential causes of autoimmune disease when such mechanisms fail. In the final section, the effector limb of the immune response will be highlighted, with particular reference to autoreactive phenomena leading to tissue injury.

Antigen presentation

The classical antigen presenting cells (APC) are the macrophages and the function of these cells serves as a useful starting point for considering the immune response. There are three sequential steps in antigen handling by the macrophage: (i) antigen uptake, (ii) processing and (iii) presentation to the T cell (Fig. 1.1). The macrophage also secretes soluble mediators which enhance the effects of antigen presentation on T cells.

Antigen uptake

A soluble foreign antigen may be taken up by phagocytosis or pinocytosis, but for the induction of a productive immune response, the antigen must enter the APC via a receptor (Lorenz, Blum & Allen, 1990). This allows foreign antigens to be taken up in preference to potentially competing self antigens, thus preventing the mass of self proteins swamping the APC. Such receptors include those specific for mannose, complement and the Fc portion of immunoglobulins which may have bound to antigen, as well as low affinity lectin-like receptors that augment uptake of aggregated or precipitated antigen.

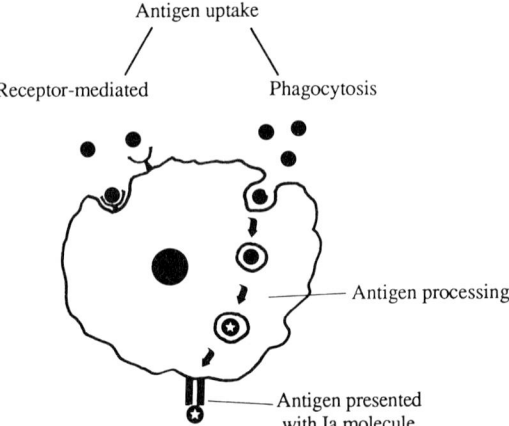

Fig. 1.1   The three steps of antigen presentation. Antigen is interna-
lised by the APC, in many cases by means of surface receptors, and
processed into peptide fragments which associate with Ia (or MHC class
II) molecules. The peptide/Ia complexes expressed on the APC surface
stimulate antigen-specific T cells.

Antigen processing

T cells only recognise peptide fragments of antigens. These determinants, or
epitopes, are around 12 amino acids in size, contrasting with the epitopes
recognised by B cells which usually comprise conformational determinants
depending on the tertiary structure of the intact antigen. The APC must
produce these peptide fragments by processing, a requirement dissected *in
vitro* by the use of lysosomotropic drugs like chloroquine (which make acid
vesicles alkaline) and by fixing macrophages with formaldehyde. These
techniques showed that the lysosome was an important site of antigen
processing and that this was complete within an hour, fixation thereafter
having no effect on APC function (Unanue, 1984). The exact mechanisms
involved in processing have not yet been identified, but lysosomes may be
particularly important for phagocytosed antigens, whereas endosomes may
contain proteases capable of degrading antigen taken up by receptor-
mediated endocytosis. Fusion of endocytic vesicles with others capable of
producing degradation is a further possibility (Lanzavecchia, 1990).

Antigen presentation to the T cell

Antigenic peptides must be associated with molecules encoded by the major
histocompatibility complex (MHC) before their recognition by T cells.

MHC molecules can be divided into two kinds: class I, encoded by the HLA-A, -B and -C regions of the MHC in man and class II, encoded by the HLA-DR, -DQ and -DP regions (discussed further in Chapter 2). This dichotomy in antigen presenting molecules is reflected by the existence of two subsets of T cells identifiable by their surface markers: CD8, for class I recognising T cells, and CD4, for class II recognising T cells (CD stands for cluster of differentiation, an expression given to certain phenotypic structures on the lymphocyte surface). After uptake and processing, soluble antigens are presented exclusively by class II MHC molecules (these are also called Ia molecules or antigens, a term derived from their original identification as *I*mmune response-*a*ssociated molecules). Presentation can even be mimicked *in vitro;* proteolytic fragments of an antigen (but not the intact molecule) will interact with class II molecules on a lipid monolayer and stimulate appropriate T cells (Babbitt *et al.*, 1986).

Analysis at a molecular level has demonstrated that there is physical binding of the antigenic peptide to the Ia molecule; these binding sites on the class II molecule for the peptide have been termed agretopes (Fig. 1.2; Heber-Katz, Hansburg & Schwartz, 1983). This was originally shown using a fluorescently labelled antigenic peptide, derived from hen egg lysozyme, which bound in a saturable and homogenous fashion to appropriate murine Ia molecules by equilibrium dialysis, whereas native lysozyme and peptides

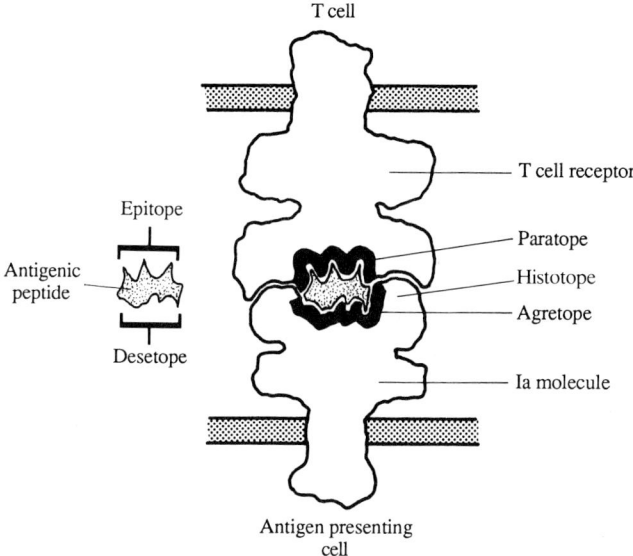

Fig. 1.2   Interaction of peptide/Ia complex with the T cell receptor. To the left is the peptide fragment alone indicating the epitope and desetope regions.

whose amino acids were altered did not bind (Babbitt *et al.*, 1985). Similar findings have been made in several other systems, which have also indicated that binding is rather slow. Ia may therefore exist in a storage compartment after synthesis to allow sufficient time to form a complex with antigenic peptide (Buus, Sette & Grey, 1987). The dissociation time is also long but is decreased by acidic pH; Ia may be recycled through lysosomes or acidic endosomal vesicles to remove peptides. The exact mechanisms and intracellular kinetics involved in Ia/peptide association and dissociation are unknown, but the non-polymorphic invariant chain linked to class II molecules seems essential to this process. The invariant chain may serve to transport the class II molecules (either nascent or derived from recycling) to the antigen processing compartment (Stockinger *et al.*, 1989).

As alluded to earlier, the APC can take up self antigens and peptides from self antigens can bind to class II molecules, thus competing with foreign antigens for presentation. However, self peptides capable of binding to free Ia molecules on the APC surface seem to be an insignificant source of interference and the uptake of foreign rather than self antigens for processing may be preferential. In addition, endogenous self peptides may be prevented from extensive Ia binding by compartmentalisation or by protection of the binding site by the invariant chain (Unanue *et al.*, 1989). Recent evidence suggests that this safeguard may not hold for all antigens, as endogenously synthesised influenza peptides can complex with Ia molecules in a pre-Golgi network compartment (Nuchtern, Biddison & Klausner, 1990).

The immunogenetic consequences of peptide/Ia interactions are considered in the next chapter. In the present context, it is evident that the amount of Ia expressed by an APC will be one key determinant of CD4$^+$ T cell stimulation; the concentration of antigenic peptide achieved after uptake and processing is another (Matis *et al.*, 1982). Macrophage Ia expression is not constitutive. For example, in the mouse it is confined to monocytes and young macrophages whereas mature cells become Ianegative (Unanue, 1984). However, a number of factors induce Ia expression and γ-interferon (γ-IFN) derived from stimulated T cells is the key lymphokine responsible (Steeg *et al.*, 1982). Several other modulators of macrophage Ia have been identified. In particular prostaglandins and hydrocortisone down-regulate Ia expression, which may have important consequences in inflammation and immunity (Unanue, 1984). Other inhibitors of macrophage Ia are α-fetoprotein, which could contribute to the immunological hyporesponsiveness required to protect the fetal allograft from rejection during pregnancy (Lu, Changelian & Unanue, 1984) and α- and β-IFN which are produced by macrophages and may thus act in an autocrine fashion to regulate Ia expression (Inaba *et al.*, 1986).

Costimulator release

Two other sets of molecules facilitate the interaction between APC and T cells: those involved in adhesion, which for convenience will be discussed in the context of T cell stimulation and the cytokines, which are required to drive activation and stimulation of T cells whose receptors have been triggered by antigen plus Ia. In fact, the archetypal leucocyte-derived cytokine or interleukin (IL), IL-1, was originally identified via the ability of stimulated macrophage supernatants to enhance T cell proliferation (Table 1.1; Gery, Gershon & Waksman, 1972). By modulating macrophage Ia or surface bound IL-1, an additive effect of these two molecules on antigen presentation to T cells can be shown (Kurt-Jones, Virgin & Unanue, 1985). Although macrophages are the main source of IL-1, it is now recognised that most cells can make this molecule (Di Giovine & Duff, 1990). Molecular cloning has identified at least two species, IL-1α and IL-1β, with dissimilar primary structures. These probably have different biological activities and in particular it may be that IL-1β acts in the fluid phase, whereas IL-1α is cell bound, but how cell-associated IL-1 relates to released IL-1 remains controversial. Proteolytic fragments of IL-1 may also have biological activity.

IL-1 displays an impressive collection of immunological and non-immunological actions (Le & Vilček, 1987; Di Giovine & Duff, 1990), but T cell activation remains the most distinctive. After triggering antigen receptors, T cell division is mediated exclusively by autocrine IL-2 release and IL-2 receptor expression (Meuer *et al.*, 1984) and both of these are stimulated by IL-1. This cytokine is central to the activation of resting T cells, those T cells already activated being variably dependent on IL-1 for optimal proliferation (Chu *et al.*, 1985). Other T cell activities, such as lymphokine release, may have less requirement for IL-1.

Macrophage IL-1 synthesis is stimulated by phagocytosis of micro-organisms. Uptake of soluble protein antigens has no direct effect, but their presentation to the T cell leads to release of T cell cytokines such as tumour necrosis factor (TNF), which indirectly stimulate production of IL-1. There is evidence that T cell–APC contact is also stimulatory (Weaver & Unanue 1986; Weaver, Duncan & Unanue, 1989). Further regulation of IL-1 synthesis could result from prostaglandin release or from specific IL-1 antagonists which are now being characterised (Larrick, 1989).

A second costimulator may have potentially greater importance than IL-1, based on the findings in adult mice that a subset of CD4$^+$ T cells fails to respond to an antigen after exposure to a high-dose intravenous injection of the antigen or antigen coupled to syngeneic spleen cells. This phenomenon could be due to stimulation of suppressor T cells or to the inactivation of

Table 1.1. *Major immunological effects of cytokines*

Cytokine[a]	Main Immune Effect[b]
IL-1	T cell activation (by IL–2 receptor expression and lymphokine release)
	Costimulates B cell growth and differentiation
	Enhanced NK cell activity
IL-2	T cell growth and lymphokine release
	B cell growth and differentiation
	Enhanced NK and cytotoxic T cell activity
IL-3	Stem cell growth
IL-4	B cell growth
	T cell growth
IL-5	B cell growth and differentiation (mouse)
	Eosinophil growth and differentiation (man)
IL-6	B cell differentiation
	T cell activation
IL-7	Early B cell growth
	Costimulates T cell growth
γ-IFN	Enhanced MHC class II (Ia) molecule expression
	Cofactor with other cytokines for multiple immune actions
TNF (from monocytes) and lymphotoxin (from T cells)	Enhanced MHC class I and class II molecule expression
	Stimulates IL-1 release and macrophage activation
TGF-β	Inhibits T cell and B cell proliferation
	Activates monocytes

[a]IL = interleukin, IFN = interferon, TNF = tumour necrosis factor, TGF = transforming growth factor.
[b]Only certain key activities are listed; many cytokines, particularly IL-1 and IL-6, have multiple non-immunological actions. Macrophages are the principal source of IL-1, TNF and TGF-β; T cells release the remaining cytokines.

responder T cells. *In vitro* experiments have favoured the latter explanation, mouse (and human) T cells remaining unresponsive in culture for up to eight days after exposure to high concentrations of peptide antigen or antigen-coupled splenocytes (Lamb & Feldmann, 1984; Jenkins & Schwartz, 1987). Similar unresponsiveness has been noted in T cells exposed to antigen on a class II-bearing planar lipid membrane (Quill & Schwartz, 1987).

IL-1 and a variety of other cytokines fail to reverse this T cell paralysis and it seems likely that an unidentified costimulator, which could be a soluble cytokine or an accessory molecule present on the macrophage cell surface, is required to activate a T cell once the peptide/Ia complex interacts with the T

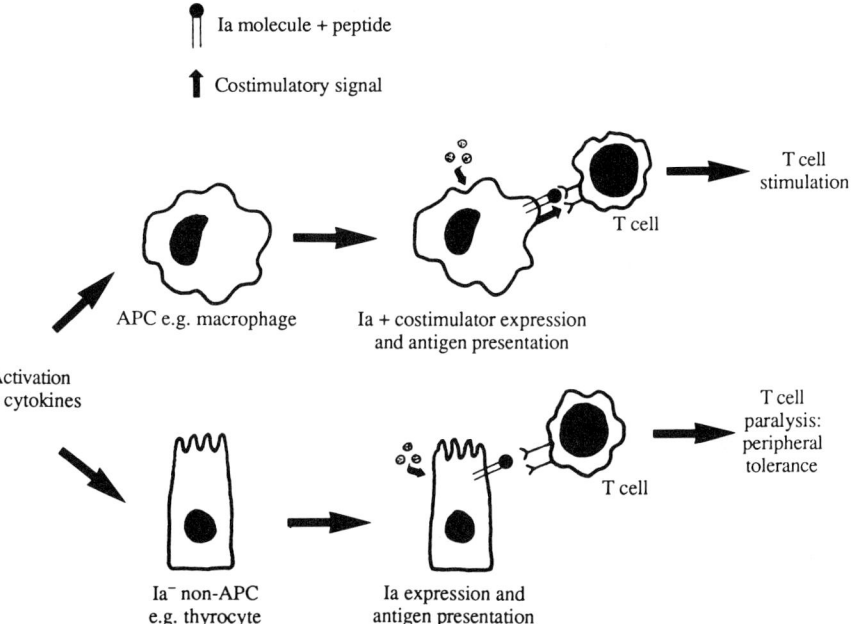

Fig. 1.3   Two forms of antigen presentation. The upper half shows conventional antigen presentation by an APC such as a macrophage, which can deliver a costimulatory signal to the T cell. Ia expression and antigen presentation by a non-classical APC, such as a beta cell or thyrocyte, may lead to T cell tolerance if the costimulator is not provided.

cell receptor (Fig. 1.3). In the absence of this costimulator, the T cell not only fails to divide but also becomes unresponsive to subsequent stimulation by APC. The biochemical events resulting in unresponsiveness are unknown, though they require active protein synthesis and depend on changes in intracellular calcium (Mueller, Jenkins & Schwartz, 1989). These changes are presumably reversed by the costimulator, which also may affect the IL-2 gene directly.

Antigen presentation by other cells

It is now clear that many other Ia^+ cells besides macrophages can present antigen. Lymphoid dendritic cells are of major importance in certain primary immune responses, considerably exceeding monocytes and macrophages in APC function (Van Voorhis *et al.*, 1983). In experiments testing other cell populations for APC function, even minor contamination with these potent dendritic cells can be a problem. Dendritic cells are widely dispersed throughout the body although they may form only a minor proportion of the lympho-reticular cells present in tissues (Austyn, 1987). It seems likely that many primary and memory T cell responses require dendritic cells as APC for initiation; thereafter, other APC, including macrophages, can induce T cell proliferation and lymphokine secretion (Inaba, Koide & Steinman, 1985). A second level of APC preference may also exist, since individual T cell clones respond to antigen presented either by dendritic cells or macrophages, but not both (Katz *et al.*, 1986). Moreover, dendritic cells may be unable to activate antigen-specific T helper cell responses to soluble antigens (Ramila *et al.*, 1985). Thus APC heterogeneity could be a selective mechanism determining T cell responses at the clonal level.

B cells can also present antigen (Chesnut & Grey, 1981; Lanzavecchia, 1985). Uniquely for APC, B cells have an inbuilt antigen specificity resulting from their cell surface immunoglobulins, which act as receptors for specific proteins. This allows efficient internalisation and processing of a considerable concentration of antigen for subsequent presentation to the T cell. In turn, the T cell will stimulate the same B cell, because of its proximity, to synthesise antibodies of the same specificity as the immunoglobulin receptor for antigen. B cell APC function can be enhanced by cytokines such as γ-IFN or TNF and this effect is not due to increased Ia expression or IL-1 synthesis; a reasonable assumption is that such cytokines stimulate expression of the costimulator signal (Hawrylowicz & Unanue, 1988). Resting B cells are inefficient APC which may relate to differences between these and activated B cells in the glycosylation of Ia molecules (Krieger *et al.*, 1988).

A variety of other cells may function as APC, including endothelial cells, fibroblasts transfected with genes to express Ia and activated T cells (Wagner, Vetto & Burger, 1985; Germain & Malissen, 1986; Lanzavecchia *et al.*, 1988). However, the effectiveness of these cells *in vivo* may be limited by their ability to capture sufficient antigen and differences in processing abilities between these cells and macrophages may also contribute to relative inefficiency. An added dimension here is the possible division of processing and presentation between cell populations. For instance, lymph node macrophages may process an antigen which is subsequently presented by germinal centre B cells (Szakal, Kosco & Tew, 1988). Finally, it is clear that Ia expression alone is not sufficient to enable a cell to present antigen. Keratinocytes express Ia molecules after γ-IFN treatment but are unable to activate T cells, inducing instead a state of T cell unresponsiveness (Gaspari, Jenkins & Schwartz, 1988). Once again, this has been related to the inability of these cells to provide a costimulator signal.

T cell stimulation

CD4$^+$ T cells recognise processed antigenic peptide combined with an Ia molecule by means of a T cell receptor specific for both antigen and Ia. This section describes the T cell receptor and the other accessory molecules which stabilise this interaction. The events following T cell stimulation are then discussed and finally the activation requirements for the CD8$^+$ T cell subset are considered.

The T cell receptor

More than 90% of mature T cells in man (including almost all those which are CD4$^+$ or CD8$^+$) express a clone-specific T cell receptor comprising an α and β glycoprotein chain, while the remaining T cells express a receptor comprising a γ and a δ chain (Davis, 1988). It is important to note that the receptor is not simply specific for antigenic peptide. It is also MHC-restricted, meaning that it will only be triggered by peptide plus a particular MHC molecule, which could be one of the many polymorphic class II molecules in the case of CD4$^+$ T cells (Rosenthal & Shevach, 1973). Both $\alpha\beta$ and $\gamma\delta$ forms of receptor are non-covalently linked to a complex of peptides with extracellular and intracellular domains termed CD3, which is responsible for signal transduction after receptor–ligand binding (Terhorst *et al.*, 1988). Besides CD3, transfection experiments have confirmed that both chains of the receptor are required for recognition of antigen (Saito *et al.*, 1987).

The T cell receptor, like the MHC class I and II molecules, is a member of the immunoglobulin supergene family (Williams & Barclay, 1988). This group of molecules usually has a cell surface recognition role and shares in common an immunoglobulin-like domain. In the case of the T cell receptor, there are two extracellular immunoglobulin-related domains on each chain, the distal variable (V) region and the more proximal constant (C) region. These are linked to a hydrophobic transmembrane region and a short intracytoplasmic tail. There are from 50 to 100 Vα and 75 to 100 Vβ gene segments which contribute to the diversity of T cell receptors. This heterogeneity is increased by the presence of α and β junctional (J) and β diversity (D) segments which rearrange during T cell differentiation to form the contiguous gene. Thus a huge repertoire of specific T cell receptors can be produced to recognise the peptide/Ia complex, using all the mechanisms available to B cells to generate immunoglobulin diversity, with the exception of somatic mutation (Table 1.2; Fink *et al.*, 1986).

T cells expressing $\gamma\delta$ T cell receptors are usually CD4$^-$, CD8$^-$ ('double-negative') but can express a wide variety of other T cell-related surface

Table 1.2. *Sequence diversity generated by human T cell receptor (TCR) genes*

	$\alpha\beta$ TCR		$\gamma\delta$ TCR	
	α	β	γ	δ
V segments	50–100	75–100	9	6
D segments	–	2	–	3
J segments	60–80	13	5	3
N segments	V-J	V-D, D-J	V-J	V-D, D_3-J plus D_1-D_2 and D_2-D_3

molecules and in man are distributed throughout the lymphoid system (Groh *et al.*, 1989). In the mouse, however, these cells seem particularly localised to epithelia and display restricted receptor heterogeneity at these sites (Augustin, Kubo & Sim, 1989). The V domains of the γ and δ chains are not as diverse as those of the $\alpha\beta$ receptor, with only nine Vγ and six Vδ gene segments, and there are also a smaller number of Jγ and Jδ segments (Strominger, 1989). However, imprecision of joining, the presence of three D regions and the addition of nucleotides (N region addition) between the V, D and J segments generate considerable δ chain diversity.

The function of T cells expressing the $\gamma\delta$ receptor is unknown. There is some evidence that they are restricted to the recognition of antigen presented by MHC-encoded molecules with limited polymorphism, termed class Ib (Bonneville *et al.*, 1989; Vidovic *et al.*, 1989), but this has been called into question by the finding of normal $\gamma\delta$ T cell numbers in transgenic mice incapable of making class I MHC molecules (Zijlstra *et al.*, 1990). One suggestion is that these T cells recognise a limited number of autologous 'indicator peptides', the best examples of which are the heat shock proteins (Born *et al.*, 1990). These highly conserved proteins occur in all organisms. They can be released from cells by diverse stresses including inflammation and are immunodominant antigens in certain infective organisms, especially mycobacteria. Thus recognition of autologous heat shock proteins by $\gamma\delta^+$ T cells could be important in the immune surveillance of epithelia and the regulation of other lymphocytes, while their response to heterologous heat shock proteins would provide a defence against particular micro-organisms.

Accessory molecules

Several other molecules augment the interaction of T cell receptor with Ia plus peptide by facilitating adhesion (Fig. 1.4; Springer *et al.*, 1987;

Makgoba, Sanders & Shaw, 1989). The major contributors are CD2 and its ligand lymphocyte function-associated antigen-3 (LFA-3), and LFA-1 and its ligands intercelluar adhesion molecule-1 (ICAM-1) and ICAM-2. LFA-1 (or CD11a/CD18) is a member of the integrin molecular family and is widely expressed by bone marrow-derived cells. The other three adhesion molecules belong to the immunoglobulin supergene family. CD2 is restricted to T cells whereas LFA-3 is found on almost all cells, independent of their state of activation. ICAM-1 has a restricted tissue distribution, mainly confined to APC, lymphocytes and endothelium, but its expression can be enhanced and induced on other cells by a variety of cytokines. Less is known currently about the distribution and regulation of ICAM-2.

The key feature of these molecules is that they facilitate the binding of a T cell to its target, which could be an APC like a macrophage, or a virally infected cell destined for killing by a cytotoxic cell. The adhesion between T cell and APC precedes the interaction between T cell receptor and the Ia/peptide complex. This initial adherence is unstable, but if the T cell receptor does engage the appropriate ligand, the LFA-1 molecule on the T cell is converted to a high avidity state which favours stable LFA-1/ICAM-1 adhesion. In the absence of T cell receptor ligation, LFA-1 remains in a low avidity state and this allows the T cell to become mobile again, free to seek its appropriate antigen trigger (Dustin & Springer, 1989). Another outcome of adhesion molecule interactions is to amplify the T cell response, the binding of CD2 and LFA-1 to their ligands providing activation signals, which for CD2, but not LFA-1, are independent of CD3 (Hunig et al., 1987; Wacholtz, Patel & Lipsky, 1989).

A subsidiary group of adhesion molecules exists, originally thought to mediate lymphocyte homing to certain organs. These include the complement receptor CR3 (CD11b), another leucocyte integrin which may bind to ICAM-1, and the VLA-4 and MEL-14 antigens whose ligands are unknown (Kuypers & Roos, 1989; Makgoba et al., 1989). CD44, previously known (amongst other names) as the Hermes molecule, is widely distributed but is acquired by T cells during differentiation and may augment T cell–target cell binding, as well as modulate CD2-LFA-3 interactions (Haynes et al., 1989).

The T cell-associated molecule CD4 is yet another member of the immunoglobulin supergene family, in this case a 55 kd single chain glycoprotein with four extracellular domains. CD4 almost certainly binds to a non-polymorphic region of the APC Ia molecule (Fig. 1.4), thus stabilising the interaction with the T cell receptor, although this has not been shown directly (Bierer et al., 1989). The function of CD4 as an accessory molecule may be more complex than this, however, since there is evidence that engagement of CD4 triggers a particular tyrosine kinase which could be important in modifying the subsequent T cell response (Robey & Axel,

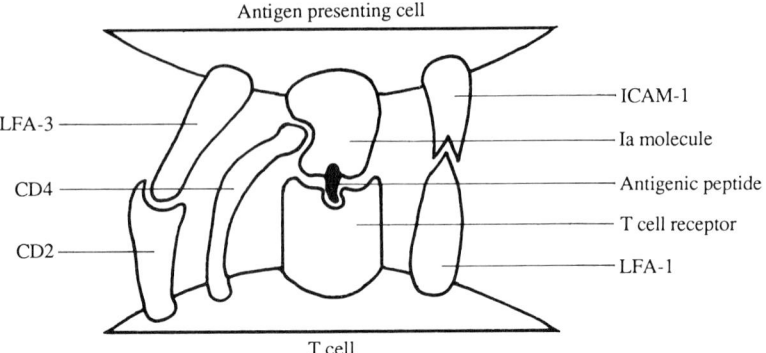

Fig. 1.4   Major adhesion molecules in APC-CD4⁺ T cell interaction. Cytolytic CD8⁺ T cells use the same molecules, except that CD8 replaces CD4 and stabilises the T cell receptor interaction with class I MHC molecules, which present endogenous peptide on a target cell.

1990). It is likely that CD4 and CD8 have evolved to allow the immune system to develop two distinct types of response, helper and killer, broadly restricted by the class II and class I molecules respectively. This division arises intrathymically during ontogeny, but it is not clear whether CD4 and CD8 direct separate differentiation pathways, or whether T cells are selected within the thymus by their ability to recognise a particular class of MHC molecules and this subsequently dictates function.

CD4⁺ T cell function

CD4⁺ T cells are often equated with helper T cells but while this is often the case, there is compelling evidence for the existence of suppressor and cytotoxic CD4⁺ T cells (Krensky *et al.*, 1982; Silver, Scott & Quill, 1989). Instead, CD4 expression should be thought of as the class II MHC restriction molecule of the T cell. Experiments on cloned murine T cells suggest a functional dichotomy in the CD4⁺ population, 'helper' cells effectively stimulating B cell antibody production and 'inflammatory' cells providing protection against micro-organisms (Mosmann & Coffman, 1989). The two CD4⁺ subsets produce discrete sets of cytokines which account for these functional differences (Table 1.3). In particular, helper T cells produce IL-4, IL-5 and IL-6, which cause murine B cell proliferation and differentiation, whereas the other subset produces γ-IFN, lymphotoxin and TNF which may mediate delayed type hypersensitivity reactions and killing of intracellular pathogens. However, it is not yet clear whether a similar dichotomy exists in man, and many human and murine CD4⁺ T cell clones appear capable of producing a mixed pattern of cytokine release. One possible explanation for this anomaly is that CD4⁺ T cells begin with one phenotype and function

Table 1.3. *Cytokine release by murine T helper cell subsets*

	TH1 (Inflammatory T cells)	TH2 (B helper T cells)
IL-2	++	−
IL-3	++	++
IL-4	−	++
IL-5	−	++
IL-6	−	++
γ-IFN	++	−
TNF	++	+
Lymphotoxin	++	−

and that some of these mature to become one of several potential CD4$^+$ subsets; the density of ligand binding to the T cell receptor could modulate this development (Bottomly *et al.*, 1989).

A second type of functional subdivision of human CD4$^+$ T cells has been proposed based on monoclonal antibodies which define surface markers, 'suppressor-inducer' CD4$^+$ T cells staining with the 2H4 monoclonal antibody and 'helper-inducer' CD4$^+$ T cells staining with the 4B4 antibody (Morimoto *et al.*, 1985). It is now known that 2H4 recognises the RA isoform of CD45, the leucocyte common (or T200) antigen. Another isoform, CD45R0, is recognised by the monoclonal antibody UCHL1 and stains the reciprocal CD4$^+$ subset, identical to that defined by the 4B4 reagent (which recognises CD29, one of the β chains of the integrin family of molecules). There is now strong evidence that the CD45RA$^+$ subset represents naïve CD4$^+$ T cells, whereas the CD45R0$^+$, CD29$^+$ subset comprises both memory and activated CD4$^+$ T cells (Sanders, Makgoba & Shaw, 1988; Beverley, Merkenschlager & Wallace, 1989). As would be expected, the latter population expands from birth to maturity and this process can also be observed *in vitro* upon stimulation of naïve T cells. Thus these apparently discrete subsets of inducer cells are in fact different maturational stages of the CD4$^+$ population, expressing different functions at different times (Table 1.4). Whether other markers (e.g. Leu 8, which occurs on non-helper T cells) identify subsets within the mature population that represent developmental stages or stable lineages is unclear.

CD8$^+$ T cell activation and function

As already mentioned, CD8$^+$ T cells recognise antigen presented by class I MHC molecules, and are often termed the cytotoxic (and suppressor) T cell

Table 1.4. *Properties of naïve and memory CD4$^+$ T cells*

	Naïve cells	Memory/Activated cells
1. Phenotype		
CD45RA	+ +	− or +
CD45R0 (UCHL1)	−	+ +
CD29	−	+ +
Ia	−	± to + +
2. Lymphokine production		
IL-2	+ +	+ +
IL-3	+	+ +
IL-4	−	+
γ-IFN	±	+ +
3. Function		
Proliferation to:		
(i) Recall antigens	±	+ +
(ii) Lectins	+ +	+
(iii) CD3 cross-linking	+	+ +
Effect on B cells		
(i) Help for antibody production	−	+ +
(ii) Induction of suppressors after mitogen stimulation	+ +	−

lineage. As for the CD4$^+$ subset, this equation of phenotype with function is by no means absolute. The α and β T cell receptor genes used by CD8$^+$ T cells are the same as those used by the CD4$^+$ population, emphasising that these are two highly homologous, overlapping subpopulations. The prime role of CD8$^+$ T cells seems to be reactivity against endogenous antigens whose epitopes are synthesised in the cytoplasm of the cellular target.

The archetypal example of such a target is a cell infected with a virus; the viral antigens are synthesised intracellularly, partially degraded to peptides at an undefined site and complexed with MHC class I molecules. Once expressed on the cell surface, this antigen/MHC class I complex will be recognised by a specific CD8$^+$ T cell and the infected cell then killed (Zinkernagel & Doherty, 1975; Townsend *et al.*, 1988). The ability of class II MHC molecules to use this endogenous pathway, in addition to their more usual pathway for recognising exogenous antigens, has already been mentioned. A dramatic feature of the process is the apparent ability of antigenic peptides with binding sites for class I molecules to determine the correct folding of the α chains of these molecules, as well as their association with β2-microglobulin and their transport to the cell surface (Townsend *et al.*,

1989). Thus there seem to be two main responses in the immune system: (i) helper, leading to antibody formation and mediated because an exogenous antigen is presented by class II molecules and (ii) cytotoxic, leading to killing of the target cell and usually mediated because endogenously synthesised antigen is presented by class I molecules.

Like CD4, CD8 is required to produce efficient antigen recognition by the T cell receptor, probably dependent on the association of the CD8 intra-cellular domain with the same tyrosine kinase as CD4 (Robey & Axel, 1990). CD8 may still transduce different signals to CD4 by using an alternative kinase substrate, or by stimulating an additional pathway. It is now clear that CD8 does act as a co-receptor for the MHC class I molecule, and the binding site has been mapped to the third domain on the α chain (Salter et al., 1990). By generating point mutants of a class I gene transfected into a target, it was also shown that cytotoxic T cell recognition of the transfectants correlated with the degree of CD8 binding, and that CD8 and the T cell receptor bound to the same class I molecule.

While cytotoxic function seems generally agreed on, the phenomenon of T cell-mediated suppression has become a matter of extreme controversy. Various levels of $CD8^+$ T cell-mediated immunoregulation that suppress delayed type hypersensitivity in the mouse have been analysed in great detail (Dorf & Benacerraf, 1984). On the other hand, some have gone so far as to question the very existence of suppressor cells (Möller, 1988) and certainly the cause of T suppressor cells was not helped by the fact that their apparently MHC-encoded marker in mice, I-J, is now known not to exist within the MHC (Murphy, 1987). However, this enigma has been remedied to a certain extent by the biochemical identification of I-J as a novel dimer which is expressed by helper as well as suppressor T cell clones, although its ligand remains unknown (Nakayama et al., 1989).

Recent developments in cloning techniques have led to the isolation of several T cell clones with suppressor function. In particular a distinct suppressor cell growth factor derived from monocytes (plus prostaglandin E_2 and γ-IFN) appears to be necessary for differentiation of human $CD8^+$ suppressor cells, following their initial stimulation by $CD4^+$ inducer cells and IL-2 (Rich, ElMasry & Fox, 1986; ElMasry, Fox & Rich, 1987). Suppressor cells generated in this fashion can inhibit the proliferative response of $CD4^+$ T cells to pokeweed mitogen, a non-specific stimulus causing division of all $CD4^+$ T cells.

Antigen-specific $CD8^+$ suppressor cell clones have been established from patients with leprosy, capable of inhibiting $CD4^+$ T cell proliferation induced by Mycobacterium leprae (Modlin et al., 1987). These clones appear to use the normal $\alpha\beta$ T cell receptor. Furthermore, the suppressor cells appear to recognise specific antigen in a MHC-restricted fashion, but their effect is not necessarily specific or MHC-restricted; they appear to induce

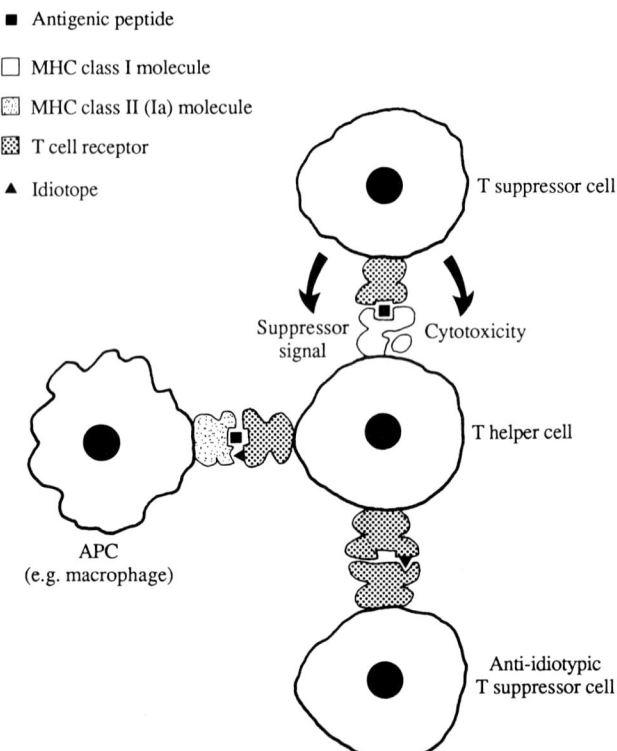

■ Antigenic peptide

☐ MHC class I molecule

▨ MHC class II (Ia) molecule

▩ T cell receptor

▲ Idiotope

T suppressor cell

Suppressor signal   Cytotoxicity

T helper cell

APC
(e.g. macrophage)

Anti-idiotypic
T suppressor cell

Fig. 1.5   Three possible modes of suppressor cell action. The upper CD8$^+$ suppressor cell is stimulated by peptide presented in the context of a MHC class I molecule by the CD4$^+$ T helper cell. This may trigger release of specific or non-specific suppressor factors. Alternatively, the suppressor cell may be cytotoxic and kill the helper cell in a specific and MHC-restricted fashion. The T cell receptor of lower suppressor cell interacts anti-idiotypically with an idiotope on the helper T cell receptor and may thus inhibit T helper function. Support for this mechanism comes from attenuation of experimental autoimmune disease by anti-idiotypic T cells, generated in response to immunisation with peptides which correspond to idiotypic determinants on the helper T cell receptor.

inactivation or anergy in the CD4$^+$ population by an unknown mechanism (Salgame, Modlin & Bloom, 1989). Other explanations for T suppressor cell effects include: (i) release of antigen-specific suppressor factors (Asherson, Colizzi & Zembala, 1986), (ii) cytotoxicity to helper cells (Lanzavecchia, 1989) and (iii) reactivity of the suppressor cells against the variable region (idiotype) of the T cell receptor on the target clone (Fig. 1.5), thus behaving as anti-idiotypic cells (Batchelor, Lombardi & Lechler, 1989). However, *in vitro* experiments on T suppressor cells are fraught with problems providing more trivial explanations for inhibitory effects, such as cell crowding and competition for growth factors (Palacios & Möller, 1981). It is also apparent that either CD4$^+$ or CD8$^+$ T cells may become suppressor cells, and that there is considerable leeway for changing function during an individual cell's development, depending on ambient conditions (Melchers & Rzepka, 1988; Batchelor *et al.*, 1989). These difficulties make the molecular analysis of T suppressor cell function exceedingly difficult, although there can be little doubt of the phenomenon of suppression itself.

B cells and antibody production

Each B cell expresses a novel surface immunoglobulin or antibody, capable of unique binding to an antigen and generated by a variety of mechanisms to induce diversity. The regulation of B cell development, from a resting state to a plasma cell secreting immunoglobulin, generally depends upon antigen recognition (via surface immunoglobulin) followed by proliferation and differentiation in response to cytokines. This sequence will be considered in detail below.

Immunoglobulin structure and function

A typical immunoglobulin molecule, the prototype product of the immuno-globulin supergene family, consists of two identical heavy chains and two identical light chains linked by disulphide bonds. The amino terminus in both sets of chains contains a V region domain (analogous to the T cell receptor). These form the antigen binding site and thus create the specificity of the antibody. Each light chain has a single C domain, whereas the heavy chain has three such C domains: these determine the effector function of the molecule.

The control of immunoglobulin genomic rearrangements and the mech-anisms involved in generating the huge diversity of the antibody repertoire have been defined in detail (Alt, Blackwell & Yancopoulos, 1987). In essence this is achieved by (i) recombination between the already diverse V, D and J gene segments (Table 1.5), (ii) N-region sequence heterogeneity at the heavy chain VDJ and light chain VJ junctions, (iii) pairing of different heavy and light chains and (iv) somatic mutation which changes nucleotides within the V region. The latter is an active process that characteristically generates antibodies of altered affinity and occurs late in the immune response, during immunoglobulin class switching. Similar mechanisms, with

Table 1.5. *Sequence diversity generated by human immunoglobulin genes*

	Heavy chain	Light chain (kappa)[a]
V segments[b]	100–200	90–100
D segments	30	–
J segments	6	5
N segments	V-D, D-J	V-J

[a]Less information available for lambda light chains.
[b]Diversity is increased by somatic mutation within the hypervariable regions.

the exception of somatic mutation, are used to generate T cell receptor diversity. Both molecules exhibit tremendous heterogeneity, but the emphasis appears to be on the generation of V region diversity for B cells and J region diversity for T cells, which may in turn relate to different sites of antigen interaction.

There are two types of light chain, kappa (κ) and lambda (λ), which vary in their C domains. Greater variability in the heavy chain C domains produces a number of different isotypes or immunoglobulin classes and subclasses (Table 1.6): both κ and λ light chains associate with each isotypic heavy chain. These isotypes serve different biological functions. For instance, IgM is produced typically during the primary phase of an immune response to an antigen and IgG is the main class of antibody in a secondary response. The four IgG subclasses show major differences in biological properties and this heterogeneity within the IgG may also be important in a secondary response, determining complement fixation and binding to cell surface Fc receptors (Burton, Gregory & Jefferis, 1986). For the heavy chain isotypes (except the δ chain of IgD), class switching is produced by means of a unique switch region preceding each C gene segment. This allows more distal 3' end C genes to link to VDJ genes, instead of the most proximal 3' gene: Cμ and intervening C region genes are lost in the process. Class switching is at least in part controlled by T cell-derived cytokines, although the clearest definition of this is in the mouse rather than man (Finkelman *et al.*, 1990).

Idiotypes and anti-idiotypes

An idiotype is a set of antigenic determinants, or idiotopes, on the V region of an antibody, usually involving both heavy and light chains. Because of the extensive diversity of immunoglobulins, the immune system has antibodies in its repertoire which bind these idiotopes, so called anti-idiotypic antibodies. These in turn can generate the formation of anti-anti-idiotypes (Fig.

Table 1.6. *Major characteristics of the human immunoglobulin isotypes*

Isotype	Approx MW (kd)	Serum concentration (g/l)	Function
IgG_1	145	10	Secondary immune response to T cell-dependent antigens; opsonise, fix complement (in the order $IgG_3 > IgG_1 > IgG_2 \gg IgG_4$) and bind to Fc receptors ($IgG_1 = IgG_3 > IgG_4 \gg IgG_2$)
IgG_2	145	3	
IgG_3	170	1	
IgG_4	145	0.5	
		(Total IgG 7–19)	
IgA_1	160	3	Mucosal immunity, when secreted with a secretory component; present in colostrum.
IgA_2	160	0.5	
		(Total IgA 0.8–5.0)	
IgM	970	115 (0.5–2.0)	Primary immune response; fix complement
IgD	185	0.03	Unknown: cell surface receptor?
IgE	190	<0.0001	Protection against parasites; mediates Type I acute hypersensitivity

1.6). The result is a network maintaining a steady state of antibody interaction (Jerne, 1974; Geha, 1981). Introduction of antigen leads to stimulation of idiotypic antibody synthesis, which, in the simplest case, then stimulates anti-idiotype formation and restores the equilibrium.

As already discussed, similar idiotypic–anti-idiotypic interactions may operate for T cells via their receptors and anti-idiotypic antibodies may modulate T cell as well as B cell function by interacting with T cell receptor idiotopes. There are two main types of anti-idiotypic antibodies, those which actually interact with the antigen binding site (or paratope) on the idiotype and those which interact with other idiotopes on the V region that are not associated with antigen binding. These will have different immuno-regulatory properties and roles in disease.

B cell activation

Although certain antigens like lipopolysaccharide can activate B cells directly, antibody responses to the great majority of antigens require the

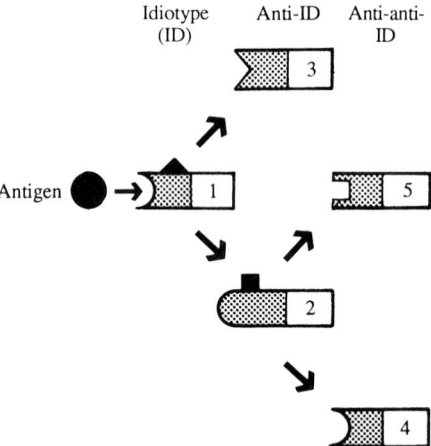

Fig. 1.6 Antibody idiotype network. Antigen stimulates the production of an idiotype (ID), antibody 1. This example has two idiotopes
or antigenic determinants in the variable region (dotted area). One is in
the antigen binding site (or paratope) and this may lead to the formation
of an anti-ID, antibody 2, which thus has an internal image of the
antigen in its paratope. The second idiotope is outside the paratope and
is shown as a triangle. The anti-ID against this idiotope, antibody 3, has
a paratope which does not resemble the antigen. The anti-IDs, 2 and 3,
can give rise to further antibodies called anti-anti-IDs. Antibodies 4 and
5 are anti-anti-IDs for antibody 2 and again these may recognise
structures inside or outside the paratope.

participation of helper T cells. This constitutes the initial step in B cell
activation and depends upon intimate contact between the T and B cell,
which is probably due to interaction between the helper T cell receptor and
B cell-processed antigen plus Ia molecule (Howard, 1985; Lanzavecchia,
1985). After initial interaction with antigen, progress of the B cell through
the sequential stages of proliferation and differentiation is antigen-
independent and results from non-specific lymphokine secretion by the
helper T cell (Fig. 1.7). Local lymphokine delivery to the appropriate,
specific B cell results from conjugate formation between the two cells (Swain
& Dutton, 1987).

Several model systems have been used *in vitro* to investigate the regulation of B cell development. These have bypassed the initial requirement
for antigen by using mitogens, in particular those which mimic the action of
antigens by cross-linking the B cell surface immunoglobulin (Kehrl et al.,
1984). Although such studies originally suggested the existence of discrete
factors controlling the separate stages of B cell development, recent work
with recombinant products has shown considerable overlap in the activities

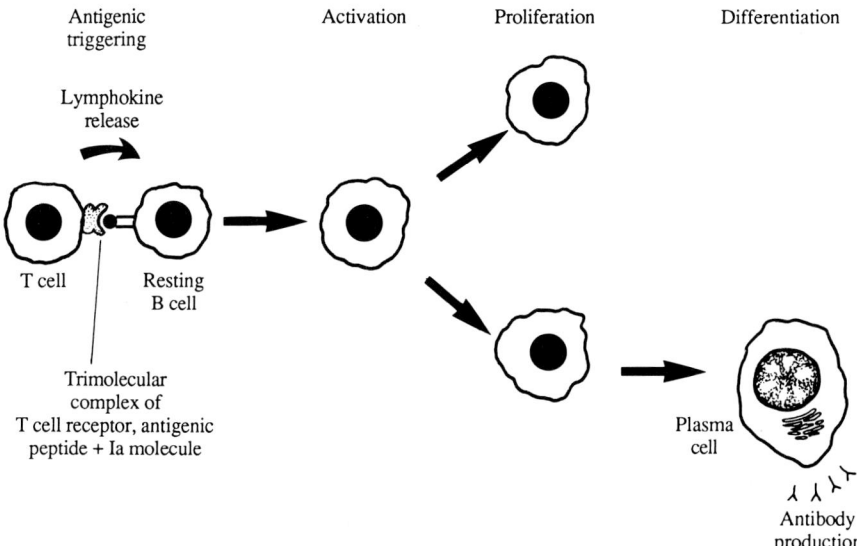

Fig. 1.7 B cell stimulation. Resting B cells require activation by antigen as the first step in becoming mature plasma cells. Local delivery of lymphokines, especially IL-4 and IL-6, by conjugated T cells drives the B cell through the stages of proliferation and differentiation to become capable of antibody production. The requirements for antigen and T cells can be overcome *in vitro* by cross-linking B cell surface immunoglobulins and supplying the necessary lymphokines.

of these lymphokines, which act at more than one point in the activation pathway and can modulate other cell types besides the B cell (Kishimoto & Hirano, 1988). This lack of specificity may not be a problem in the case of localised delivery mentioned above.

The principal cytokines produced by T cells and monocytes are detailed in Table 1.1 and indeed most have some effect on B cells (Balkwill & Burke, 1989). There are certain important species differences (for instance, IL-5 in man causes eosinophil activation, but stimulates murine B cells). Activated human B cells proliferate in response to IL-4 and this is enhanced by γ-IFN; many other cytokines costimulate this, including IL-1, IL-2, IL-6, TNF, lymphotoxin and several uncharacterised growth factors. Differentiation seems primarily dependent on IL-6 but this too is costimulated by IL-1, IL-2 and γ-IFN. Transforming growth factor-β inhibits both proliferation and differentiation.

Thus the normal B cell population comprises cells at a variety of developmental stages. In addition, two subsets exist which, in the mouse at least, are separate lineages. The majority of peripheral B cells in the adult mouse derives from progenitors in the spleen and bone marrow, but a minor subset, found mainly in the peritoneum, strangely expresses the T cell marker Lyt-1 and this cell type is highly enriched in neonates (Hayakawa, Hardy & Herzenberg, 1985). There is a corresponding subset in man which also expresses a typically T cell-associated marker, CD5, and these comprise up to 20% of the circulating B cells (Casali & Notkins, 1989). This population of cells produces mainly low affinity, polyreactive IgM antibodies directed against a variety of self and foreign antigens, including so-called natural autoantibodies, which may remove damaged cell components (Grabar, 1975) or act as a first line of defence against pathogens. In certain circumstances, such as rheumatoid arthritis or murine models of systemic lupus erythematosus, these self-reactive antibodies may contribute to the pathogenesis of autoimmune disease (Casali & Notkins, 1989). However, most autoimmune diseases result in the production of high affinity, monoreactive IgG autoantibodies derived from CD5$^-$ B cells, which have been positively selected for antigen after V region somatic mutation.

Discrimination between self and non-self

Ideally an animal should mount a response against each and every foreign antigen yet fail to react to self antigens. Originally it was thought that the possibility of self reactivity could not exist (the 'horror autotoxicus' of Ehrlich) but it is now clear that self recognition provides the very basis for the induction of tolerance to autoantigens during ontogeny and that this process continues throughout life in various networks of immunoregulation which maintain self tolerance. Paradoxically, it is the failure of appropriate self recognition which results in autoimmune disease. The mechanisms producing T cell tolerance acquisition in the developing thymus have become clearer recently, particularly through experiments on transgenic mice. By stably transferring new or altered genes into mouse embryos, lineages of adult animals can be analysed to determine how the immune system deals with these novel antigens, as discussed below. Tolerance produced in the thymus is probably incomplete in all animals and in any case may be bypassed, for instance by pathogens. However, back-up mechanisms exist which operate to prevent autoreactivity and these will be treated separately.

Tolerance induction in the thymus

T or B cell tolerance is produced in one of two ways: deletion and the imposition of a state of unresponsiveness or anergy. T cells are mainly subject to the first of these and B cells to the second (Nossal, 1989; Schwartz, 1989). The thymus has a fundamental role in selecting and tolerising T cells and this function is probably invested in both the thymic epithelium and the accessory cells of bone marrow origin (Salaün *et al.*, 1990). It is believed that the recognition of self peptides plus self MHC in ontogeny deletes what would otherwise be autoreactive T cells.

Two lines of evidence support this. The first depends on the analysis of the T cell receptor repertoire using monoclonal antibodies. T cells whose receptors express a particular β chain V segment (Vβ17a) are found in strains of mice which do not have the I-E MHC class II molecule, whereas Vβ17a$^+$ T cells are scarce in F_1 crosses with mice expressing I-E. Staining T cells for Vβ17a showed that these cells were lost in the F_1 animals as they matured in the thymus, and this resulted from tolerisation to I-E plus some unknown self peptide (Marrack *et al.*, 1988). Confirmation of this phenomenon has come from transgenic experiments. Transgenic mice were created whose cytotoxic T cells should preferentially express a receptor recognising the male transplantation antigen H-Y. In female animals about 15% of the peripheral CD8$^+$ T cells express the transgenic receptor for H-Y whereas such T cells are exceedingly rare in male mice (Kisielow *et al.*, 1988). In the male mice (which, unlike the females, will constitutively express the H-Y antigen), the cytotoxic transgenic cells which would respond to H-Y are deleted in the thymus. A few cells in fact escape this process, but these have low levels of surface CD8, which may compromise their self reactivity.

This process of negative selection occurs at a precursor stage when the T cells express both CD4 and CD8. As a result, class II MHC molecules in the fetal thymus can influence the repertoire of cells which will become CD8$^+$, as well as those destined to be CD4$^+$ (Fowlkes, Schwartz & Pardoll, 1988; Kisielow *et al.*, 1988). Because of deletion, the vast majority of immature small cortical thymocytes do not survive and this process of activation-driven cell death may depend upon expression of new gene products which are associated with genome fragmentation (Ucker, Ashwell & Nickas, 1989). Intrathymic elimination of self-reactive T cells also applies to $\gamma\delta$ receptor-bearing T cells (Dent *et al.*, 1990).

Experiments on transgenic mice have also demonstrated a second, positive selection process for T cells, biasing them towards recognition of particular MHC products. Proof of this comes from mice whose transgenic T cell receptor recognises antigen presented by a particular MHC molecule. In such animals there is considerable enrichment of T cells expressing this receptor if they develop in a thymic environment which also expresses the MHC molecule (Sha *et al.*, 1988). For instance, the MHC molecule H-2D^b is a class I restricting element for the H-Y antigen recognised by the cytotoxic T cell receptor in the transgenic mice described above. These cytotoxic T cells are positively expanded in females which are H-2D^b-positive, whereas in mice of other strains, expressing a different MHC molecule, this does not occur (Teh *et al.*, 1988).

Added complexity is provided by the existence within the thymus of a non-deletional mechanism for inducing tolerance, namely clonal anergy. This has been clearly demonstrated for a strain-specific group of murine self antigens called Mls (minor lymphocyte-stimulating). T cells reacting against these utilise particular $V\beta$ receptor gene segments. The Mls–1[a] antigen is recognised by T cells expressing the $V\beta6$ receptor; immunising Mls–1[b] mice with Mls–1[a] expressing cells induces anergy (rather than deletion) in the $V\beta6^+$ T cells of the recipient (Rammensee, Kroschewski & Frangoulis, 1989). The creation of chimeric animals has shown that a similar process of anergy in $V\beta6^+$ cells can be produced intrathymically (Ramsdell, Lantz & Fowlkes, 1989).

One dilemma still to be resolved is how the thymus, through a combination of these processes, not only allows the development of a complete repertoire of responses against an as yet unseen universe of foreign antigens, but also functionally deletes T cells reacting against all self antigens. There is some evidence that thymic presentation of novel self peptides, or peptides presented in a non-physiological manner, may select T cells capable of subsequent reactivity against foreign peptides (Schild *et al.*, 1990). Covering reactivity against all possible self peptides seems too much of a task for the thymus. As already mentioned, even abundant self antigens like H-Y in male mice do not induce complete deletion of reactive T cells and rare, tissue-specific autoantigens would seem unlikely to be any better at this (Smith *et al.*, 1989). Some such antigens may be shed by developing tissues and reach the thymus to induce tolerance, while others appear to evade this need by sequestration from the immune system. However the results of accidental exposure will clearly be disastrous if this latter strategy fails, as in sympathetic ophthalmia induced when lens protein is released by trauma. The immune system has developed two extrathymic, fail-safe mechanisms to deal with self-reactive T cells which have escaped either intrathymic tolerance or the induction of anergy: peripheral tolerance and suppression.

Peripheral tolerance and suppression

Strong support for the notion of peripheral tolerance has come from the creation of transgenic mice whose pancreatic beta cells alone express the I-E MHC class II molecule, to test the hypothesis that this property would convert the beta cells into APC. However, the opposite happened. These animals, which were otherwise I-E$^-$, did not delete their $V\beta17a^+$ T cells and did not destroy their islets, indicating that the T cells were tolerised peripherally (Lo *et al.*, 1988). Further studies *in vitro* showed that these I-E$^+$ beta cells induced I-E-specific T cell unresponsiveness, rather than stimulation (Markmann *et al.*, 1988). Such findings are in accord with the hypothesis, already described, that Ia expression alone is insufficient to confer APC function on a cell and furthermore, in the absence of an essential costimulator, presentation of antigen by a class II molecule can actually inactivate a T cell (Fig. 1.3). This mechanism for T cell tolerance seems well suited for preventing T cell reactivity against peripheral tissues, which will express class II MHC antigens in response to inflammatory cytokines and thus prevent the fortuitous activation of any non-deleted autoreactive T cells in the vicinity.

Tolerance to a transgenic class I (rather than class II) MHC antigen expressed by beta cells also occurs extrathymically, but this can be reversed *in vitro* by supplying a critical amount of antigen and IL-2 (Morahan, Allison & Miller, 1989). These results suggest that $CD8^+$ cytotoxic T cells reactive against extrathymic self antigens may be less demanding of intrathymic tolerance than $CD4^+$ cells, posing little threat provided there is complete inactivation of the helper cells which could provide IL-2. However, if these untolerised cytotoxic T cells were to be supplied with appropriate antigen plus IL-2, for instance during an inflammatory response, there is obvious potential for the initiation of autoimmune destruction.

A final mechanism to control thymically untolerised, self-reactive T cells is their active suppression. Arguments for and against the importance of T suppressor cells have been reviewed above, and in the subsequent chapters some of the evidence for active suppression as a means of controlling endocrine autoimmunity will be reviewed. One possible mode of suppressor cell action is essentially similar to that of peripheral tolerance, namely blocking a necesssary second signal to helper cells (Salgame *et al.*, 1989), and in turn suggesting a commonality in the operation of these processes which reinforce central tolerance.

B cell tolerance

Self-reactive B cells exist in the adult and this observation led to the original suggestion of clonal anergy as a mechanism for control of autoimmunity (Nossal & Pike, 1980). The possession of such B cells can be indulged in, provided autoantigen-specific T helper cells are deleted, but this is a risky strategy which may result in autoantibody formation. Once again, transgenic mice have provided insights into how self-reactive B cells are tolerised and prevented from autoreactivity.

For these experiments two types of animals were mated, one producing a transgenic antigen, hen egg lysozyme (HEL) and the other expressing a transgenic anti-HEL immunoglobulin on the surface of the majority of B cells. In the doubly transgenic progeny, the anti-HEL B cells were *not* deleted, yet did not respond to antigens or mitogens and this corresponded with the retention of surface IgD but the loss of IgM (Goodnow *et al.*, 1989). The presence of a similar surface phenotype in mature, non-transgenic B cells suggests that this may be an important mechanism for preventing autoantibody formation, although the biochemical events involved in anergy induction have not been identified.

Complete deletion of certain self-reactive B cells also appears possible. In crosses of H-2^k mice with H-2^d mice producing a transgenic H-2^k antibody, B cells expressing the transgene could not be detected. This implies that the B cells were deleted by contact with the H-2^k MHC class I molecule (Nemazee & Burki, 1989) although this may be difficult to distinguish from anergy. Possibly both mechanisms operate, multivalent antigens inducing deletion and univalent antigens anergy.

Breaking tolerance and the initiation of autoimmunity

The foregoing discussion of tolerance to self antigens has already hinted at possible break points which could lead to autoimmunity. In essence these are as follows:

1. Autoreactive cells fail to be deleted or rendered anergic.
2. Neonatally untolerised T cells fail to be kept in check by peripheral tolerance and suppression mechanisms in adult life.
3. Cross-reactive foreign antigens induce a response against a normally 'silent' self antigen (e.g. drug-induced haemolytic anaemia or myocarditis after streptococcal infection in rheumatic fever).
4. Sequestered autoantigens are exposed in adult life (e.g. lens protein).

The last of these seems unlikely to apply to the majority of self antigens, and most autoimmune disorders do not follow an obvious insult involving exposure to a foreign antigen, although it may be difficult to determine the initiating point in these diseases. The first two possibilities seem very plausible origins for autoimmunity. It is now apparent that intrathymic self tolerance for T cells is generally incomplete. Indeed, neonatal thymectomy in mice results in organ-specific autoimmune disease by enhancing this imperfect clonal deletion (Smith *et al.*, 1989). Furthermore, the production of cytokines as a result of local inflammation could expand non-tolerised, self-reactive B cells and CD8$^+$ cytolytic T cells, while ineffective peripheral tolerance, suppressor cell dysfunction or aberrant provision of costimulator signals could allow stimulation of autoreactive CD4$^+$ T cells. The existence of so many potential sources of self reactivity suggests that autoimmune diseases will probably have complex, multifactional causes. This is mirrored

Table 1.7. *Criteria for establishing an autoimmune aetiology for a disease (Rose & Bigazzi, 1978)*

1. Demonstration of autoantibodies (either circulating or cell-bound) or cell-mediated autoreactivity in patients with the disease.
2. Isolation of the autoantigen against which the autoreactivity is directed.
3. Production of autoantibodies or cell-mediated autoreactivity in animals using the same antigen.
4. Appearance of pathological changes in sensitised animals analogous to those in the human disease.

by the diverse effector mechanisms producing target organ damage, which will be discussed next.

Effector mechanisms in autoimmune disease

This final section considers the potential mechanisms causing tissue injury in autoimmune disease. Of course, there is nothing unique about such responses compared to those directed against foreign antigens and pathogens and much of our understanding of the pathogenesis of autoimmune disease has been based on the effector components of the normal immune response. The traditional distinction between humoral and cell-mediated mechanisms is still a convenient division and this is recognised in the criteria originally proposed for establishing an autoimmune aetiology of a disease (Rose & Bigazzi, 1978; Table 1.7). However, there are many soluble factors besides antibodies which act as intermediaries in pathogenesis, blurring this dichotomy.

Autoantibodies

In several autoimmune conditions there is unequivocal evidence that autoantibodies mediate disease. Placental transfer of these pathogenic antibodies can lead to transient neonatal illness, as in Graves' disease and myasthenia gravis and often disease can be transferred to and between animals by serum. Antibodies may affect tissue structure and function directly. Thus thyrocyte adenylate cyclase stimulation in Graves' disease appears to be the result of autoantibodies binding to the thyroid stimulating hormone (TSH) receptor and mimicking the action of TSH (Burman & Baker, 1985). In myasthenia gravis, muscle weakness is due to the loss of acetylcholine receptors from muscle end-plates caused by autoantibodies which can physically block access of acetylcholine to its receptor and accelerate internalisation of receptors cross-linked by antibody. However, another major, antibody-dependent mechanism also contributes to myasthenia, namely complement-mediated injury (Engel & Fumagalli, 1982) and this is the characteristic mode of antibody-mediated damage in many autoimmune diseases.

The complement system comprises a complex group of proteins whose activation leads to the production of biologically active molecules with several discrete functions (Whaley, 1987). Activation of complement occurs by two distinct pathways, classical and alternative, both of which will lead to splitting of the C3 and C5 components and the formation of a membrane attack complex (MAC) capable of producing cell lysis (Fig. 1.8). The classical pathway is usually activated by immune complexes of antigen and antibody of the IgM, IgG_1, IgG_2 or IgG_3 isotypes, although bacterial lipopolysaccharide, viral membranes and other non-immunological signals can also act as initiators. Immunoglobulins bound to antigen as immune complexes undergo conformational changes which expose a C1q binding region in the CH_2 domain of the Fc portion, and thus stimulate classical

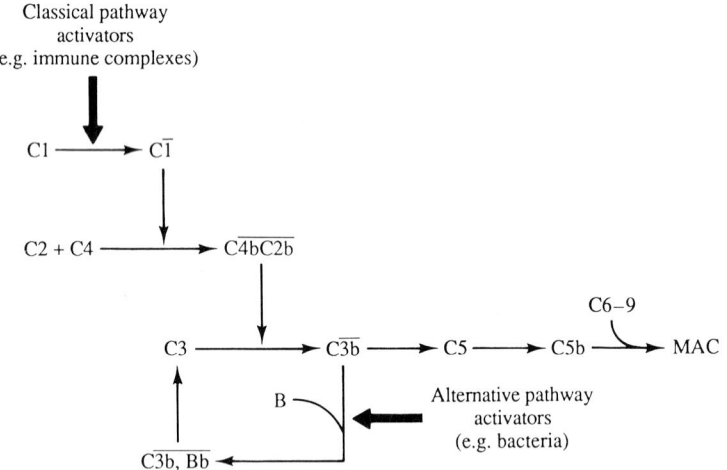

Fig. 1.8   Complement cascade. This enzyme system can be activated by the classical or alternative pathways at the points shown. In general, complement components are split to form small 'a' fragments and large 'b' fragments. The b fragments act as enzymes to stimulate the next step in the cascade: when active, these are designated by a line above the components. Regulatory components which control the level of activation are not shown. Both activation pathways lead to the formation of the membrane attack complex (MAC) which can lyse cells and mediate other forms of sublethal injury.

pathway activation. This region of the IgG_4 molecule is not readily accessible to C1q because of the short hinge region in this isotype and so IgG_4
subclass antibodies do not fix complement. The alternative pathway is
activated by many stimuli including bacterial and fungal pathogens and
lipopolysaccharides; immune complexes may enhance such activation.

There are several pathogenic effects of complement activation. The C3a
and C5a fragments (anaphylotoxins) cause histamine release and vasodila-
tion and attract neutrophils. C3b and C4b act as opsonins, coating immune
complexes or foreign particles and thus facilitating their phagocytosis by
complement receptor-mediated uptake. The MAC mediates the characteristic cytolytic function of complement, but it is now clear that most nucleated
cells are in fact relatively resistant to lysis by homologous complement,
owing to the existence of mechanisms for clearing MACs from the cell
surface, and the presence of several MAC-inhibitory proteins (Morgan,
1989). This defence requires energy and sustained complement attack, with
incomplete cell recovery, will ultimately be lethal to the cell. However,
formation of MACs can induce several other, non-lethal effects, which may
be important in mediating tissue injury under limiting conditions. These
include the release of reactive oxygen metabolites, prostaglandins, thromb-
oxanes and leukotrienes.

MAC formation has been implicated in many autoimmune disorders. As
already mentioned, loss of acetylcholine receptors in myasthenia gravis
seems dependent on complement-mediated injury and oligodendrocytes
appear to be a target for MAC attack in multiple sclerosis (Scolding et al.,
1989). Inflammatory mediators released by synoviocytes in response to
MACs may be involved in the pathogenesis of rheumatoid arthritis (Morgan
et al., 1988) and renal injury in various types of glomerulonephritis could
have a similar cause (Cybulsky et al., 1986).

Cell-mediated cytotoxicity

Four types of cell-mediated cytotoxicity may be important in autoimmunity.
Firstly, cytotoxic T cells can kill target cells after recognition of specific
surface antigen plus MHC molecule. Natural killer (NK) cells have no
antigen receptors and typically react against a variety of tumour targets.
However, a degree of specificity may be achieved if these cells identify
targets coated with antibody which interacts with the Fc receptor on the NK
cell, so-called antibody-dependent cell mediated cytotoxicity (ADCC).
Finally, monocytes and macrophages can release a wide variety of cytotoxic
and phlogistic mediators which may exacerbate autoimmune responses.

Cytotoxic T lymphocytes are characteristically $CD8^+$, recognising antigen associated with class I MHC molecules, but $CD4^+$ cytotoxic T cells do
occur. Target cell lysis requires close contact with the cytotoxic T cell for

only a few minutes before damage is irreversible and this binding depends on adhesion molecules (Nabholz & MacDonald, 1983). One mechanism for target cell killing is degranulation of the cytotoxic T cell, which is thought to lead to the release of a calcium-dependent pore forming protein or perforin. This molecule shares many structural and functional features with complement components C8 and C9, suggesting that there may be a family of molecules capable of producing cell lysis by membrane disruption. A great deal of circumstantial evidence has accumulated supporting the role of perforin in mediating cytotoxicity (Young & Liu, 1988; Tschopp & Nabholz, 1990) but calcium-independent and perforin-free target cell killing may also occur, indicating the existence of alternative pathways (Clark, 1988). At least one possibility is that cytotoxicity can be mediated by lymphotoxin, a T cell-derived cytokine structurally homologous to TNF and competing for the same cell surface receptor (Paul & Ruddle, 1988). There may also be heterogeneity in the lytic mechanism used, depending both on the stage of cytotoxic T cell development and on the target cell susceptibility to lysis. It is as yet unclear how the cytotoxic T cell protects itself from self-destruction.

NK cells were originally identified in normal, healthy individuals who nonetheless have lymphocytes which kill a variety of allogeneic tumour cell targets spontaneously. These cytotoxic cells are therefore neither MHC nor antigen restricted. NK cells are usually large, granular lymphocytes which are CD3$^-$ but may express other surface markers, such as CD2 and CD8, shared with T cells. They can be induced to express IL-2 receptors and respond to IL-2 (Ortaldo & Herberman, 1984; Jondal, 1987). There is good evidence that NK cells also mediate ADCC, by expressing a cell surface receptor for the Fc portion of IgG (CD16), although originally this was a phenomenon ascribed to a separate population of so-called killer (K) cells (De Landazuri et al., 1979). NK cell-mediated cytotoxicity is dependent, at least in part, on perforin (Liu et al., 1986) but the secretion of other cytokines, like lymphotoxin, may also be important. Heterogeneity exists within the NK cell pool; this may reflect different stages of development rather than clonally separate subpopulations. An additional complicating feature in the evaluation of NK cells is the ability of T cells to develop NK cell-like characteristics, particularly unrestricted tumour cell killing, after lymphokine stimulation (lymphokine-activated killer or LAK cells). Induction of LAK cell activity with IL-2 is currently being explored as a form of immunotherapy for tumours.

NK cells are probably important as a primitive immune surveillance system. Their absence as a result of rare genetic defects (e.g. the beige mouse strain, or the Chediak–Higashi syndrome in man) leads to a high incidence of lymphomas. Besides their anti-tumour activity, NK cells may play roles in regulating normal lymphocyte and stem cell proliferation, in defence against viruses and in other immunological responses by the production of an array of lymphokines similar to T cells. Altered NK cell function occurs in many disorders, reflecting the wide variety of factors, including hormones, which influence NK cells. A major problem in dissecting a role for these cells in autoimmunity is to envisage how NK cells can produce specific tissue injury, unless it is by mediating ADCC.

Finally, macrophages and other phagocytic cells may be important effectors of autoimmune damage. During the process of phagocytosis, these cells release proteases, reactive oxygen metabolites and cytokines, all of which can contribute to inflammation and organ damage (Fantone & Ward, 1982; Balkwill & Burke, 1989). In particular, the cytokines IL-1 and TNF may modulate target cell metabolism, and may synergise with injurious T cell-derived lymphokines like γ-IFN and lymphotoxin.

Summary

This very brief overview has attempted to integrate the basic features of the normal immune response with the initiating and effector mechanisms resulting in autoimmune disease. Our understanding of how the immune system concatenates has been advanced enormously by the elucidation of cellular interactions at a molecular level, giving functional meaning to surface molecules originally characterised by antibodies. In turn this has led to a rounded picture of how autoimmunity is normally prevented, although many details remain to be filled in. It seems naïve to expect that the aetiology of a particular autoimmune condition will depend on a single factor, given the numerous controls built in to the immune system to prevent autoreactivity. Indeed, even the proximal events in initiating autoimmune disease seem, in almost all cases, to depend upon an appropriate combination of genetic and environmental factors, as discussed in the next chapter.

References

Alt, F.W., Blackwell, T.K. & Yancopoulos, G.D. (1987). Development of the primary antibody repertoire. *Science*, **238**, 1079–87.

Asherson, G.L., Colizzi, V. & Zembala, M. (1986). An overview of T-suppressor cell circuits. *Annual Review of Immunology*, **4**, 37–68.

Augustin, A., Kubo, R.T. & Sim G.K. (1989). Resident pulmonary lymphocytes expressing the $\gamma\delta$ T-cell receptor. *Nature*, **340**, 239–41.

Austyn, J.M. (1987). Lymphoid dendritic cells. *Immunology*, **62**, 161–70

Babbitt, B.P., Allen, P.M., Matsueda, G., Haber, E. & Unanue, E.R. (1985). Binding of immunogenic peptides to Ia histocompatibility molecules. *Nature*, **317**, 359–60.

Babbitt, B.P., Matsueda, G., Haber, E., Unanue, E.F. & Allen, P.M. (1986). Antigenic competition at the level of peptide-Ia binding. *Proceedings of the National Academy of Science, USA*, **83**, 4509–13.

Balkwill, F.R. & Burke, F. (1989). The cytokine network. *Immunology Today*, **10**, 299–304.

Batchelor, J.R., Lombardi, G. & Lechler, R.I. (1989). Speculations on the specificity of suppression. *Immunology Today*, **10**, 37–40.

Beverley, P.C., Merkenschlager, M. & Wallace, D.L. (1989). Identification of human naive and memory T cells. In *Progress in Immunology VII*, ed.-in-chief F. Melchers, pp. 432–38. Berlin: Springer-Verlag.

Bierer, B.E., Sleckman, B.P., Ratnofsky, S.E. & Burakoff, S.J. (1989). The biologic roles of CD2, CD4 and CD8 in T-cell activation. *Annual Review of Immunology*, **7**, 579–99.

Bonneville, M., Kouichi, I., Krecko, E.G., Itohara, S., Kappes, D., Ishida, I., Kanagawa, O., Janeway, C.A., Murphy, D.B. & Tonegawa, S. (1989). Recognition of a self major histocompatibility complex TL region product by $\gamma\delta$ T-cell receptors. *Proceedings of the National Academy of Science, USA*, **86**, 5928–32.

Born, W., Happ, M.P., Dallas, A., Reardon, C., Kubo, R., Shinnick, T., Brennan, P. & O'Brien, R. (1990). Recognition of heat shock proteins and $\gamma\delta$ cell function. *Immunology Today*, **11**, 40–3.

Bottomly, K., Lugman, M., Murray, J., West, J., Woods, A. & Carding, S. (1989). Clonal expansion and differentiation to effector function in normal CD4 T cell subpopulations. In *Progress in Immunology VII*, ed.-in-Chief, F. Melchers, pp. 593–7. Berlin: Springer-Verlag.

Burman, K.D. & Baker, J.R. (1985). Immune mechanisms in Graves' disease. *Endocrine Reviews*, **6**, 183–232.

Burton, D.R., Gregory, L. & Jefferis, R. (1986). Aspects of the molecular structure of IgG subclasses. *Monographs in Allergy*, **19**, 7–35.

Buus, S., Sette, A. & Grey, H.M. (1987). The interaction between protein-derived immunogenic peptides and Ia. *Immunological Reviews*, **98**, 115–41.

Casali, P. & Notkins, A.L. (1989). $CD5^+$ B lymphocytes, polyreactive antibodies and the human B cell repertoire. *Immunology Today*, **10**, 364–8.

Chesnut, R.W. & Grey, H.M. (1981). Studies on the capacity of B cells to serve as antigen-presenting cells. *Journal of Immunology*, **126**, 1075–9.

Chu, E.T., Lareau, M., Rosenwasser, L.J., Dinarello, C.A. & Geha, R.S. (1985). Antigen presentation by EBV-B cells to resting and activated T cells: role of interleukin 1. *Journal of Immunology*, **134**, 1676–81.

Clark, W.R. (1988). Perforin – a primary or auxiliary lytic mechanism? *Immunology Today*, **9**, 101–4.

Cybulsky, A.V., Rennke, H.G., Feintzeig, I.D. & Salant, D.J. (1986). Complement-induced glomerular epithelial cell injury. Role of the membrane attack complex in rat membranous nephropathy. *Journal of Clinical Investigation*, **77**, 1096–107.

Davis, M.M. (1988). T cell antigen receptor genes. In *Molecular Immunology*, ed. B. D. Hames & D. M. Glover, pp. 61–79. Oxford: IRL Press.

De Landazuri, M.O., Silva, A., Alvarez, J. & Herberman, R.B. (1979). Evidence that natural cytotoxicity and antibody-dependent cellular cytotoxicity are mediated in humans by the same effector cell populations. *Journal of Immunology*, **123**, 252–8.

Dent, A.L., Matis, L.A., Hooshmand, F., Widacki, S.M., Bluestone, J.A. & Hedrick, S.M. (1990). Self-reactive $\gamma\delta$ T cells are eliminated in the thymus. *Nature*, **343**, 714–19.

Di Giovine, F.S. & Duff, G.W. (1990). Interleukin 1 : the first interleukin. *Immunology Today*, **11**, 13–20.

Dorf, M.E. & Benacerraf, B. (1984). Suppressor cells and immunoregulation. *Annual Review of Immunology*, **2**, 127–57.

Dustin, M.L. & Springer, T.A. (1989). T-cell receptor cross-linking transiently stimulates adhesiveness through LFA–1. *Nature*, **341**, 619–24.

ElMasry, M.N., Fox, E.J. & Rich, R.R. (1987). Sequential effects of prostaglandins and interferon-γ on differentiation of $CD8^+$ suppressor cells. *Journal of Immunology*, **139**, 688–94.

Engel, A.G. & Fumagalli, G. (1982). Mechanisms of acetylcholine receptor loss from the neuromuscular junction. In *Receptors, Antibodies and Disease*, CIBA Foundation Symposium 90, pp. 197–219. London: Pitman.

Fantone, J.C. & Ward, P.A. (1982). Role of oxygen-derived free radicals and metabolites in leukocyte-dependent inflammatory reactions. *American Journal of Pathology*, **107**, 397–418.

Fink, P.J., Matis, L.A., McElligott, D.L., Bookman, M. & Hedrick, S.M. (1986). Correlations between T-cell specificity and the structure of the antigen receptor. *Nature*, **321**, 219–26.

Finkelman, F.D., Holmes, J., Katona, I.M., Urban, J.F., Beckman, M.P., Park, L.S., Schooley, K.A., Coffman, R.L., Mosmann, T.R. & Paul, W.E. (1990). Lymphokine control of in vivo immunoglobulin isotype selection. *Immunology Today*, **8**, 303–33.

Fowlkes, B.J., Schwartz, R.H. & Pardoll, D.M. (1988). Deletion of self-reactive thymocytes occurs at a CD4$^+$8$^+$ precursor stage. *Nature*, **334**, 620–3.

Gaspari, A.A., Jenkins, M.K. & Katz, S.I. (1988). Class II MHC-bearing keratinocytes induce antigen-specific unresponsiveness in hapten-specific TH1 clones. *Journal of Immunology*, **141**, 2216–19.

Geha, R.S. (1981). Regulation of the immune response by idiotypic-antiidiotypic interactions. *New England Journal of Medicine*, **305**, 25–8.

Germain, R.N. & Malissen, B. (1986). Analysis of the expression and function of class-II major histocompatibility complex-encoded molecules by DNA-mediated gene transfer. *Annual Review of Immunology*, **4**, 281–315.

Gery, I., Gershon, R.K. & Waksman, B. (1972). Potentiation of T lymphocyte responses to mitogens. I The responding cell. *Journal of Experimental Medicine*, **136**, 128–42.

Goodnow, C.C., Crosbie, J., Jorgensen, H., Brink, R.A. & Basten, A. (1989). Induction of self-tolerance in mature peripheral B lymphocytes. *Nature*, **342**, 385–90

Grabar, P. (1975). Hypothesis. Auto-antibodies and immunological theories: an analytical review. *Clinical Immunology and Immunopathology*, **4**, 453–66.

Groh, V., Porcelli, S., Fabbi, M., Lanier, L., Picker, L.J., Anderson, T., Warnke, R.A., Bhan, A.K., Strominger, J.L. & Brenner, M.B. (1989). Human lymphocytes bearing T cell receptor $\gamma\delta$ are phenotypically diverse and evenly distributed throughout the lymphoid system. *Journal of Experimental Medicine*, **169**, 1277–94.

Hawrylowicz, C.M. & Unanue, E.R. (1988). Regulation of antigen presentation 1. IFN-γ induces antigen-presenting properties on B cells. *Journal of Immunology*, **141**, 4083–8.

Hayakawa, K., Hardy, R.R. & Herzenberg, L.A. (1985). Progenitors for Ly-1 B cells are distinct from progenitors for other B cells. *Journal of Experimental Medicine*, **161**, 1554–68.

Haynes, B.F., Telen, M.J., Hale, L.P. & Denning S.M. (1989). CD44 – a molecule involved in leukocyte adherence and T-cell activation. *Immunology Today*, **10**, 423–8.

Heber-Katz, E., Hansburg, D. & Schwartz, R.H. (1983). The Ia molecule of the antigen-presenting cell plays a critical role in immune response gene regulation of T cell activation. *Journal of Molecular and Cellular Immunology*, **1**, 3–14.

Howard, J. (1985). Immunological help at last. *Nature*, **314**, 494–5

Hunig, T., Tiefenthaler, G., Meyer zum Buschenfolde, K.H. & Meuer, S.C. (1987). Alternative pathway activation of T cells by binding of CD2 to its cell-surface ligand. *Nature*, **326**, 298–301.

Inaba, K., Koide, S. & Steinman, R.M. (1985). Properties of memory T lymphocytes isolated from the mixed leukocyte reaction. *Proceedings of the National Academy of Science, USA*, **82**, 7686–90.

Inaba, K., Kitaura, M., Kato, T., Watanabe, Y., Kawade, Y. & Muramatsu, S. (1986). Contrasting effect of α/β and γ-interferons on expression of macrophage Ia antigens. *Journal of Experimental Medicine*, **163**, 1030–5.

Jenkins, M.K. & Schwartz, R.H. (1987). Antigen presentation by chemically modified splenocytes induces antigen-specific T cell unresponsiveness in vitro and in vivo. *Journal of Experimental Medicine*, **165**, 302–19.

Jerne, N.K. (1974). Towards a network theory of the immune system. *Annales de l'Institut Pasteur/Immunology*, **125c**, 373–89.

Jondal, M. (1987). The human NK cell – a short over-view and an hypothesis on NK recognition. *Clinical and Experimental Immunology*, **70**, 255–62.

Katz, D.R., Feldmann, M., Tees, R. & Schreier, M.H. (1986). Heterogeneity of accessory cells interacting with T-helper clones. *Immunology*, **58**, 167–72.

Kehrl, J.H., Muraguchi, A., Butler, J.L., Falkoff, R.J.M, & Fauci, A.S. (1984). Human B cell activation, proliferation and differentiation. *Immunological Reviews*, **78**, 75–96.

Kishimoto, T. & Hirano, T. (1988). Molecular regulation of B lymphocyte response. *Annual Review of Immunology*, **6**, 485–512.

Kisielow, P., Blüthmann, H., Staerz, U.D., Steinmetz, M. & von Boehmer, H. (1988). Tolerance in T-cell-receptor transgenic mice involves deletion of nonmature CD4$^+$8$^+$ thymocytes. *Nature*, **333**, 742–6.

Kreiger, J., Jenis, D.M., Chesnut, R.W. & Grey, H.M. (1988). Studies on the capacity of intact cells and purified Ia from different B cell sources to function in antigen presentation to T cells. *Journal of Immunology*, **140**, 388–94.

Krensky, A.M., Reiss, C.S., Mier, J.W., Strominger, J.L. & Burakoff, S.J. (1982). Long-term human cytolytic T-cell lines allospecific for HLA-DR6 antigen are OKT4$^+$. *Proceedings of the National Academy of Science, USA*, **79**, 2365–9.

Kurt-Jones, E.A., Virgin, H.W. & Unanue, E.R. (1985). Relationship of macrophage Ia and membrane IL-1 expression to antigen presentation. *Journal of Immunology*, **135**, 3652–4.

Kuypers, T.W. & Roos, D. (1989). Leukocyte membrane adhesion proteins LFA-1, CR3 and p150,95: a review of functional and regulatory aspects. *Annales de l'Institut Pasteur/Immunology*, **140**, 461–86.

Lamb, J.R. & Feldman, M. (1984). Essential requirement for major histocompatibility complex recognition in T-cell tolerance induction. *Nature*, **308**, 72–4.

Lanzavecchia, A. (1985). Antigen-specific interaction between T and B cells. *Nature*, **314**, 537–9.

Lanzavecchia, A. (1989). Is suppression a function of class II-restricted cytotoxic T cells? *Immunology Today*, **10**, 157–9.

Lanzavecchia, A. (1990). Receptor-mediated antigen uptake and its effect on antigen presentation to class II-restricted T lymphocytes. *Annual Review of Immunology*, **8**, 773–93.

Lanzavecchia, A., Roosnek, E., Gregory, T., Berman, P. & Abrignani, S. (1988). T cells can present antigens such as HIV gp120 targeted to their own surface molecules. *Nature*, **334**, 530–2.

Larrick, J.W. (1989). Native interleukin 1 inhibitors. *Immunology Today*, **10**, 61–6.

Le, J. & Vilček. J. (1987). Tumor necrosis factor and interleukin 1: cytokines with multiple overlapping biological activities. *Laboratory Investigation*, **56**, 234–47.

Liu, C.-C., Perussia, B., Cohn, Z.A. & Young, J.D. (1986). Identification and characterization of a pore-forming protein of human peripheral blood natural killer cells. *Journal of Experimental Medicine*, **164**, 2061–76.

Lo, D., Burkly, L.C., Widera, G., Cowing, C., Flavell, R.A., Palmiter, R.D. & Brinster, R.L. (1988). Diabetes and tolerance in transgenic mice expressing class II MHC molecules in pancreatic beta cells. *Cell*, **53**, 159–68.

Lorenz, R.G., Blum, J.S. & Allen, P.M. (1990). Constitutive competition by self proteins for antigen presentation can be overcome by receptor-enhanced uptake. *Journal of Immunology*, **144**, 1600–6.

Lu, C.Y., Changelian, P.S. & Unanue, E.R. (1984). α-fetoprotein inhibits macrophage expression of Ia antigens. *Jounal of Immunology*, **132**, 1722–7.

Makgoba, M.W., Sanders, M.E. & Shaw, S. (1989). The CD2-LFA-3 and LFA-1-ICAM pathways: relevance to T cell recognition. *Immunology Today*, **10**, 417–22.

Markmann, J., Lo, D., Naji, A., Palmiter, R.D., Brinster, R.L. & Heber-Katz, E. (1988). Antigen presenting function of class II MHC expressing pancreatic cells. *Nature*, **336**, 476–9.

Marrack, P., Lo, D., Brinster, R., Palmiter, R., Burkly, L., Flavell, R.H. & Kappler, J. (1988). The effect of thymus environment on T cell development and tolerance. *Cell*, **53**, 627–34.

Matis, L.A., Jones, P.P., Murphy, D.B., Hedrick, S.M., Lerner, E.A., Janeway, C.A., McNicholas, J.M. & Schwartz, R.H. (1982). Immune response gene function correlates with the expression of an Ia antigen. *Journal of Experimental Medicine*, **155**, 508–23.

Melchers, I. & Rzepka, R. (1988). Plasticity of T cell function. Cloned EL-4 lymphoma cells may help or suppress a primary antibody response depending on their own concentration and the assay system. *Journal of Immunology*, **141**, 2873–81.

Meuer, S.F., Hussey, R.E., Cantrell, D.A., Hodgdon, J.C., Schlossman, S.F., Smith, K.A. & Reinherz, E.L. (1984). Triggering of the T3-Ti antigen-receptor complex results in clonal T-cell proliferation through an interleukin 2-dependent autocrine pathway. *Proceedings of the National Academy of Science, USA*, **81**, 1509–13.

Modlin, R.L., Brenner, M.B., Krangel, M.S., Duby, A.D. & Bloom, B.R. (1987). T-cell receptors of human suppressor cells. *Nature*, **329**, 541–4.

Möller, G. (1988). Do suppressor T cells exist? *Scandinavian Journal of Immunology*, **27**, 247–50.

Morahan, G., Allison, J. & Miller, J.F.A.P. (1989). Tolerance of class I histocompatibility antigens expressed extrathymically. *Nature*, **339**, 622–4.

Morgan, B.P. (1989). Complement membrane attack on nucleated cells: resistance, recovery and non-lethal effects. *Biochemistry Journal*, **264**, 1–14.

Morgan, B.P., Daniels, R.H., Watts, M.J. & Williams, B.D. (1988). *In vivo* and *in vitro* evidence of cell recovery from complement attack in rheumatoid synovium. *Immunology*, **73**, 467–72.

Morimoto, C., Letvin, N.L., Boyd, A.W., Hagan, M., Brown, H.M., Kornacki, M.M. & Schlossman, S.F. (1985). The isolation and characterization of the human helper inducer T cell subset. *Journal of Immunology*, **134**, 3762–9.

Mosmann, T.R. & Coffman, R.L. (1989). TH1 and TH2 cells: different patterns of lymphokine secretion lead to different functional properties. *Annual Review of Immunology*, **7**, 145–73.

Mueller, D.L., Jenkins, M.K. & Schwartz, R.H. (1989). Clonal expansion versus functional clonal inactivation: a costimulatory signalling pathway determines the outcome of T cell antigen receptor occupancy. *Annual Review of Immunology*, **7**, 445–80.

Murphy, D.B. (1987). The I-J puzzle. *Annual Review of Immunology*, **5**, 405–28.

Nabholz, M. & MacDonald H.R. (1983). Cytolytic T lymphocytes. *Annual Review of Immunology*, **1**, 273–306.

Nakayama, T., Kubo, R.T., Kishimoto, H., Asano, Y. & Tada, T. (1989). Biochemical identification of I-J as a novel dimeric surface molecule on mouse helper and suppressor T cell clones. *International Immunology*, **1**, 50–8.

Nemazee, D.A. & Burki, K. (1989). Clonal deletion of B lymphoctyes in a transgenic mouse bearing anti-MHC class I antibody genes. *Nature*, **337**, 562–6.

Nossal, G.J.V. (1989). Immunologic tolerance: collaboration between antigen and lymphokines. *Science*, **245**, 147–53.

Nossal, G.J.V. & Pike, B.L. (1980). Clonal anergy: persistence in tolerant mice of antigen-binding B lymphocytes incapable of responding to antigen or mitogen. *Proceedings of the National Academy of Science, USA*, **77**, 1602–6.

Nuchtern, J.G., Biddison, W.E. & Klausner, R.D. (1990). Class II MHC molecules can use the endogenous pathway of antigen presentation. *Nature*, **343**, 74–6.

Ortaldo, J.R. & Herberman, R.B. (1984). Heterogeneity of natural killer cells. *Annual Review of Immunology*, **2**, 359–94.

Palacios, R. & Möller, G. (1981). T cell growth factor abrogates concanavalin A-induced suppressor cell function. *Journal of Experimental Medicine*, **153**, 1360–5.

Paul, N.L. & Ruddle, N.H. (1988). Lymphotoxin. *Annual Review of Immunology*, **6**, 407–38.

Quill, H. & Schwartz, R.H. (1987). Stimulation of normal inducer T cell clones with antigen presented by purified Ia molecules in planar lipid membranes. Specific induction of a long-lived state of proliferative nonresponsiveness. *Journal of Immunology*, **138**, 3704–12.

Ramila, G., Sklenar, I., Kennedy, M., Sunshine, G.H. & Erb, P. (1985). Evaluation of accessory cell heterogeneity. II. Failure of dendritic cells to activate antigen-specific T helper cells to soluble antigens. *European Journal of Immunology*, **15**, 189–92.

Rammensee, H.-G., Kroschewski, R. & Frangoulis, B. (1989). Clonal anergy induced in mature $V\beta 6^+$ T lymphocytes on immunizing Mls–1^b mice with Mls–1^a expressing cells. *Nature*, **339**, 541–5.

Ramsdell, F., Lantz, T. & Fowlkes, B.J. (1989). A nondeletional mechanism of thymic self tolerance. *Science*, **246**, 1038–41.

Rich, R.R., ElMasry, M.N. & Fox, E.J. (1986). Human suppressor T cells: induction, differentiation, and regulatory functions. *Human Immunology*, **17**, 369–87.

Robey, E. & Axel, R. (1990). CD4: collaborator in immune recognition and HIV infection. *Cell*, **60**, 697–700.

Rose, N.R. & Bigazzi, P.E. (1978). *The Autoimmune Diseases*. CRC Handbook Series in Clinical Laboratory Science. Cleveland, Ohio: CRC.

Rosenthal, A.S. & Shevach, E.M. (1973). Function of macrophages in antigen recognition by guinea pig T lymphocytes. I Requirement for histocompatible macrophages and lymphocytes. *Journal of Experimental Medicine*, **138**, 1194–212.

Saito, T., Weiss, A., Miller, J., Norcross, M.A. & Germain, R.N. (1987). Specific antigen-Ia activation of transfected human T cells expressing murine Ti $\alpha\beta$-human T3 receptor complexes. *Nature*, **325**, 125–30.

Salgame, P., Modlin, R. & Bloom, B.R. (1989). On the mechanism of human T cell suppression. *International Immunology*, **1**, 122–9.

Salaün, J., Bandeira, A., Khazaal, I., Calman, F., Coltey, M., Coutinho, A. & Le Douarin, N.M. (1990). Thymic epithelium tolerizes for histocompatibility antigens. *Science*, **247**, 1471–5.

Salter, R.D., Benjamin, R.J., Wesley, P.K., Buxton, S.E., Garrett, T.P.J., Clayberger, C., Krensky, A.M., Norment, A.M., Littman, D.R. & Parham, P. (1990). A binding site for the T-cell co-receptor CD8 on the $\alpha 3$ domain of HLA-A2. *Nature*, **345**, 41–5.

Sanders, M.E., Makgoba, M.W. & Shaw, S. (1988). Human naive and memory T cells: reinterpretation of helper-inducer and suppressor-inducer subsets. *Immunology Today*, **9**, 195–8.

Schild, H., Rötzschke, O., Kalbacher, H. & Rammensee, H.-G. (1990). Limit of T cell tolerance to self proteins by peptide presentation. *Science*, **247**, 1587–9.

Schwartz, R.H. (1989). Acquisition of immunologic self-tolerance. *Cell*, **57**, 1073–81.

Scolding, N.J., Morgan, B.P., Houston, A., Linington, A., Campbell, A.K. & Compston, D.A.S. (1989). Vesicular removal by oligodendrocytes of membrane attack complexes formed by activated complement. *Nature*, **339**, 620–2.

Sha, W.C., Nelson, G.A., Newberry, R.D., Kranz, D.M., Russell, J.H. & Loh, D.Y. (1988). Positive and negative selection of an antigen receptor on T cells in transgenic mice. *Nature*, **336**, 73–6.

Silver, L.S., Scott, D.W. & Quill, H. (1989). Suppression of antibody sythesis by $CD4^+$ T cell clones and normal T cells stimulated with monoclonal anti-CD3 antibody. *Journal of Immunology*, **143**, 3448–54.

Smith, H., Chen, I-M., Kubo, R. & Tung, K.S.K. (1989). Neonatal thymectomy results in a repertoire enriched in T cells deleted in adult thymus. *Science*, **245**, 749–52.

Springer, T.A., Dustin, M.L., Kishimoto, T.K. & Marlin, S.D. (1987). The lymphocyte function-associated LFA-1, CD2 and LFA-3 molecules: cell adhesion receptors of the immune system. *Annual Review of Immunology*, **5**, 223–52.

Steeg, P.S., Moore, R.N., Johnson, H.M. & Oppenheim, J.J. (1982). Regulation of murine Ia antigen expression by a lymphokine with immune interferon activity. *Journal of Experimental Medicine*, **156**, 1780–93.

Stockinger, B., Pessara, U., Lin, R.H., Habicht, J., Grez, M. & Koch, N. (1989). A role of Ia-associated invariant chains in antigen processing and presentation. *Cell*, **56**, 683–9.

Strominger, J.L. (1989). The γδ T cell receptor and class Ib MHC-related proteins: enigmatic molecules of immune recognition. *Cell*, **57**, 895–8.

Swain, S.L. & Dutton, R.W. (1987). Consequences of the direct interaction of helper T cells with B cells presenting antigen. *Immunological Reviews*, **99**, 263–80.

Szakal, A.S., Kosco, K.H. & Tew, J.G. (1988). A novel in vivo follicular dendritic cell-dependent iccosome-mediated mechanism for delivery of antigen to antigen-processing cells. *Journal of Immunology*, **140**, 341–53.

Teh, H.S., Kieselow, P., Scott, B., Kishi, H., Nematsu, Y., Bluthmann, H. & von Boehmer, H. (1988). Thymic major histocompatibility complex antigens and the αβ T-cell receptor determine the CD4/CD8 phenotype of T cells. *Nature*, **335**, 229–33.

Terhorst, C., Alarcon, B., de Vries, J. & Spits, H. (1988). T lymphocyte recognition and activation. In *Molecular Immunology*, ed. B.D. Hames & D.M. Glover, pp. 145–88. Oxford: IRL Press.

Townsend, A., Bastin, J., Gould, K., Brownlee, G., Andrews, M., Coupar, B., Boyle, D., Chan, S. & Smith, G. (1988). Defective presentation to class I-restricted cytotoxic T lymphocytes in vaccinia-infected cells is overcome by enhanced degradation of antigen. *Journal of Experimental Medicine*, **168**, 1211–24.

Townsend, A., Öhlen, C., Bastin, J., Ljunggren, H.-G., Foster, L. & Kärre, K. (1989). Association of class I major histocompatibility heavy and light chains induced by viral peptides. *Nature*, **340**, 443–8.

Tschopp, J. & Nabholz, M. (1990). Perforin-mediated target cell lysis by cytolytic T lymphocytes. *Annual Review of Immunology*, **8**, 279–302.

Ucker, D., Ashwell, J.D. & Nickas, G. (1989). Activation-driven T cell death. I. Requirements for de novo transcription and translation and association with genome fragmentation. *Journal of Immunology*, **143**, 3461–9.

Unanue, E.R. (1984). Antigen presenting functions of the macrophage. *Annual Review of Immunology*, **2**, 395–428.

Unanue, E.R., Harding, C.V., Larescher, I.F. & Roof, R.W. (1989). Further analysis of the role of MHC molecules in antigen presentation. In *Progress in Immunology VII*, ed.-in-chief F. Melchers, pp. 52–9. Berlin: Springer-Verlag.

Van Voorhis, W.C., Valinsky, J., Hoffman, E., Luban, J., Hair, L.S. & Steinman, R.M. (1983). Relative efficacy of human monocytes and dendritic cells as accessory cells for T cell replication. *Journal of Experimental Medicine*, **158**, 174–91.

Vidovic, D., Roglic, M., McKune, K., Guerder, S., MacKay, C. & Dembic, S. (1989). Qa-1 restricted recognition of foreign antigen by a γδ T-cell hybridoma. *Nature*, **340**, 646–50.

Wacholtz, M.C., Patel, S.S. & Lipsky, P.E. (1989). Leukocyte function-associated antigen 1 is an activation molecule for human T cells. *Journal of Experimental Medicine*, **170**, 431–48.

Wagner, C.R., Vetto, R.M. & Burger, D.R. (1985). Subcultured human endothelial cells can function independently as fully competent antigen-presenting cells. *Human Immunology*, **13**, 33–47.

Weaver, C.T. & Unanue, E.R. (1986). T cell induction of membrane IL-1 on macrophages. *Journal of Immunology*, **137**, 3868–73.

Weaver, C.T., Duncan, L.M. & Unanue, E.R. (1989). T cell induction of macrophage IL–1 during antigen presentation. Characterization of a lymphokine mediator and comparison of TH1 and TH2 subsets. *Journal of Immunology*, **142**, 3469–76.

Whaley, K. (ed.). (1987). *Complement in Health and Disease*. Lancaster: MTP Press.

Williams, A.F. & Barclay, A.N. (1988). The immunoglobulin superfamily – domains for cell surface recognition. *Annual Review of Immunology*, **6**, 381–405.

Young, J.D.E. & Liu, C.C. (1988). Multiple mechanisms of lymphocyte mediated killing. *Immunology Today*, **9**, 140–4.

Zijlstra, M., Bix, M., Simister, N.E., Loring, J.M., Raulet, D.H. & Jaenisch, R. (1990). β2-microglobulin deficient mice lack $CD4^-8^+$ cytolytic T cells. *Nature*, **344**, 742–6.

Zinkernagel, R.M. & Doherty, P.C. (1975). H-2 compatibility requirement for T-cell-mediated lysis of target cells infected with lymphocytic choriomeningitis virus. Different cytotoxic T-cell specificities are associated with structures coded for in H-2K or H-2D. *Journal of Experimental Medicine*, **141**, 1427–36.

−2−
Immunogenetics and autoimmunity

What triggers the initiation of the autoimmune processes described in the last chapter? It seems that for almost all types of autoimmunity a combination of genetic predisposition and environmental factors is decisive. It is clear that relations of affected individuals have a higher than random risk of developing these disorders, although strong evidence for an environmental component in aetiology comes from studies on monozygotic twins, highlighted in subsequent chapters, showing less than 50% concordance for thyroiditis and type 1 diabetes mellitus. Such environmental factors, many of which remain hypothetical, will probably be diverse and unique to each disorder and the available information on these will be discussed under individual headings. However, it is worth considering in a more general manner how genetic influences may operate in autoimmunity, to make clear why MHC and other candidate genes have been studied in such detail in the autoimmune endocrinopathies.

Immunogenetics began with a chance observation: the synthetic polypeptide (T,G)-A-L induced an antibody response in Dutch or Himalayan but not Sandylop breeds of rabbit and similar observations were later made in various mouse strains (McDevitt *et al.*, 1966). Subsequent work showed that (i) a single dominant genetic factor was responsible for determining whether or not a mouse responded to this peptide, and (ii) the response to a modified peptide, (H,G)-A-L, in which tyrosine was replaced by histidine, again depended on strain, but these were separate to the responder strains for (T,G)-A-L (McDevitt & Sela, 1967). Parallel findings were made in guinea pigs and it was in these animals that it first became clear that the immune response genes operate by encoding MHC class II molecules on macrophages (Rosenthal & Shevach, 1973; Shevach & Rosenthal, 1973). At the same time, the role of MHC class I molecules in determining presentation of viral antigens to cytotoxic T cells (Zinkernagel & Doherty, 1974) became established. From these and many similar observations came the rapid developments in understanding the structure and function of MHC-encoded molecules. Their key role as restriction elements for presenting peptide antigens to T cells was described in Chapter 1. The next section considers the polymorphism of MHC-encoded molecules and how this influences the immune response.

MHC class I and II molecules

Molecular genetics and polymorphism

Terminology

Because so many experimental models of autoimmunity rely on mice, it is worth describing the organisation of the murine MHC as well as detailing the human counterpart (Fig. 2.1). The symbols used to describe MHC genes and their products may repel the uninitiated. In essence, the MHC is called H-2 in mice (an historical term, derived from the recognition of the antigens by antibody II from rabbits) and HLA in man (standing for human leucocyte antigen). Both contain genes encoding three classes of molecules. Class I molecules, as previously described, restrict the response of $CD8^+$ T cells, whereas class II or Ia molecules restrict the response of $CD4^+$ T cells (Ia comes from murine studies, indicating that these molecules are *I*mmune response *a*ssociated). Both class I and class II genes are members of the

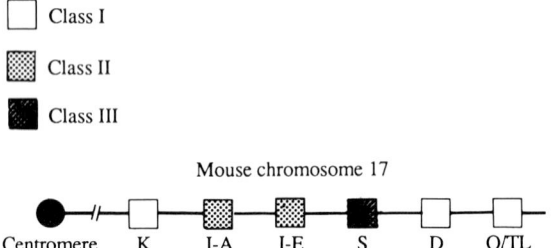

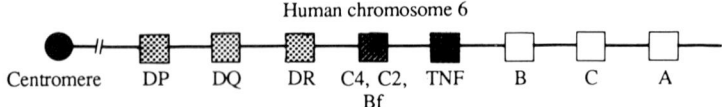

Fig. 2.1 The murine H-2 and human HLA MHC complexes. The sequence of loci is shown but this is not to scale; the entire human HLA complex occupies over 3000 kb. C4, C2 and Bf are complement components which are encoded by human class III genes. The genes encoding tumour necrosis factor (TNF) and lymphotoxin lie telomeric to the complement loci.

immunoglobulin supergene family. Class III molecules are heterogeneous, some being immunologically active, like TNF and complement components, and others having nothing to do with immunity, like the 21-hydroxylase cytochrome P-450.

The genes for these three classes of molecules are grouped in regions, which are divided into subregions encoding related but distinct and allelic molecules. For instance, in mice the class I gene subregions are termed H-2D and H-2K, with a further group of class I-like molecules in the TL/Q complex. In man there are three established class I loci; HLA-A, HLA-B and HLA-C. The class I and II genes are generally highly polymorphic. The combination of particular alleles within a continuous length of the chromosome is called the haplotype and, because recombination is not random, certain stretches of the chromosome may be inherited *en bloc*. This gives rise to distinctive extended HLA haplotypes which occur more often than would be expected by chance alone (e.g. the frequent occurrence of the HLA-A1, -B8,-DR3 haplotype in Caucasians), a phenomenon called linkage disequilibrium. As indicated by this example, the different HLA alleles are identified by numerals, sometimes preceded by a w standing for workshop, meaning a tentative assignation not yet fully delineated. Mouse haplotypes are identified by lower case letters as superscripts, e.g. strain B10.A (5R) has the MHC haplotype $H-2K^b$, $H-2I-A^b$, $H-2I-E^k$, $H-2D^d$.

The class II molecules comprise an α and β chain and the genes encoding these chains are termed A and B respectively. Class I molecules are also dimers, but only the α chain is encoded in the MHC. The class I β chain is an invariant polypeptide termed $\beta2$-microglobulin encoded on a separate chromosome. Pseudogenes have sequences very similar to normal genes but lack the segments necessary for expression of the gene; the MHC has a large number of these.

Chromosomal organisation

H-2 lies on chromosome 17 and HLA on chromosome 6. The arrangement of genes within these complexes is shown in Fig. 2.1. It will be noted that the class I MHC region in mouse contains an enigmatic group of non-classical or class Ib genes termed Q and TL. These have limited polymorphism and variable tissue expression. There are additional genes in the human class I region but these share little sequence homology with the Q and TL genes. A third group of MHC-like class Ib molecules, termed CD1, exists in man and mouse, which is not linked to the MHC (Strominger, 1989a). It is possible that these class Ib molecules restrict some $\gamma\delta$ receptor-bearing T cells.

The class Ia genes have variable polymorphism, HLA-C being the least polymorphic in man. A typical class I gene consists of six to eight exons, encoding a leader peptide, three extracellular domains $\alpha1$, $\alpha2$ and $\alpha3$, a

transmembrane region and one to three exons encoding the intracytoplasmic tail. There are multiple hypervariable positions at which MHC
allelic differences arise, in contrast to most other allelic systems in which
only one or two positions may alter. This gives rise to 50–100 different class I
alleles in man and mouse, most variations being concentrated in the $\alpha 1$ and
$\alpha 2$ regions. A variety of mechanisms have been proposed to explain the
evolution of such polymorphism at certain loci, coupled to the retention of
very high sequence homology elsewhere in this family of genes (Strachan,
1987). Besides random point mutation, blocs of nucleotides may have been
exchanged at recombination or by gene conversion. The evolutionary
pressure to do this has probably been the need within a species to maintain
an adequate pool of class I molecules, capable of binding diverse viral
peptides.

Class II genes and their products are rather more complex than class I
(Trowsdale *et al.*, 1987; Guillemot *et al.*, 1988). Both chains of these
molecules are encoded in the MHC. There are three expressed families in
man (HLA-DP, HLA-DQ and HLA-DR) and two in the mouse (I-A,
homologous to HLA-DQ and I-E, homologous to HLA-DR). Within the
HLA-D region, there are several pseudogenes, including DRB2 and DN/
DO. Another pair of genes, DXA and DXB, has no obvious structural
defect, but is not transcribed. The exact structure of the class II region varies
between individuals. In particular, subjects with HLA-DR1 express only
one of the two DRB genes expressed by non-DR1 individuals. The chromo-
somal order of the human class II genes shown in Fig. 2.2 has been
established by restriction fragment analysis and pulsed field gel electrophoresis (Hardy *et al.*, 1986).

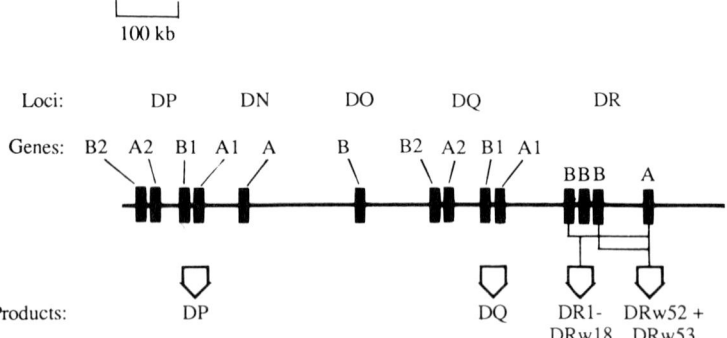

Fig. 2.2   Organisation of the human MHC class II region. Only some
genes give rise to expressed product; the remainder are pseudogenes,
e.g. DPA2 and DPB2, or are not transcribed for reasons which are not
clear, e.g. DQA2 and DQB2 (formerly called DX). The number of
DRB genes varies in different haplotypes.

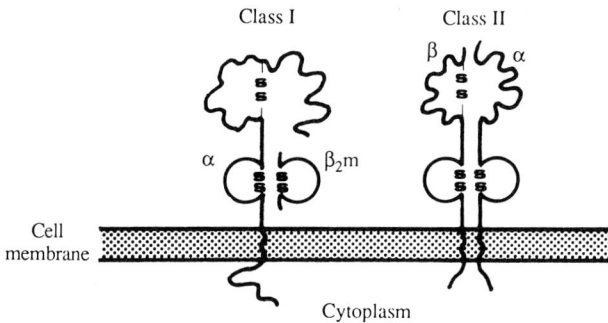

Fig. 2.3   Structure of class I (left) and class II (right) MHC molecules. β2m is β2-microglobulin: disulphide bonds are shown S–S. The α3 plus β2m (class I) and α2 plus β2 domains (class II) are those most proximal to the membrane, shown as almost circular regions. The α1 and β1 domains of the class II molecule lie distally and contain the polymorphic regions involved in antigen binding. These domains are analogous to the α1 and α2 domains of the class I molecule.

All of the expressed genes have a similar structure, resembling that of class I genes, with two exons for the external domains on each α or β chain. HLA-DRA genes have only one polymorphic residue, a property shared with the genes encoding murine I-Eα chains. HLA-DPA genes show limited polymorphism while HLA-DQA are very diverse, and HLA-DRB and -DQB genes are more polymorphic than HLA-DPB. Most allelic variations are found in the exon encoding the outer or first domains of the α or β chain. As for class I molecules, the allelic differences are particularly due to three or four hypervariable regions. Similar mechanisms of genetic information exchange and evolutionary pressures probably generated and maintain this extensive polymorphism.

Structure

The overall structures of the class I and II MHC molecules are similar (Strominger, 1987). The class I α chain is 44 kd and non-covalently linked to β2-microglobulin which is 12- kd (Fig. 2.3). The α2, α3 and β domains contain intrachain disulphide bonds and the α chain is glycosylated. Class II molecules comprise a non-covalently linked α and β chain, with β1, β2 and α2 intradomain disulphide bonds (Fig. 2.3). Both chains are glycosylated. Usually an α chain forms a pair with a β chain encoded by the same subregion, e.g. DRα with DRβ. This can involve both *cis* and *trans* complementation, that is, the α chain can be encoded either on the same chromosome or on the opposite homologous chromosome as the β chain. However, a cell line has been described expressing a hybrid molecule

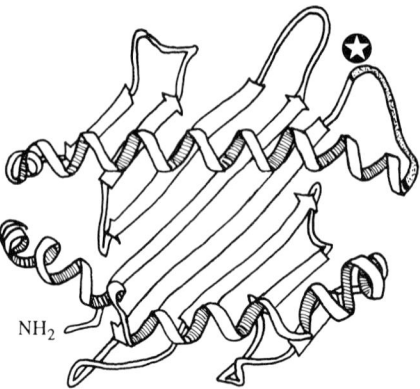

Fig. 2.4 Model of the HLA-A2 model (after Bjorkman *et al.*, 1987a,b). The antigen binding groove is shown, made up of two α helices with a β-pleated sheet floor. Class II MHC molecules are very likely to have a similar structure but, instead of comprising the continuous α_1 and α_2 domains of a class I molecule, the components of the groove will be the α_1 and β_1 domains, i.e. two separate chains. The probable site of the NH_2 terminal of the second chain involved in forming a class II antigen binding groove is shown by the asterisk; in this case, the dotted sequence would no longer be present.

comprising a DRα chain and DQβ chain and similar mismatched hetero-dimers have been created by transfecting certain cells with murine class II genes (Lotteau *et al.*, 1987). The frequency of such mismatching, and of T cells recognising heterodimeric class II molecules are unknown, but this type of pairing could greatly increase the class II repertoire of diversity.

Crystallisation and X-ray diffraction have revealed that in HLA-A2, and presumably all other class I molecules, the α1 and α2 domains form an anti-parallel β-pleated sheet, above which are two α helices (Bjorkman *et al.*, 1987a,b). Antigenic peptide is thought to lie in the groove between the α helices, resting on the floor of the β-pleated sheet (Fig. 2.4). The key feature here is that most of the HLA-A2 polymorphic residues lie around this groove, either on the α helices and pointing inward or on the β-pleated sheet and pointing up. Thus the ability of peptides to bind to class I molecules is governed by the conformation of the antigen-binding groove (the agretope: Fig. 1.2) which in turn depends on the particular allele encoded by the class I gene. Conversely, modifying peptides by single amino acids can impair their ability to bind to any given groove and this will be discussed in detail later. Computer predictions suggest that both the α and the β chains of the T cell receptor interact with HLA-A2. The first and second domains of each receptor chain bind to residues on the class I α1 and α2 domain α-helices (the histotope: Fig. 1.2), while the third domain of the receptor interacts with the antigenic peptide between (Davis & Bjorkman, 1988; Claverie, Prochnicka-Chalufour & Bougueleret, 1989).

It seems certain that class II molecules will have a similar overall structure (Brown *et al.*, 1988). The techniques of site-directed mutagenesis and gene transfer have been employed to create panels of murine Ia genes with single or multiple amino acid substitutions in the $\alpha1$ and $\beta1$ domains. These mutant genes have been expressed in normally Ia-negative cells and the effects on antigen presentation to Ia restricted T cell clones have been tested to determine which class II polymorphic residues are involved in antigen binding and T cell recognition (Cohn *et al.*, 1986; Lechler *et al.*, 1986; Brett *et al.*, 1989). The results show that T cells require both chains of the class II molecules for triggering. Different peptides may bind in separate parts of the groove, as certain substitutions abolish the binding of some peptides but not others. The same peptide may also bind in more than one way to a particular groove. These two features presumably increase the chance of a peptide producing an immune response and explain why it is difficult to predict the allele-specific binding of peptides simply from their sequences.

In the course of characterising the structure of HLA-A2, it was found that the majority of molecules in the crystals contained peptides already sited in the binding groove (Bjorkman *et al.*, 1987a,b). Together with the known slow dissociation of peptide/MHC complexes, this suggests that most cell surface MHC molecules usually contain peptides. Some of these may be foreign, but the bulk are probably derived from endogenous self proteins. Indeed it seems that the presence of peptide may be a necessary requirement for the transport of class I molecules to the cell surface (Townsend *et al.*, 1989).

As discussed in Chapter 1, selective processing and presentation of foreign antigens with new MHC molecules occurs during an immune response, but binding of self peptides seems to predominate under basal conditions. Such MHC/self peptide complexes are probably responsible for positive selection of T cells within the fetal thymus, perhaps because certain endogenous peptides are structurally related analogues of the yet-to-be-experienced universe of foreign peptides, whereas other endogenous peptides lead to negative selection and the deletion or anergy of potentially autoreactive T cells (Germain, 1990). The details of thymic selection which handle these antithetical events remain unclear.

Another feature explained by the regular presence of self peptides in MHC molecules is the mixed lymphocyte reaction. When lymphocytes from two unrelated (allogeneic) individuals are mixed, there is reciprocal stimulation dependent on recognition of MHC molecules and the frequency of such alloreactive T cells is surprisingly high. It has been difficult to explain why the body maintains so many alloreactive cells, when their only role seems to be the frustration of transplant attempts. However, it now seems that alloreactivity involves recognition of donor foreign MHC plus donor self peptide complexes by responder T cells (Strominger, 1989b; Lechler *et al.*,1990). *In vivo*, the responder T cells are tolerant of the same self peptides but only when presented by self MHC. The donor self peptides may be the same as the responder, but bind differently to the allogeneic MHC molecule, thus presenting a novel conformation to the responder T cell receptor. Alternatively, the donor and recipient MHC may bind different sets of self peptides derived from the same endogenous proteins, which would also result in a new conformation being presented to responder T cells by donor MHC plus peptide. Alloreactivity could also depend on the allogeneic MHC molecule, which may either provoke a response alone (because it is treated as foreign) or bind with various affinities to the T cell receptor as a result of variations in the histotope. Even mixing T cells (which do not express class II molecules under basal conditions) with class II-positive cells from the same (autologous) donor will provoke weak stimulation of the T cells. In this autologous mixed lymphocyte reaction the T cells are presumably recognising some foreign peptides already complexed to the MHC molecules. Of course, during such experiments there is also the potential for this to occur anyway, due to processing of proteins present in the culture medium.

MHC immune response gene function

Because class II molecules present peptides from soluble proteins to helper T cells, the MHC genes encoding them are likely to be involved in determining immune responsiveness to these antigens. This applies equally to foreign and self antigens. There are three potential mechanisms by which the class II loci could operate as immune response genes: determinant selection, clonal deletion and immune suppression. It is worth considering the first two possibilities together.

Determinant selection means that an immune response to a protein is permitted only if the class II molecule can bind the appropriate protein-derived peptide. As already indicated, the great polymorphism of the antigen-binding groove ensures that only some peptides can bind to the MHC molecule, so that antigenic determinants are selected by the groove (hence its alternative designation, agretope, from *a*ntigenic *r*ecognition : Fig. 1.2). Clonal deletion simply means that certain T cell clones are missing from the repertoire of an individual because the particular MHC genes have deleted, or failed to positively select, these clones. The essential difference between the two mechanisms is that determinant selection leaves the animal with a complete array of T cells, whereas the T cell repertoire is attenuated after clonal deletion.

A considerable effort has been made to delineate which of these accounts for the immune response gene effect of class II molecules, but detailed analysis has shown that both are likely to operate for multideterminant antigens (Schwartz, 1986). Unequivocal evidence for the phenomenon of determinant selection was provided by the demonstration of specific peptide binding to purified class II molecules only when the latter were derived from a responder haplotype (Babbitt *et al.*, 1985). Conversely, if the class II molecules came from mice which would not respond to the peptide *in vivo*, then no binding was seen with the peptide *in vitro*. To determine how frequently clonal deletion operates in life, multiple substitutions have been made in only those regions of an immunogenic peptide recognised by T cells, so that peptide binding to the agretope was still permitted. In all cases T cells capable of recognising these modified peptides were found in responder mice (Ogasawara, Maloy & Schwartz, 1987). Such observations suggest that the T cell clonal repertoire is huge and clonal deletion uncommon. Nonetheless, holes in the T cell repertoire do exist if a sufficient array of possibilities is tested (Guillet *et al.*, 1987). Overall, clonal deletion may be less important than determinant selection as an immune response gene effect of the MHC with regard to determining reactivity to protein antigens.

Immune suppression gene effects are also a possible mechanism influencing responder status, as a result of MHC regulation of T suppressor cell activation. Although an effect resembling clonal deletion may be produced, in this situation T helper cells should exist in low-responder animals, their failure to respond being the result of active suppression. Certainly a wide array of antigens seem to induce T suppressor cells in low-responder strain mice (Jensen, Kapp & Pierce, 1987). For complex proteins, there are many potential antigenic determinants or epitopes and responder status is determined by a balance between the number of epitopes recognised and the extent of suppression induced. In this context, it is important to note that certain determinants on antigens may actually induce suppression rather than help (Wicker *et al.*, 1984).

The nature of the MHC loci controlling the suppressor response is unclear but there is accumulating evidence that class II genes may be the most important, particularly H-2I-E in mice and HLA-DQ in man (Oliveira & Mitchison, 1989). As an example of this type of MHC effect, family studies and *in vitro* analysis have shown that responsiveness to a streptococcal cell wall antigen is controlled by HLA-DQ genes in a dominant fashion and that low responders generate streptococcal antigen-specific suppressor T cells *in vitro* (Nishimura & Sasazuki, 1983). However, much remains to be learned concerning the exact cell interactions involved and the mechanisms by which suppression is actually induced. It is also possible that non-MHC genes may modulate suppressor cell function.

While this section has concentrated on class II genes, class I loci are equally important in determining the immune response, only in this case to endogenous peptides, which are typically derived from viruses and other intracellular parasites. Thus, the ability to respond to these pathogens depends on the class I repertoire as sadly evident in the cheetah, a species in which overhunting and subsequent inbreeding has resulted in a diminished pool of class I genes and enhanced susceptibility to viral infections. Manipulation of residues around the binding site on HLA-A2 has confirmed that this alters presentation of viral peptides to cytotoxic T cells (Strominger, 1989b).

The MHC in autoimmune disease

In the subsequent chapters, MHC genetic associations with autoimmune endocrinopathies will be described both in experimental animals and in man. Many similar associations of MHC antigens with diverse diseases have been described (Tiwari & Terasaki, 1985), but while some of these are clearly related to the function of immune response genes within the MHC as discussed above, other associations have no such obvious relationship. For instance, narcolepsy is strongly associated with HLA-DR2. In certain disorders, like 21-hydroxylase deficiency, the reason is definitely non-immunological, the association being with the class III MHC gene encoding the particular P-450 cytochrome for this enzyme. Studies on MHC-encoded susceptibility to autoimmune conditions are relatively straightforward in the mouse and other animals because the MHC genes can be defined by use of inbred strains. These MHC effects can be tested further by appropriate crosses, especially between high and low responder strains. The next section discusses the far greater problems encountered when assessing the influence of the MHC on autoimmunity in man.

Methods for determining HLA haplotypes

HLA antigen identification, commonly called tissue typing, originally depended on the reactivity of these antigens with antisera from the multiparous women who have produced antibodies against paternal antigens shed by the fetus (Payne, 1957). Individuals who have received a blood transfusion or rejected a renal transplant are other sources of antibodies against HLA antigens. However, all such sera usually contain several different antibodies, making analysis difficult and much effort has gone into standardising these reagents now in world-wide use. To detect an individual's HLA antigens, his lymphocytes (or B cells in the case of DR antigens) are used as targets in a microlymphocytotoxicity assay (Terasaki & McClelland, 1974). The cells are incubated with a panel of antisera covering all known HLA determinants plus complement and cell death recorded. By determining which antisera produce killing, it is possible to assign the MHC haplotype. As well as antiserum definition, problems have arisen because certain antigens are more difficult to type than others. This originally applied to DR antigens as a whole, which were detected instead by cellular methods. Moreover, it is possible that some HLA antigens remain to be identified, particularly those with restricted ethnic distribution. A major advance has been the development of monoclonal antibodies against discrete MHC antigens (particularly class II) and the specificity of these is now known in considerable detail (Marsh & Bodmer, 1989). This knowledge should make it possible to immunise animals with transfected cells bearing mutated MHC antigens, so that a complete panel of useful typing antibodies can be produced.

In the mixed lymphocyte reaction, the main response is mounted by T cells against allogeneic class II antigens. This reaction was originally used to distinguish HLA-D region-encoded molecules. Serological testing for the DR group of antigens, identified primarily on the B cell (rather than T cell) fraction of peripheral blood, was developed later (Bodmer, Pickbourne & Richards, 1977). The technique of typing D antigens by mixed lymphocyte culture depends upon the use of standard cell lines known to be homozygous for a particular antigen; when mixed with the lymphocytes to be typed, the latter will not proliferate if the individual has the same D antigen as the homozygous typing cells. It became apparent that other D antigens besides DR stimulated this response, because two sets of cells serologically identical for DR often produced a proliferative response (Stastny et al., 1983). Originally termed SB, MT and MB, it is now known that these antigens correspond to HLA-DQ and HLA-DP. Another important consequence of work on mixed lymphocyte cultures was the definition of several subsets within some serologically defined DR molecules. This is because the T cells recognise different antigenic determinants to the antisera. For instance, several T cell-defined antigens associated with DR4 (called Dw4, Dw10, Dw13 and Dw14) were denoted in Caucasians and further analysis has enabled serological splitting of DR4, with subtypes analogous to these Dw types (Festenstein & Ollier, 1987).

Although serological HLA typing is now a robust technique, it remains complicated and time consuming. Many early studies on disease associations were only able to test for a limited number of class I and II molecules and occasionally a poorly standardised reagent has given spurious results. A crucial development in the study of HLA and disease has been the application of molecular techniques to define the genes rather than their expressed products. The extensive genomic polymorphisms that exist particularly in first exons of the DR, DQ and DP B genes and to a lesser extent the first exons of DQ and DP A genes were studied initially by restriction fragment analysis. This method relies on the existence of polymorphisms in genomic DNA sequences that are targets for a group of microbially derived enzymes called restriction endonucleases. These are used to digest DNA and the fragments are then size-fractionated on a gel before denaturation of the double-stranded DNA and transfer by Southern blotting to a membrane support or filter. The immobilised fragments are visualised with a radio-labelled homologous and D subregion-specific probe. Fragment sizes will vary according to distribution of polymorphic sites 'cut' by the enzyme. By choosing the correct probes and 'informative' restriction enzymes, a strong correlation has been found between alleles identified by such restriction fragment length polymorphism (RFLP) patterns and serologically charac-terised alleles (Carlsson *et al.*, 1987; Bidwell, 1988). In particular, it is usually possible to assign unambiguous DR types by RFLP analysis using *Taq* I digested DNA hybridised sequentially with DRβ, DQα and DQβ genomic cDNA probes. DQ probes are useful in typing DR genes because there is close linkage disequilibrium between these subregions. For in-stance, detection of a DQw2a RFLP pattern with DQα and DQβ probes implies the existence of a DR3 allele.

This type of analysis has revealed several 'splits' within DR types that are not detectable by serological typing. For example, DR3 RFLP patterns can be divided into those associated with the HLA-B8 haplotype (DR3[1]) and those associated with HLA-B18 (DR3[2]). Splits of the DQ alleles can be recognised but serological subtypes of DQw3, associated with DR4, have proved less amenable to RFLP analysis. Novel RFLP patterns have also been detected that appear to be related to autoimmune disease. These include polymorphisms within non-expressed genes like DX (Hitman *et al.*, 1987) and polymorphisms uncovered by less common restriction endonu-cleases, such as a DQβ *Hinc* II restriction fragment which is frequently found in patients with myasthenia gravis (Bell *et al.*, 1986). Another polymorphism, revealed by *Rsa* I digestion and DQβ hybridisation, is associated with coeliac disease, although this now appears to be the result of cross-hybridisation of the DQβ probe with DP sequences (Howell *et al.*, 1988). Besides pointing to possible involvement of DP as well as DR and DQ genes in autoimmune disease, the last example illustrates the problem of cross-hybridisation in RFLP analysis, resulting from the high level of homology between loci.

One way of overcoming this has been the use of allele-specific oligonucleo-tide probes. Once the complete sequence of the class II genes was known, it was possible to define sequences within the hypervariable region specific for each allele and to synthesise short stretches of about 20 nucleotide bases (oligonucleotides) complementary to these sequences. By using allele-specific oligonucleotide probes on Southern blotted DNA digests, the DR4 associated DQw3 alleles could be split into DQ3.1 and DQ3.2 by their independent hybridisation patterns (Holbeck & Nepom, 1986).

However, there are inherent problems in the use of such short probes, related to the transfer of sufficient enzyme-digested genomic DNA to a filter for detection, particularly because oligonucleotides are difficult to radiolabel to a high specific activity. The polymerase chain reaction (PCR) has been a key technique in overcoming this, because the method produces large amounts of amplified DNA from the region of interest (Saiki *et al.*, 1985). The PCR requires synthesis of two oligonucleotides (termed primers) complementary to genomic DNA sequences which flank the target sequence and, for the purposes of HLA typing, these flanking primers need to bind to regions which show no allelic variation.

In a typical cycle of the reaction, genomic DNA is denatured at high temperature (95 °C) and then the oligonucleotide primers are allowed to anneal to their complementary sequences by lowering the temperature to 40–55 °C. To complete the reaction, the temperature is raised to around 70 °C which activates a thermostable DNA polymerase *Taq* (derived from the bacterium *Thermus aquaticus*), that extends the primer sequence using added nucleotides and the flanked genomic DNA as template (Saiki *et al.*, 1988). Thus the amount of the DNA segment of interest is doubled by this cycle. Since the extension products are complementary to the primers, they too can participate in a second PCR cycle. As more cycles are completed, there is an exponential increase in the target DNA sequence. Typically 30 cycles are performed using an automatic thermal cycler to vary the temperatures.

PCR amplification of DNA sequences from the HLA-D region has been invaluable in the rapid characterisation of polymorphisms, particularly because the amplified sequences can be blotted directly onto a filter and probed with allele-specific oligonucleotides that are capable of detecting single base changes within the target segment. This technique was originally used to distinguish DQB1 alleles in diabetes (Todd, Bell & McDevitt, 1987) and the same approach has been employed to determine DP types (Bugawan *et al.*, 1988). The PCR amplified material can also be used for efficient, direct sequencing. These new methods for HLA typing represent a considerable advance over previous assays based on antibodies or cell interactions, not only in precision but also in rapidity and cost, and their application has already made a fundamental contribution to autoimmunity. This is most obvious in the analysis of genetic susceptibility to diabetes, as detailed in Chapter 4.

Statistical analysis

The analysis of results obtained by any of these methods for HLA typing in autoimmunity is centred around proving an association with the disease under study. This is well reviewed by Mathews (1984). There are two basic

Table 2.1. *Methods used in population studies to determine the significance and strength of associations between disease and genetic markers (Svejgaard, Platz & Ryder, 1983)*

1. 2 × 2 Contingency table

	Marker present	Marker absent
Patients	N1	N3
Normals	N2	N4

2. Frequency of marker in patients (F)

$$F = \frac{N_1}{N_1 + N_3}$$

3. Relative risk (RR)

$$RR = \frac{N_1 \times N_4}{N_2 \times N_3}$$

4. Aetiological fraction (AF)

$$AF = \left[\frac{RR - 1}{RR}\right]\left[\frac{N_1}{N_1 + N_3}\right] = \left[\frac{RR - 1}{RR}\right]F$$

5. Preventive fraction (PF)

$$PF = \frac{[1 - RR]F}{RR[1 - F] + F}$$

N = number of subjects.

experimental approaches: (i) the population study, in which the frequency of HLA types is compared in controls and unrelated individuals with the disease and (ii) the family study, in which HLA haplotype sharing between related, affected individuals is tested. Of course, similar statistical treatment is appropriate in testing for disease associations with other genes besides those in the MHC.

In the simplest form of population studies, the frequency of various alleles tested in controls and disease groups is compared by multiple 2 × 2 contingency tables, using the X^2 test to assess statistical significance (Table 2.1). If numbers are small, Yates' correction is applied or Fisher's exact test is performed instead. It is necessary to use a two-tailed significance test unless there is reason *a priori* to suspect that the observation of an association may be correct (e.g. if the study is designed to confirm a preliminary report). A special problem also arises from analysing multiple alleles, because the potential association of each allele with disease leads to a series of null hypotheses. For instance, if 20 alleles are examined, it is no longer reasonable simply to use $P < 0.05$ as a significance level for a disease association with one of these alleles, since this P value means simply that 1 out of every 20 'significant' observations could have arisen by chance alone, a quite likely occurrence if the influence of 20 variables is assessed. It is usual to apply a correction factor to avoid wrongly accepting a P value as significant in these circumstances, the simplest being to multiply any P value obtained by the number of alleles tested. Thus, if one allele, of 20 analysed, was increased in a disease group with a P value of 0.001 when compared to controls, the *corrected* P value would be $0.001 \times 20 = 0.02$. This is still less than the generally accepted value for biological significance, 0.05, making the association statistically significant at this particular level.

Having shown an association in population studies, the next step is to determine its strength. The commonest means of expressing this is the relative risk or cross-product ratio, which is the risk of developing a disease with a particular HLA allele present compared to the risk in its absence (Table 2.1). Typically, the relative risk is greater than 1.0, implying a positive association of the allele with the disease, the risk being stronger the bigger the number. A relative risk below 1.0 reflects a negative association and a decreased frequency of the allele in disease. This could be non-specific; for example, another allele may have a strong positive association and so unassociated alleles will be present at a lower than normal frequency. Alternatively, a negative association could be related to a protective effect of the allele. The method of Woolf (1955) can be used to combine information from different studies to give a pooled estimate of relative risk or to show that relative risks are heterogeneous between populations, for instance due to racial differences in susceptibility.

A less frequently used but important measure of the strength of an association is the aetiological fraction or δ statistic of Bengtsson & Thomson (1981). This expresses the attributable risk, that is, how much of a disease within a population is the result of the allele, while the relative risk refers to the risk for an individual (Table 2.1). If a genetic marker is rare in the normal population, then quite weak associations with a disease will produce a very high relative risk, whereas the aetiological fraction will give a more meaningful assessment of the strength of the association. The aetiological fraction is used only if the relative risk is greater than 1.0: values below 1.0 imply a decreased risk and the strength of this can be determined by the preventive fraction (Table 2.1).

A drawback of population-based studies is that many genes within the MHC are tightly linked. It is therefore difficult to be sure that any one allele really determines susceptibility as opposed to simply acting as a marker for a linked susceptibility gene. Linkage disequilibrium has already been discussed and is responsible for the existence of particularly frequent haplotypes in a population, e.g. HLA-A1,-B8,-DR3 in Caucasians. Many auto-immune diseases are associated with HLA-B8 and with HLA-DR3, imply-ing a susceptibility locus in close linkage with these markers. Disproportion-ate relative risk may indicate which of the two markers is nearer to the key locus.

Because classic Mendelian methods, utilising directed breeding, are obviously impossible in human genetics, statistical analysis has been used to study linkage of genes. This has been applied to naturally occurring families with autoimmunity, in essence testing disease association because the genetic marker should segregate with the disease in multiple cases within a family. Although the marker will be associated with such familial disease if linkage is proven, this does not mean that the same marker will necessarily be associated with disease expression in another family. However, because MHC linkage disequilibrium tends to keep alleles in similar linkages within the whole population, family to family variation usually does not occur in studies of HLA genes.

A major problem of family studies in autoimmune diseases is incomplete penetrance: one cannot be sure that an individual, unaffected at the time of study, will not develop disease subsequently. This has been circumvented by an adoption of Penrose's sib-pair method (Thomson & Bodmer, 1977). At least two disease-affected sibs are required and these are genotyped by reference to their parents. Considering one extreme of no linkage between an HLA haplotype and disease, one would expect a quarter of such sibs to be identical, a half to share one haplotype and a quarter to share neither haplotype. On the other hand, if a haplotype conferred complete susceptibi-lity to disease, then all affected sibs would be identical for the haplotype if there was recessive transmission, while half would be identical and half would share a single (disease-related) haplotype if the transmission was dominant. Family studies of HLA genes in autoimmunity have revealed significant linkages somewhere between the two extremes of linkage or not: it will be noted that the method provides additional information on the likely mode of inheritance if HLA linkage is proved. It is possible that a similar type of analysis of polymorphic DNA markers suitably spaced throughout the genome could localise candidate genes in polygenic diseases, including autoimmune diseases (Bodmer, 1987).

The strength of the linkage between two genes in family studies is estimated with the aid of lod (*l*ogarithm of the *od*ds ratio) scores. These express the ratio of two likelihoods, L1 and L2, L1 being the probability that the data are the result of two loci linked under a specific recombination fraction (θ) and L2 being the probability that the same data show no linkage, in which case $\theta = 0.5$ (Cavalli-Sforza & Bodmer, 1971). The lod score is the logarithm of this ratio, with a value of 3 or greater implying linkage. The calculation is usually made by computer to define the maximum likelihood estimate of θ. Ideal families for studies of linkage beween two genes are those with one double heterozygote and one double homozygote parent, as well as a large kindred with three generations; if both parents are double heterozygotes then linkage analysis cannot be performed.

The mechanism of association

As will be seen in the subsequent chapters, the association of autoimmune diseases with particular MHC alleles is incomplete. Detailed analysis suggests both the impact of other genes that determine susceptibility and the importance of additional environmental factors. For many endocrine disorders it is believed that HLA associations reflect the influence of immune response genes within the MHC, but it is not known whether the particular genes responsible are those chosen for testing or instead are genes in close linkage disequilibrium with the marker gene. Analysis at a molecular level now makes it feasible to determine exactly which functional genes are involved.

An example of the potential for extended haplotypes obscuring the true genetic relationship is provided by systemic lupus erythematosus (SLE). In Caucasians with SLE there is an increased frequency of HLA-A1,-B8, -DR3-positive individuals, but the association is almost certainly the result of this haplotype being in strong linkage disequilibrium with the null allele of C4A, which is encoded in the class III region between HLA-B and HLA-D (Fig. 2.1). SLE is, broadly speaking, an immune complex disorder with a very high prevalence in certain rare, homozygous forms of complement deficiency. In these unusual patients, the resulting inability to form soluble immune complexes (C3 and C4 inhibit lattice formation between antibody and antigen) and the reduced clearance of immune complexes (because reticulo-endothelial complement receptors will not be engaged) accounts for this association. However, the much commoner case of partial deficiency of complement components, resulting from a C4 null allele in a heterozygote, for example, also provides a powerful predisposition to the development of the more typical form of SLE (Lachmann & Walport, 1987). Thus a major reason for the association of HLA-DR3 with SLE is the class III genes in linkage disequilibrium.

It remains possible that DR3 may contribute additional susceptibility to SLE, as in so many other autoimmune diseases. Considerable evidence now suggests that even normal, healthy DR3-positive subjects differ from other controls in a variety of immune functions. These include (in the DR3 subjects) delayed Fc receptor-mediated clearance of immune complexes (Lawley et al., 1981), reduced degradation rate and increased persistence of antigen endocytosed by macrophages (Legrand et al., 1982), altered lymphocyte responsiveness to mitogens (Ambinder et al., 1982) and decreased

IL-1 production *in vitro* (Hashimoto *et al.*, 1990). Overall, these findings suggest a non-specific enhancer effect of HLA-DR3 on the immune response, whether normal or autoimmune.

Finally, it is possible that other genes lie within the MHC that influence disease. Some of these are not associated with immune function, including two which are associated with conditions of endocrine interest: HLA markers have proved invaluable in determining the genetic locus for 21-hydroxylase deficiency causing congenital adrenal hyperplasia (White & New, 1988) and idiopathic haemochromatosis behaves as an HLA-linked recessive disease but the gene product is so far unknown (Tiwari & Terasaki, 1985). The location of the genes encoding TNF and lymphotoxin between the HLA-B and class III regions of the human MHC suggests another mechanism for disease associations within HLA, depending on the genetic control of lymphokines.

Non-MHC genes and autoimmune disease

In many autoimmune disorders the association with HLA genes is weak and, even in those in which it is reasonably strong, HLA-identical siblings show a much lower concordance for the presence of disease than monozygotic twins. This indicates the influence of other genes of which there are at least three broad candidates: (i) genes influencing an autoantigen or its expression, (ii) immunoglobulin genes and (iii) T cell receptor genes. Little progress has been made so far with the first of these since few autoantigens have been fully characterised until quite recently. As yet, there are no obvious indications that genetically determined self-antigen variability plays a key role in autoimmune disease. However, there is some evidence that the other two sets of candidate genes contribute to disease susceptibility, as indeed might be predicted from their involvement in antigen recognition.

Immunoglobulin genes

Two major types of genetic variation in immunoglobulin genes could influence autoimmunity. The first involves the idiotype or antigen-binding region (Fig. 1.8). It is an attractive idea that autoantibodies may arise because an individual has genes encoding autoreactive heavy and light chain V regions while a healthy person does not (Adams, 1978), but direct testing of this has not yet been possible. Examination of the immunoglobulin repertoire of mice with SLE-like diseases has failed to reveal any defect in germline immunoglobulin genes or their rearrangement, suggesting instead that the autoantibodies in these animals arise from normal, germline-

Table 2.2. *Allotypes of human immunoglobulins*

	Location	Allotype	Alphameric	Numeric	Previous
Light chain	kappa	Km	1, 2 or 3[a]	1, 2 or 3	InV
Heavy chain	γ1	G1m	a, f, x or z	1, 3, 2 or 17	Gm
	γ2	G2m	n	23	Gm
	γ3	G3m	b0, b1, b3, b4, b5, c3, c5, g, g5, s, t, u, or v	11, 5, 13, 14, 10, 6, 24, 21, 28, 15, 16, 26, or 27	Gm
	α2	A2m	1 or 2	1 or 2	Am2
	ε	Em	1	1	

[a]Only a few allotypes are mutually exclusive. Allotypes are transmitted as haplotypes, often characterised simply by using the G1m and G3m allotypes alone. The three most common haplotypes in Caucasians are G1m(1,17); G3m(21), G1m(1,2,17); G3m(21) and G1m(3); G3m(5,13,14).

encoded V genes (Kofler, Dixon & Theofilopoulos, 1987). However, more detailed RFLP analysis has demonstrated subtle kappa chain V gene differences between normal and autoimmune mice (Bona, 1988). The genes encoding several human autoantibodies (rheumatoid factors, anti-DNA and anti-Sm) have been sequenced and generally appear to be germline-encoded: this remains to be tried with organ-specific autoantibodies because of the difficulty in obtaining suitable monoclonal B cells (Sanz & Capra, 1988).

The second set of immunoglobulin genes to be studied in relation to autoimmunity is that encoding allotypes (Schanfield & Van Loghem, 1986). These are highly polymorphic determinants found on the constant region of γ1, γ2, γ3, α2 and ε heavy chains and the κ light chain, arising as a result of only one or two amino acid substitutions (Table 2.2). The nomenclature for the different allotypes has changed several times, which can make comparisons between studies difficult. Few allotypes are mutually exclusive or antithetical and, because all immunoglobulin isotypes are usually represented in an individual, whole serum therefore contains a number of different allotypes. Heavy chain allotypes are clustered together as a haplotype, with particularly tight linkage between the Gm and Am genes.

These ethnically stable haplotypes have been useful in anthropological research but allotypes have also been used as polymorphic markers in studies of the immune responses. Certain Gm allotypes are associated with the serum level of immunoglobulin isotypes (Morell *et al.*, 1972) and with the magnitude of an antibody response to bacterial antigens (Wells, Fudenberg & Mackay, 1971). Such analysis has been extended to autoimmune diseases and a number of associations have been found which appear more impressive when account is taken of interaction with HLA genes (Whittingham, Mackay & Mathews, 1984). The mechanism for these associations and the additive effect of HLA is unclear, although it is tempting to speculate on linkage of constant region allotypic markers with genes controlling antibody formation.

Allotypic markers have usually been detected by the serological method of haemagglutination inhibition, using Rhesus antibodies of known allotype to coat human Rhesus-positive red cells. These coated cells are then reacted with an anti-allotype (often raised in animals) which will produce red cell agglutination. However, if a test serum is added (in excess) in which the immunoglobulins share the allotype of the Rhesus antibody, the anti-allotype reacts with the test sample and so the antibody-coated red cells do not agglutinate. By determining which types of coated cells do not agglutinate in the presence of the test sample, it is possible to delineate the allotypic haplotype of the sample donor. As with HLA analysis, molecular techniques are now being applied to the analysis of immunoglobulin polymorphisms. RFLP patterns have been defined which are linked to allotypic markers and to immunoglobulin switch regions, although a much larger number of alleles has now been identified than using serological allotyping alone (Migone *et al.*, 1983; Johnson, De Lange & Cavalli-Sforza, 1986). These markers should allow a more precise association with disease; susceptibility associated with particular IgG RFLP patterns has already been shown in multiple sclerosis (Gaiser *et al.*, 1987).

T cell receptor genes

T helper cells have paramount importance in the immune response, their activation being initiated by the formation of the trimolecular complex between MHC class II molecule, antigenic peptide and T cell receptor. The T cell receptor repertoire is therefore likely to have far-reaching consequences in modulating the autoimmune response and recent findings have confirmed this hypothesis in some disorders. The best characterised animal model of autoimmune disease is experimental autoimmune encephalomyelitis (EAE), in which immunisation of rats or mice with myelin basic protein (MBP) produces a demyelinating condition resembling multiple sclerosis. The sequences within MBP recognised by pathogenic T cells are known and the MHC partly determines the susceptibility of a particular strain to develop EAE. In PL/J mice the majority of encephalitogenic T cell clones which recognise the N-terminal MBP peptide utilise the Vβ8 gene element in their T cell receptors. This limited heterogeneity can be utilised to prevent or reverse disease by administration of Vβ8-specific monoclonal antibodies (Acha-Orbea *et al.*, 1988; Wraith *et al.*, 1989a).

Similarly restricted T cell heterogeneity has been found in other mouse strains and in rats with EAE, the latter using $V\beta$ segments 80% homologous with the $V\beta8$ segment used by murine T cells. A curious feature is that the same T cell receptor ($V\alpha2/V\beta8$) recognises several separate MBP peptides in association with different Ia molecules. However, T cell oligoclonality is not an absolute feature of EAE, since the SJL mouse strain recognises at least three epitopes on MBP in a polyclonal fashion. Collagen-induced arthritis in mice is another experimental autoimmune disorder in which a particular $V\beta$ allele is important: recent data have suggested that there is complementation between an MHC allele and the $V\beta6$ allele in determining susceptibility, together with an influence from further, as yet unidentified genetic factors (Smith et al., 1990).

Besides suggesting an influence of T cell receptor genes in autoimmunity, these observations have triggered the development of several novel approaches to therapy, again using EAE as a model. The beneficial effect of T cell receptor antibodies has already been mentioned. Another manoeuvre has involved modifying the encephalitogenic MBP peptide by amino acid substitutions so that these bind strongly to the MHC molecule but do not stimulate pathogenic T cells (Urban, Horvath & Hood, 1989; Wraith et al., 1989b). When given with the native peptide, EAE is no longer induced, possibly because of competition between the peptides for the Ia agretope. An alternative, active approach has been to immunise animals with synthetic peptides corresponding to idiotypic determinants on the T cell receptor (Howell et al., 1989; Vandenbark, Hashim & Offner, 1989). This seems to induce $CD8^+$ T cells which can protect against EAE, presumably through an idiotypic–anti-idiotypic interaction (Fig. 1.5).

Evidence for similar T cell receptor involvement in human autoimmune disease is now being assembled. Genetic susceptibility to some conditions may be determined in part by T cell receptor genes. As an example, various polymorphisms in the receptor α and β chain genes have been associated with multiple sclerosis in population and family studies (Oksenberg et al., 1989; Seboun et al., 1989). While such findings clearly suggest a role for these genes in susceptibility, a skewed distribution of receptor usage by the T cell population responsible for autoimmunity, associated with oligoclonality, would not necessarily be revealed by this approach.

Restricted clonality of autoreactive T cells has been suggested within the cerebrospinal fluid in multiple sclerosis and in the synovium of patients with rheumatoid arthritis (Hafler et al., 1988; Stamenkovic et al., 1988). However, methodological problems concerning artefactual clonal selection may have influenced the results in the rheumatoid patients, since a subsequent study found only minimal evidence for clonal restriction in this disease (Duby et al., 1989). On the other hand, clear evidence of restricted $V\alpha$ gene expression by T cells infiltrating central nervous system plaques in multiple sclerosis has been obtained by PCR amplification and probing of post-mortem brain samples (Oksenberg *et al.*, 1990). This has been extended by the identification of limited Vβ usage by human T cell lines derived from patients with multiple sclerosis which are reactive with immunodominant regions of MBP (Wucherpfennig *et al.*, 1990).

Further analysis of the influence of the T cell receptor repertoire on human autoimmune disease will depend upon the application of sequence analysis techniques like these to the identification of the rearranged genes used by autoreactive T cell clones of clearly defined specificity. It is also worth mentioning that the random nature of T cell receptor (and immuno-globulin) gene rearrangements may explain some of the discordant heritabi-lity of autoimmune disease in family studies. For instance, although mono-zygotic twins are regarded as genetically identical, the stochastic rearrangement of these genes will produce different receptor and antibody repertoires in the two individuals. If one twin happens to make a receptor with autoreactive potential and the other does not, then obviously there will be a difference between them in the risk of developing an autoimmune disease. How much such a mechanism, rather than environmental factors, contributes to familial disease incidence is unclear and elucidating this will require analysis of the repertoire in affected and unaffected individuals.

Summary

This brief review of immunogenetics has concentrated on the human MHC and in particular the class II genes since these have been the most frequently studied in autoimmune endocrinopathies. The development of new, mol-ecular techniques for analysing HLA-D region genes has greatly extended our knowledge of the nature of the associations with disease at a structural level, although the functional correlates are less clearly understood. In addition, it is apparent that non-MHC genes contribute to autoimmune disorders and further progress, especially in analysing T cell receptor gene usage by autoreactive T cells, could lead to specific and effective immuno-therapy for these conditions.

References

Acha-Orbea, H., Mitchell, D.J., Timmermann, L., Wraith, D.C., Tausch, G.S., Waldor, M.K., Zamvil, S.S., McDevitt, H.O. & Steinman, L. (1988). Limited heterogeneity of T cell receptors from lymphocytes mediating autoimmune encephalomyelitis allows specific im-mune intervention. *Cell*, **54**, 263–73.

Adams, D.D. (1978). The V gene theory of inherited autoimmune disease. *Journal of Clinical and Laboratory Immunology*, **1**, 17–24.

Ambinder, J.M., Chiorazzi, N., Gibofsky, A., Fotino, M. & Kunkel, H.G. (1982). Special characteristics of cellular immune function in normal individuals of the HLA-DR3 type. *Clinical Immunology and Immunopathology*, **23**, 269–74.

Babbitt, B.P., Allen, P.M., Matsueda, G., Haber, E. & Unanue, E.R. (1985). Binding of immunogenic peptides to Ia histocompatibility molecules. *Nature*, **317**, 359–60.

Bell, J., Smoot, S., Newby, C., Toyka, K., Rassenti, L., Smith, K., Hohlfeld, R., McDevitt, H. & Steinman, L. (1986). HLA-DQ beta-chain polymorphism linked to myasthenia gravis. *Lancet*, **i**, 1058–60.

Bengtsson, B.O. & Thomson, G. (1981). Measuring the strength of associations between HLA antigens and diseases. *Tissue Antigens*, **17**, 356–63.

Bidwell, J. (1988). DNA-RFLP analysis and genotyping of HLA-DR and DQ antigens. *Immunology Today*, **9**, 18–23.

Bjorkman, P.J., Saper, M.A., Samraoui, B., Bennett, W.S., Strominger, J.L. & Wiley, D.C. (1987a). Structure of the human class I histocompatibility antigen HLA-A2. *Nature*, **329**, 506–12.

Bjorkman, P.J., Saper, M.A., Samraoui, B., Bennett, W.S., Strominger, J.L. & Wiley, D.C. (1987b). The foreign antigen binding site and T cell recognition regions of class I histocompatibility antigens. *Nature*, **329**, 512–18.

Bodmer, J.G., Pickbourne, P. & Richards, S. (1977). Ia serology. In *Histocompatibility Testing*, ed. W.F. Bodmer, J.R. Batchelor, J.G. Bodmer, H. Festenstein & P.J. Morris, pp. 35–84. Copenhagen: Munksgaard.

Bodmer, W.F. (1987). The human genome sequence and the analysis of multifactorial traits. In *Molecular Approaches to Human Polygenic Disease*, CIBA Foundation Symposium No. 130, pp. 215–28. Chichester: Wiley.

Bona, C. (1988). V genes encoding autoantibodies: molecular and phenotypic characteristics. *Annual Review of Immunology*, **6**, 327–58.

Brett, S.J., McKean, D., York-Jolley, J. & Berzofsky, J.A. (1989). Antigen presentation to specific T cells by Ia molecules selectively altered by site-directed mutagenesis. *International Immunology*, **1**, 130–9.

Brown, J.H., Jardetzky, T., Saper, M.A., Samraoui, B., Bjorkman, P. & Wiley, D.C. (1988). A hypothetical model of the foreign antigen binding site of class II histocompatibility molecules. *Nature*, **332**, 845–50.

Bugawan, T.L., Horn, G.T., Long, C.M., Mickelson, E., Hansen, J.A., Ferrara, G.B., Angelini, G. & Erlich, H.A. (1988). Analysis of HLA-DP allelic sequence polymorphism using the in vitro enzymatic DNA amplification of DP-α and DP-β loci. *Journal of Immunology*, **141**, 4024–30.

Carlsson, B., Wallin, J., Böhme, J. & Möller, E. (1987). HLA-DR-DQ haplotypes defined by restriction fragment analysis. Correlation to serology. *Human Immunology*, **20**, 95–113.

Cavalli-Sforza, L.L. & Bodmer, W.F. (1971). *The Genetics of Human Populations*. San Francisco: Freeman.

Claverie, J.-M., Prochnicka-Chalufour, A. & Bougueleret, L. (1989). Implications of a Fab-like structure for the T cell receptor. *Immunology Today*, **10**, 10–14.

Cohn, L.E., Glinicher, L.H., Waldmann, R.A., Smith, J.A., Ben-Nun, A., Seidman, J.G. & Choi, E. (1986). Identification of functional regions of the I-Aβ molecule by site-directed mutagenesis. *Proceedings of the National Academy of Science, USA*, **83**, 747–51.

Davis, M.M. & Bjorkman, P.J. (1988). T cell antigen receptor genes and T-cell recognition. *Nature*, **334**, 395–401.

Duby, A.D., Sinclair, A.K., Osborne-Lawrence, S.L., Zeldes, W., Kan, L. & Fox, D.A. (1989). Clonal heterogeneity of synovial fluid T lymphocytes from patients with rheumatoid arthritis. *Proceedings of the National Academy of Science, USA*, **86**, 6206–10.

Festenstein, H. & Ollier, B. (1987). Cellular typing and functional heterogeneity of MHC-encoded products. *British Medical Bulletin*, **43**, 122–55.

Gaiser, C.N., Johnson, M.J., de Lange, G., Rassenti, L., Cavalli-Sforza, L.L. & Steinman, L. (1987). Susceptibility to multiple sclerosis associated with an immunoglobulin gamma 3 restriction fragment length polymorphism. *Journal of Clinical Investigation*, **79**, 309–13.

Germain, R.N. (1990). Making a molecular match. *Nature*, **344**, 19–21

Guillemot, F., Auffray, C., Orr, H.T. & Strominger, J.L. (1988). MHC antigen genes. In *Molecular Immunology*, ed. B.D. Hanes & D.M. Glover, pp. 81–143. Oxford: IRL Press.

Guillet, J.-G., Lai, M.-Z., Briner, T.J., Buus, S., Sette, A., Grey, H.M., Smith, J.A. & Gefter, M.L. (1987). Immunological self, nonself discrimination. *Science*, **235**, 865–70.

Hafler, D.A., Duby, A.D., Lee, S.J., Benjamin, D., Seidman, J.G. & Weiner, H.L. (1988). Oligoclonal T lymphocytes in the cerebrospinal fluid of patients with multiple sclerosis. *Journal of Experimental Medicine*, **167**, 1313–22.

Hardy, D.A., Bell, J.I., Long, E.O., Lindsten, T. & McDevitt, H.O. (1986). Mapping of the class II region of the human histocompatibility complex by pulsed-field gel electrophoresis. *Nature*, **323**, 453–5.

Hashimoto, S., Michalski, J.P., Berman, M.A. & McCoombs, C. (1990). Mechanism of a lymphocyte abnormality associated with HLA-B8/DR3: role of interleukin–1. *Clinical and Experimental Immunology*, **79**, 227–31.

Hitman, G.A., Sachs, J., Cassell, P., Awad, J., Bottazzo, G.F., Tarn, A.C., Schwartz, G., Monson, J.P. & Festenstein, H. (1987). A DR3-related DXα gene polymorphism strongly associated with insulin-dependent diabetes mellitus. *Immunogenetics*, **25**, 609–14.

Holbeck, S.L. & Nepom, G.T. (1986). Exon-specific oligonucleotide probes localize HLA-DQβ allelic polymorphisms. *Immunogenetics*, **24**, 251–8.

Howell, M.D., Smith, J.R., Austin, R.K., Kelleher, D., Nepom, G.T., Volk, B. & Kagnoff, M.F. (1988). An extended HLA-D region haplotype associated with celiac disease. *Proceedings of the National Academy of Science, USA*, **85**, 222–6.

Howell, M.D., Winters, S.T., Olee, T., Powell, H.C., Carlo, D.J. & Brostoff, S.W. (1989). Vaccination against experimental allergic encephalomyelitis with T cell receptor peptides. *Science*, **246**, 668–70.

Jensen, P.E., Kapp, J.A. & Pierce, C.W. (1987). The role of suppressor T cells in the expression of immune response gene function. *Journal of Molecular and Cellular Immunology*, **3**, 267–75.

Johnson, M.J., De Lange, G. & Cavalli-Sforza, L.L. (1986). Ig gamma restriction fragment length polymorphisms indicate an ancient separation of Caucasian haplotypes. *American Journal of Human Genetics*, **38**, 617–40.

Kofler, R., Dixon, F.J. & Theofilopoulos, A.N. (1987). The genetic origin of autoantibodies. *Immunology Today*, **8**, 374–9.

Lachmann, P.J. & Walport, M.J. (1987). Deficiency of the effector mechanisms of the immune response and autoimmunity. In *Autoimmunity and Autoimmune Disease*, CIBA Foundation Symposium No. 129, pp. 149–71. Chichester: Wiley.

Lawley, T.J., Hall, R.P., Fauci, A.S., Katz, S.I., Hamburger, M.I. & Frank, M.M. (1981). Defective Fc-receptor functions associated with the HLA-B8/DRw3 haplotype. *New England Journal of Medicine*, **304**, 185–92.

Lechler, R.I., Ronchese, F., Braunstein, N.S. & Germain, R.N. (1986). I-A restricted T cell recognition. Analysis of the roles of Aα and Aβ using DNA-mediated gene transfer. *Journal of Experimental Medicine*, **163**, 678.

Lechler, R.I., Lombardi, G., Batchelor, J.R., Reinsmoen, N. & Bach, F.H. (1990). The molecular basis of alloreactivity. *Immunology Today*, **11**, 83–8.

Legrand, L., Rivat-Perran, L., Huttin, C. & Dausset, J. (1982). HLA-and Gm-linked genes affecting the degradation rate of antigens (sheep red blood cells) endocytosed by macrophages. *Human Immunology*, **4**, 1–14.

Lotteau, V., Teyton, L., Burroughs, D. & Charron, D. (1987). A novel HLA-class II molecule (DRα-DQβ) created by mismatched isotype pairing. *Nature*, **329**, 339–41.

McDevitt, H.O., Askonas, B.A., Humphrey, J.H. & Sela, M. (1966). The localization of antigen in relation to specific antibody producing cells. I Use of a synthetic polypeptide (T,G)-A-L labelled with iodine–125. *Immunology*, **11**, 337–51.

McDevitt, H.O. & Sela, M. (1967). Genetic control of the antibody response. II Further analysis of determinant-specific control, and genetic analysis of the response to (H,G)-A-L in CBA and C57 mice. *Journal of Experimental Medicine*, **126**, 969–78.

Marsh, S.G.E. & Bodmer, J.G. (1989). HLA-DR and -DQ epitopes and monoclonal antibody specificity. *Immunology Today*, **10**, 305–12.

Mathews, J.D. (1984). Statistical aspects of immunogenetic associations with disease. In *Detection of Immune-Associated Genetic Markers of Human Disease*, ed. M.J. Simons & B.D. Tait, pp. 106–136. Edinburgh: Churchill Livingstone.

Migone, N., Feder, J., Cann, H., Van West, B., Hwang, J., Takahashi, N., Honjo, T., Piazza, A. & Cavalli-Sforza, L.L. (1983). Multiple DNA fragment polymorphisms associated with immunoglobulin μ chain switch-like regions in man. *Proceedings of the National Academy of Science, USA*, **80**, 467–71.

Morell, A., Skvaril, F., Steinberg, A.G., Van Loghem, E. & Terry, W.D. (1972). Correlations between the concentrations of the four subclasses of IgG and Gm allotypes in normal human sera. *Journal of Immunology*, **108**, 195–206.

Nishimura, Y. & Sasazuki, T. (1983). Suppressor T cells control the HLA-linked low responsiveness to streptococcal antigen in man. *Nature*, **302**, 67–9.

Ogasawara, K., Maloy, W.L. & Schwartz, R.H. (1987). Failure to find holes in the T-cell repertoire. *Nature*, **325**, 450–2.

Oksenberg, J.R., Sherritt, M., Begovich, A.B., Erlich, H.A., Bernard, C.C., Cavalli-Sforza, L.L. & Steinman, L. (1989). T cell receptor Vα and Cα alleles associated with multiple sclerosis and myasthenia gravis. *Proceedings of the National Academy of Science, USA*, **86**, 988–92.

Oksenberg, J.R., Stuart, S., Begovich, A.B., Bell, R.B., Erlich, H.A., Steinman L. & Bernard, C.C.A. (1990). Limited heterogeneity of rearranged T-cell receptor Vα transcripts in brains of multiple sclerosis patients. *Nature*, **345**, 344–7.

Oliveira, D.B.G. & Mitchison, N.A. (1989). Immune suppression genes. *Clinical and Experimental Immunology*, **75**, 167–77.

Payne, R. (1957). Leukocyte agglutinins in human sera. *Archives of Internal Medicine*, **99**, 587–606.

Rosenthal, A.S. & Shevach, E.M. (1973). Function of macrophages in antigen recognition by guinea pig T lymphocytes. I Requirement for histocompatible macrophages and lymphocytes. *Journal of Experimental Medicine*, **138**, 1194–212.

Saiki, R., Scharf, S., Faloona, F., Mullis, K., Horn, G., Erlich, H. & Arnheim, N. (1985). Enzymatic amplification of beta-globin genomic sequences and restriction site analysis for diagnosis of sickle cell anaemia. *Science*, **230**, 1350–4.

Saiki, R.K., Gelfand, D.H., Stoffel, S., Scharf, S.J., Higuchi, R., Horn, G.T., Mullis, K.B. & Erlich, H.A. (1988). Primer-directed enzymatic amplification of DNA with a thermostable DNA polymerase. *Science*, **239**, 487–91.

Sanz, I. & Capra, J.D. (1988). The genetic origin of human autoantibodies. *Journal of Immunology*, **140**, 3283–5.

Schanfield, M.S. & Van Loghem, E. (1986). Human immunoglobulin allotypes. In *Handbook of Experimental Immunology. Vol. 3, Genetics and Molecular Immunology*, ed. D.M. Weir, pp. 94.1–94.18. Oxford: Blackwell.

Schwartz,R.H. (1986). Immune respone (Ir) genes of the murine histocompatibility complex. *Advances in Immunology*, **38**, 31–201.

Seboun, E., Robinson, M.A., Doolittle, T.H., Ciulla, T.A., Kindt, T.J. & Hauser, S.L. (1989). A susceptibility locus for multiple sclerosis is linked to the T cell receptor β chain complex. *Cell*, **57**, 1095–100.

Shevach, E.M. & Rosenthal, A.S. (1973). Function of macrophages in antigen recognition by guinea pig T lymphocytes. II Role of the macrophage in the regulation of genetic control of the immune response. *Journal of Experimental Medicine*, **138**, 1213–29.

Smith, L.R., Plaza, A., Singer, P.A. & Theofilopoulos, A.N. (1990). Coding sequence polymorphisms among Vβ T cell receptor genes. *Journal of Immunology*, **144**, 3234–7.

Stamenkovic, I., Stegagno, M., Wright, K.A., Krane, S.M., Amento, E.P., Colvin, R.B., Duquesnoy, R.J. & Kurnick, J.T. (1988). Clonal dominance among T-lymphocyte infiltrates in arthritis. *Proceedings of the National Academy of Science, USA*, **85**, 1179–83.

Stastny, P., Ball, E.J., Dry, P.J. & Nunez, G. (1983). The human immune response region (HLA-D) and disease susceptibility. *Immunological Reviews*, **70**, 113–53.

Strachan, T. (1987). Molecular genetics and polymorphism of class I HLA antigens. *British Medical Bulletin*, **43**, 1–14.

Strominger, J.L. (1987). Structure of class I and class II HLA antigens. *British Medical Bulletin*, **43**, 81–93.

Strominger, J.L. (1989a). The γδ T cell receptor and class Ib MHC-related proteins: enigmatic molecules of immune recognition. *Cell*, **57**, 895–8.

Strominger, J.L. (1989b). Structural and functional analysis of human class I and class II major histocompatibility complex proteins, with special emphasis on alloreactivity. In *Progress in Immunology VII*, ed.-in-chief F. Melchers, pp. 43–51. Berlin: Springer-Verlag.

Svejgaard, A., Platz, P. & Ryder, L.P. (1983). HLA and disease 1982 – a survey. *Immunological Reviews*, **70**, 193–218.

Terasaki, P.I. & McClelland, J.D. (1964). Microdroplet assay of human serum cytotoxins. *Nature*, **204**, 998–1000.

Thomson, G. & Bodmer, W. (1977). The genetic analysis of HLA and disease associations. In *HLA and Disease*, ed. J. Dausset & A. Svejgaard, pp. 84–93. Copenhagen: Munksgaard.

Tiwari, J.L. & Terasaki, P.I. (1985). *HLA and Disease Associations*. Berlin: Springer-Verlag.

Todd, J.A., Bell, J.I. & McDevitt, H.O. (1987). HLA-DQβ gene contributes to susceptibility and resistance to insulin-dependent diabetes mellitus. *Nature*, **329**, 599–604.

Townsend, A., Öhlen, C., Bastin, J., Ljunggren, H.-G., Foster, L. & Kärre, K. (1989). Association of class I major histocompatibility heavy and light chains induced by viral peptides. *Nature*, **340**, 443–8.

Trowsdale, J., Young, J.A.T., Kelly, A.P., Austin, P.J., Carson, S., Meunier, H., So, A., Erlich, H.A., Spielman, R.S., Bodmer, J. & Bodmer, W.F. (1987). Structure sequence and polymorphism in the HLA-D region. *Immunological Reviews*, **85**, 5–43.

Urban, J.L., Horvath, S.J. & Hood, L. (1989). Autoimmune T cells: immune recognition of normal and variant peptide epitopes and peptide based therapy. *Cell*, **59**, 257–71.

Vandenbark, A.A., Hashim, G. & Offner, H. (1989). Immunization with a synthetic T-cell receptor V-region peptide protects against experimental autoimmune encephalomyelitis. *Nature*, **341**, 541–5.

Wells, J.V., Fudenberg, H.H. & Mackay, I.R. (1971). Relation of the human antibody response to flagellin to Gm genotype. *Journal of Immunology*, **107**, 1505–11.

White, P.C. & New, M.I. (1988). Molecular genetics of congenital adrenal hyperplasia. *Ballière's Clinical Endocrinology and Metabolism*, **2**, 941–65.

Whittingham, S., Mackay, I.R. & Mathews, J.D. (1984). HLA-Gm interactions: clinical implications. *Clinics in Immunology and Allergy*, **4**, 623–40.

Wicker, L.S., Katz, M., Sercarz, E.E. & Miller, A. (1984). Immunodominant protein epitopes. I Induction of suppression to hen eggwhite lysozyme is obliterated by removal of the first three N-terminal amino acids. *European Journal of Immunology*, **14**, 442–7.

Woolf, B. (1955). On estimating the relation between blood group and disease. *Annals of Human Genetics*, **19**, 251–3.

Wraith, D.C., McDevitt, H.O., Steinman, L. & Acha-Orbea, H. (1989a). T cell recognition as the target for immune intervention in autoimmune disease. *Cell*, **57**, 709–15.

Wraith, D.C., Smilek, D.E., Mitchell, D.J., Steinman, L. & McDevitt, H.O. (1989b). Antigen recognition in autoimmune encephalomyelitis and the potential for peptide-mediated immunotherapy. *Cell,* **59**, 247–55.

Wucherpfennig, K.W., Ota, K., Endo, N., Seidman, J.G., Rosenzweig, A., Weiner, H.L. & Hafler, D.A. (1990). Shared human T cell receptor $V\beta$ usage to immunodominant regions of myelin basic protein. *Science*, **248**, 1016–19.

Zinkernagel, R.M. & Doherty, P.C. (1974). H-2 compatibility requirement for T-cell-mediated lysis of target cells infected with lymphocytic choriomeningitis virus. Different cytotoxic T-cell specificities are associated with structures coded for in H-2K or H-2D. *Journal of Experimental Medicine*, **141**, 1427–36.

–3–
Autoimmune thyroid disease

Thyroid autoimmunity leads to several different disorders, comprising the commonest clinically significant autoimmune diseases in the community. In an *annus mirabilis*, 1956, three remarkable discoveries were made. Witebsky and Rose first disproved the dogma that autoreactivity could not occur by their observations on experimental autoimmune thyroiditis (EAT), which was induced by immunisation of rabbits with thyroid extract from the same species emulsified in complete Freund's adjuvant. These animals developed both thyroglobulin (Tg) antibodies and lymphocytic infiltration of the thyroid (Rose & Witebsky, 1956), the latter resembling the histological picture of Hashimoto's thyroiditis. Secondly, Roitt, Doniach and colleagues showed that the serum of these patients also contained Tg autoantibodies and finally Adams & Purves (1956) discovered the presence of an abnormal circulating thyroid stimulator in patients with Graves' disease, although it was some years later before this was characterised as a TSH receptor autoantibody.

The two features of disease frequency and historical precedence have resulted in a vast literature on autoimmune thyroiditis. In this chapter, particular emphasis will be placed on recent developments in the study of these disorders; extensive reviews of the older literature can be found elsewhere (Volpé, 1981; Weetman & McGregor, 1984). However, before considering the thyroid diseases in man, it is worth discussing insights obtained from EAT in animals.

Experimental models

Observations in EAT and similar diseases in other target organs gave rise to the criteria by which an autoimmune disorder can be defined (Table 1.7). It is striking that Graves' disease does not strictly fulfil these in that no animal model has yet been described. The recent cloning of the TSH receptor (see below) will soon allow production of sufficient antigen to assess whether this is due to absence of lymphocytes reacting against TSH receptor in the immune repertoire of laboratory animals. EAT is a model of Hashimoto's thyroiditis and can be induced by immunisation with thyroid antigens or by manipulating T cells; a third type arises spontaneously.

Immunisation-induced EAT

Probably all species will develop EAT after immunisation with autologous or syngeneic Tg in adjuvant. The latter usually consists of a suspension of mycobacteria in oil, so-called complete Freund's adjuvant (CFA). This prolongs the duration of antigen exposure and enhances antigenicity by non-specific effects on APCs and T cells; it may also produce partial degradation of the antigen. Because of size and the extent of basic immunological knowledge, the mouse has been the species most frequently studied, although important insights have been gained from immunisation-induced EAT in the rat and both will be discussed together.

Immunogenetics

It soon became apparent that certain strains of mice were good responders and others poor responders in terms of the severity of thyroid lesions developing after Tg/CFA immunisation. This segregation was linked, by the use of inbred strains, to an effect of the murine MHC H-2 genes (Vladutiu & Rose, 1971). Of interest, H-2 genes were found to have less influence on Tg autoantibody production; mice of the k or s haplotype produced antibodies and developed thyroiditis whereas those of the b or d haplotype had little thyroiditis but could produce readily detectable levels of Tg antibody. Detailed mapping has now been carried out, using congenic strains with recombination within the MHC, to localise the exact MHC genes involved (Kong, 1986). An important methodological feature of these studies was the use of bacterial lipopolysaccharide and other agents as alternative adjuvants, to exclude the possibility that immune response gene usage was determined by a property of CFA.

These adjuvants confirmed the H-2 localisation of a thyroiditis-inducing gene subsequently mapped to the I-A^k subregion in B10.BR strain mice. Lymphocytes from this strain could be sensitised to thyroid antigens on intact thyrocytes *in vitro* which was optimal when I-A subregion genes of the two cell types were compatible (Salamero & Charriere, 1983). These findings of course make sense given the immune response gene function of the class II gene, I-A (Chapter 2). The I-A^k and I-A^s encoded molecules in good responder strains may either bind immunogenic Tg peptides more efficiently or bias the T cell repertoire in these animals compared to those found in poor responders, I-A^b or I-A^d.

However, other genes also influence susceptibility. Again using recombinant strains, it was found that thyroiditis was severe in mice with the good responder I-A^k allele and either H-2D^k or H-2D^f genes, but in strains with the same I-A^k, less severe thyroiditis occurred when the H-2D genes were the b, d or g alleles. The influence of the other main class I gene, H-2K, is more controversial; the b allele at the H-2K locus seems to lessen the severity of EAT when Tg is given with CFA but not with lipopolysaccharide (Maron & Cohen, 1979; Kong, 1986). When thyroids from high (H-2^k) and low (H-2^b) responder strains are grafted together into high responder F$_1$ (H-2^k × H-2^b) recipients, only the high responder (and host) thyroids develop thyroiditis after Tg/CFA immunisation (Ben-Nun et al., 1980). Together, these results suggest that H-2 class I genes may influence the susceptibility of the target gland to damage in EAT, presumably through presentation of antigen to cytotoxic T cells. Non-MHC genes also influence murine EAT. The type of histological change seen in the thyroiditis varies between strains and granulomatous infiltration appears in RF and SJL mice, but not other high-responder strains (Imahori & Vladutiu, 1984). The Tg autoantibody response is under partial H-2 gene control, (H-2^k animals having higher levels than H-2^d), but is further regulated by immunoglobulin heavy chain genes on murine chromosome 12, which influence subclass distribution in particular (Rose et al., 1987).

Immunisation-induced EAT in rats is also strain-dependent and expression of thyroiditis may vary independently of Tg antibody levels. There is no obvious linkage between susceptibility and genes in the rat MHC, RT1, but this has not been examined in the same detail as murine EAT (Lillehoj & Rose, 1982). Furthermore, experiments involving two-way exchanges of thyroids between high and low responders, after tolerising for allografts, showed little if any influence of the genetic source of thyroid on the development of EAT (Eishi & McCullagh, 1988).

Crude microsomal preparations can induce thyroiditis in various species but contamination with Tg complicates the interpretation of these experiments. Recently, purified porcine thyroid peroxidase (TPO), the thyroid microsomal antigen, has been used to immunise mice and this produces in EAT but only in H-2^b strain animals, which are poor responders to Tg (Kotani et al., 1990). The thyroiditis occurs independently of TPO antibody formation and can be transferred by a TPO-specific T cell line. Although using xenogeneic antigen, this study opens up the possibility of a new model of EAT which depends upon what is a key autoantigen in the human counterpart.

Environmental factors

Female mice and rats develop more severe EAT than males. This can be modified experimentally, castration or oestrogen administration increasing

Tg antibody formation in males, an effect reversed by testosterone (Okayasu, Kong & Rose, 1981). Fluctuations in thyroid hormones, including hypothyroidism, have no effect on EAT but treatment with high concentrations of thyroxine (T4) suppresses both thyroiditis and Tg antibody formation, which may be a direct immunological effect of the hormone (Hassman et al., 1985). Stimulation of the gland by TSH may also be immunomodulatory, since this leads to endogenous Tg release (Lewis, Giraldo & Kong, 1987). At an appropriate level, the rise in circulating Tg reduces thyroiditis but not Tg antibody levels. This effect operates through the induction of suppressor cells which bear the murine CD4 equivalent, L3T4 (Kong et al., 1989). Pretreatment with low-dose cyclophosphamide, which may affect T suppressor cells preferentially, converts poor responder mice to good responders (although having no effect on strains which are already high responders), showing the potential for exogenous agents to influence thyroid autoimmunity (Vladutiu, 1982).

T cell responses

The concept that complete T cell tolerance to thyroid antigens prevents autoimmunity was first challenged by the induction of EAT in good responder strain mice immunised only with syngeneic Tg; T cells must exist in these animals capable of responding to the native autoantigen (ElRehewy et al., 1981). Therefore, in addition to tolerance, active regulation appears necessary to maintain unresponsiveness to Tg, determined by an appropriate balance between helper and suppressor T cell populations (Rose et al., 1981). Disturbances in the balance will tip the animal into EAT (Fig. 3.1) and several factors which can do this have already been discussed, such as cyclophosphamide and the circulating Tg level. In addition to the effects of Tg on suppressor T cell induction, pretreatment with Tg can also induce B cell tolerance and possibly anergy in Tg-specific T helper cells (Parish et al., 1988).

Both $Lyt-2^+$ and $L3T4^+$ T cells are required for the complete development of EAT, based on depletion experiments with monoclonal antibodies against these two subsets (Flynn et al., 1989). Transfer of EAT by a predominantly $Lyt-1^+$ T cell line confirmed the central role of T cells in mediating EAT, which could have been due to class II-restricted cytotoxicity, induction of cytotoxic T cells in the recipient, or transfer of a small population of $Lyt-2^+$ cytotoxic T cells (Maron et al., 1983). However, similar transfer of EAT with $L3T4^+$ T cell clones rules out this last possibility (Romball & Weigle, 1987). Another Tg-specific effector T cell clone has been described which can be down-regulated by the generation of anti-idiotypic antibodies that recognise the paratope of an anti-Tg monoclonal

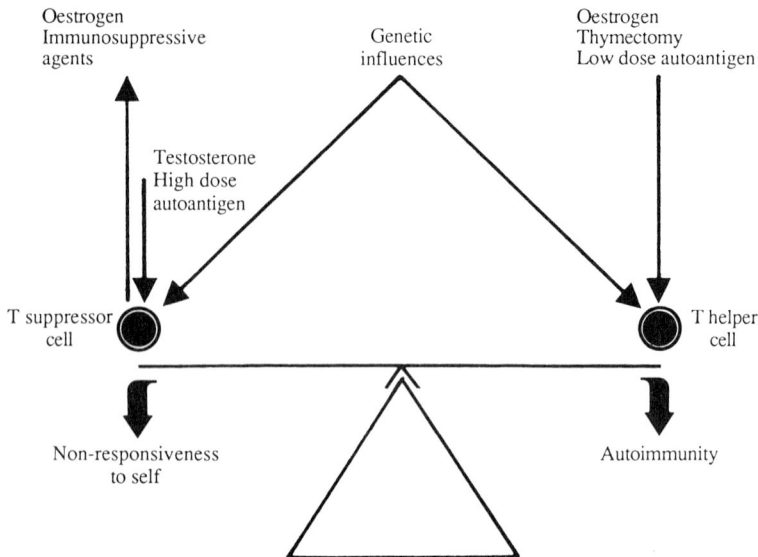

Fig. 3.1   Clonal balance and autoimmunity. Interaction of different genetic and environmental factors can shift the balance between help and suppression in favour of either autoimmunity or its prevention. Factors particularly pertinent to animal models of autoimmune thyroiditis are shown in the diagram.

antibody (Roubaty, Bedin & Charriere, 1990), indicating another mechanism for control of autoreactivity.

Helper T cell lines specific for murine Tg respond to this antigen if presented by I-A compatible dendritic cells or macrophages, but optimal proliferation depends on the presence of multiple types of APC derived from whole spleen (Champion *et al.*, 1985). Macrophages certainly take up autologous Tg *in vitro* and, when primed in this fashion, can exacerbate ongoing EAT *in vivo* (Weetman, McGregor & Hall, 1983a). Splenic B cells from mice primed with Tg *in vivo* function as efficient Tg-presenting cells *in vitro*, but this was shown with hybridoma cells formed by fusion of a Lyt-1[+], Tg-specific T cell line with an immortal partner BW 5147 as the responder population (Hutchings *et al.*, 1987). Whether non-hybridised T cells could be stimulated was not assessed.

Extending the primary sensitisation experiments mentioned above, Charriere and colleagues have produced evidence for the induction of class II antigens on thyrocytes by good responder T cells and proposed that these cells, but not macrophages, may be responsible for stimulating Tg-reactive T cells (Salamero *et al.*, 1985). However, others have found that class II-positive thyrocytes (primary cultures or lines) do not function as APC, failing to present Tg as well as other antigens, or to stimulate alloreactivity (Ebner *et al.*, 1987). It is possible that such differences could arise from variable dendritic cell contamination of the thyrocyte cultures, since these are potent APC. A clone of the rat thyroid cell line, $FRTL_5$, appears capable of stimulating mixed lymphocyte reactions when Ia expression is induced with γ-IFN (Hirose *et al.*, 1988), which would rule out a dendritic cell contribution. It is unclear how this thyroid cell clone, or indeed the parent $FRTL_5$ line, relates to normal thyroid cells in terms of costimulator release.

Given the likely requirements for such a second signal in antigen presentation (Chapter 1), it is possible that thyrocytes only function as APC when the costimulator is either supplied (by contaminating professional APC) or induced (by cloning). Support for this comes from the suppressive effect of Tg-coupled spleen cells on immunisation-induced EAT in the guinea pig (Braley-Mullen *et al.*, 1980), which suggests that Tg presented to T cells by Ia^+ cells in the absence of a second signal induces tolerance. Moreover, the major sites of autoreactive T and B cell localisation in immunisation-induced EAT are the lymph nodes and, for B cells, bone marrow, where presumably the lymphocytes are stimulated only by conventional APC (Weetman *et al.*, 1984a). Finally, Ia^+ thyrocytes are not seen in this form of thyroiditis (Cohen & Weetman, 1987). On balance, it seems unlikely that thyrocytes function as APC in immunisation-induced EAT, which most likely results from presentation of Tg by macrophages and dendritic cells.

B cell responses

Tg antibodies do not fix complement, an inherent property of the antigen whose widely spaced epitopes prevent cross-linking. In murine EAT, all four IgG subclasses are represented (Rose *et al.*, 1987). More epitopes are recognised on xenogeneic Tg and immunisation of mice with bovine Tg will induce high titres of autoantibodies but with minimal or no thyroiditis (Romball & Weigle, 1984). This is consistent with the poor correlation between Tg antibody levels and thyroiditis in the various responder strains noted above.

Effector mechanisms

The important effector cells in this form of EAT are class I-restricted $Lyt-2^+$ T cells (equivalent to CD8), which require $L3T4^+$ inducers for their expansion (Creemers, Rose & Kong, 1983). These cytotoxic cells kill autologous thyroid targets in a Tg-restricted fashion. Disease has been transferred to high-responder strain mice by serum, albeit with a low incidence and severity (Tomazic & Rose, 1975). The initial lesions suggested that this is mediated by immune complex deposition; an additional influence could have been the transfer of cytokines present in the diseased sera. Chronic treatment from birth with anti-IgM antibodies to deplete B cells prevents the formation of Tg antibodies after immunisation, but thyroiditis nonetheless occurs with the same frequency as controls (Vladutiu, 1989). Together, these results suggest the Tg antibodies are unimportant in the development of thyroid lesions in EAT.

EAT induced by T cell modulation

Altering the T cell repertoire of genetically susceptible animals results in severe thyroiditis and thyroglobulin autoantibody formation. Models of this form of EAT generally depend on thymectomy but supplementary T cell depletion has also been achieved using monoclonal antibodies, irradiation or the T cell immunosuppressive agent cyclosporin A. Rats subjected to thymectomy at three weeks old, followed by sublethal irradiation (4×200 rads), were found to develop a severe, chronic thyroiditis, resembling Hashimoto's thyroiditis and accompanied by Tg antibody formation (Penhale et al., 1973, 1975). This similarity to the human disease has been further supported by the immunohistochemical features in the thyroid and by the severity of target organ damage; other forms of EAT, including immunisation-induced thyroiditis, are less similar to Hashimoto's thyroiditis (Cohen & Weetman, 1987). Irradiation without thymectomy results in a much lower incidence of disease (Penhale et al., 1973). Radiation damage to the thyroid therefore seems an unlikely explanation for the disease, whereas a role for perturbed T cell balance is supported by the amelioration of disease after normal T cell infusions (Penhale et al., 1976).

A similar type of disease was produced in mice by neonatal thymectomy without irradiation, that also can be reversed by normal T cells (Kojima et al., 1976a,b). Neonatal thymectomy similarly induces EAT in Buffalo (Buf) strain rats (Silverman & Rose, 1974) which have a low incidence of spontaneous thyroiditis (see below): the disease is chronic but tends to ameliorate with time. Rather than rely upon the T cells remaining after thymectomy to induce EAT, more refined models have used either nude mice (which are T cell deficient) or total T cell depletion techniques in other strains, followed by reconstitution with normal T cell subsets to determine which T cells are responsible for disease induction (Sakaguchi et al., 1985; Sugihara et al., 1988). Finally, treatment of neonatal (but not adult) mice with cyclosporin A results in polyendocrine autoimmunity and the spectrum of disease can be widened to include thyroiditis when thymectomy is performed immediately after giving the drug, while it is abrogated by infusion of normal T cells (Sakaguchi & Sakaguchi, 1989).

Immunogenetics

The thymectomy and irradiation model is strain-dependent and although a clear MHC genetic influence was apparent in initial studies, wide variation in disease severity was observed in rats with the most susceptible RT1 haplotype (Penhale et al., 1975). Further analysis suggests a multigenic disorder, with one gene located in the rat MHC, RT1, another influencing the T cell repertoire and a third affecting the thyroid itself (Kotani et al., 1981). In thymectomy-induced EAT in mice, disease also appears strain-dependent, but this does not correlate with susceptibility to immunisation-induced EAT (Kojima et al., 1976a).

Environmental factors

As in immunisation-induced EAT, female animals tend to have a high incidence of thyroiditis and more severe disease after thymectomy. Castration of male animals conferred the same susceptibility as females, while progesterone augmented and oestrogen inhibited disease in females (Penhale & Ansar Ahmed, 1981; Ansar Ahmed, Young & Penhale, 1983). Infection is a major environmental factor. Rats raised under specific pathogen-free conditions until weaning were significantly less susceptible to EAT after thymectomy and irradiation, but this could be reversed by the administration of normal gastrointestinal flora (Penhale & Young, 1988). The exact micro-organism involved has not been delineated. However, these results suggest that EAT may result from microbial cross reaction with a thyroid antigen, and possibly transfer of the cross-reactive epitope from the intestine is enhanced following radiation damage.

T cell responses

The development of EAT after the manipulations listed above obviously suggests that the balance between helper and suppressor T cells has altered in favour of thyroid autoreactivity. Disease does not occur if thyroid extract is given to thymectomised rats during the course of irradiation, indicating that tolerance can be reintroduced possibly by stimulating residual suppressor cells. (Whitmore & Irvine, 1977). Although a chronic disease, thymectomy-induced EAT in the Buf rat improves with time. Tg antibody levels decline and circulating $CD8^+$ cells return to normal, supporting the idea that a suppressor population may be incompletely depleted in these models (Cohen, Dijkstra & Weetman, 1988).

The T cell subsets involved in murine forms of this disease have been delineated by reconstitution experiments. $Lyt-1^+$-depleted splenic T cells caused EAT (as well as oophoritis and gastritis) when injected into nude mice and the disease could be reversed by Lyt-1[+] cell transfer (Sakaguchi & Sakaguchi, 1989). In T cell depleted and reconstituted mice, disease appears to be induced by L3T4[+] cells weakly staining for Lyt-1; whereas, in keeping with the findings in nude mice, brightly staining Lyt-1[+] cells mediated suppression of disease, possibly by acting as inducers (Sugihara *et al.*, 1988). However, another L3T4[+] population present in thymocytes and peripheral lymphoid organs can also mediate suppression, which suggests considerable functional heterogeneity within this subset (Sugihara *et al.*, 1990).

It seems likely that neonatal thymectomy results in the maintenance of autoreactive T cell clones due to be deleted in later life; this is supported by studies of the T cell receptor repertoire in mice which develop EAT after thymectomy (H. Smith *et al.*, 1989). In mice at least, the cells which cause thyroiditis appear to be in the CD4[+] subset. Despite this incomplete tolerance, disease can be abrogated by suppressor cells, some of which may be CD4[+] (possibly inducers). In some strains, a polyendocrine disorder results, whereas in others the response appears to be thyroid-specific. This selectivity could reflect an unusually high frequency of thyroid-autoreactive T cells in incompletely tolerised animals (perhaps strain-dependent), or the importance of environmental agents such as epitopes on gut micro-organisms that cross-react with thyroid antigens.

The thyroid shows infiltration with macrophages and dendritic cells at an early stage after thymectomy in Buf rats and depletion of macrophages with silica reverses disease, so autoantigen is probably presented to autoreactive T cells by these conventional APC (Cohen *et al.*, 1988). Although class II[+] thyrocytes are seen in this form of EAT, their appearance never precedes the onset of lymphocytic infiltration, occurring instead after the peak of disease severity. These features suggest that such thyrocytes are unimportant as APC in initiating disease and it is possible that their late prominence may represent their role in establishing peripheral tolerance, as discussed in Chapter 1.

B cell responses and effector mechanisms

Thyroiditis in these animals seems primarily T cell-mediated, but Tg antibodies are readily detectable and are deposited within the thyroid gland (Noble *et al.*, 1976). The antibodies are not cytotoxic to thyroid cells *in vitro* and antibodies against other thyroid components (e.g. TPO) have not been found in the sera of thymectomised animals (Cohen & Weetman, 1990).

Spontaneous thyroiditis

The best characterised forms of spontaneous thyroiditis arise in the Obese strain (OS) chicken and the Bio Breeding (BB) and Buf strains of rat. The early work on OS chickens has been reviewed extensively (Wick *et al.*, 1982, 1985). As a result of selective breeding, more than 90% of these birds develop severe autoimmune hypothyroidism. The BB rat is best known as a model of spontaneous diabetes mellitus and this will be considered in much greater detail in the next chapter, but during the course of these studies, spontaneous thyroiditis was found in about 60% of animals (Sternthal *et al.*, 1981). The Buf rat, already mentioned, has a low incidence of spontaneous thyroiditis, which is maximal (around 25%) in multiparous females older than one year (Noble *et al.*, 1976).

Immunogenetics

Originally three genes were believed to control disease susceptibility in OS chickens: one in the MHC, another immunoregulatory locus outside the MHC and a third affecting the target organ (Rose, Bacon & Sundick, 1976). However, the effects of three genes, one at least recessive, have been detected in controlling the thyroid abnormality (Hála, 1988). The MHC may be important in outbred chickens but in the inbred, strictly selected animals used in current studies of thyroiditis this seems to play only a minor role. The major genetic determinants are those affecting the target organ and an unknown immune response gene, which may determine the hyper-responsiveness of T cells by enhancing IL-2-dependent activation (Kroemer & Wick, 1989). The cause of genetically determined thyroid abnormalities, which include increased iodine uptake before thyroiditis develops, decreased cell growth *in vitro* and enhanced susceptibility to passively transferred Tg antibody, is unknown (Trudeu *et al.*, 1983; Neu *et al.*, 1985).

The two forms of spontaneous thyroiditis in the rat are obviously genetically determined, being strain-specific. An important association between the MHC and the development of thyroiditis was shown using Buf × BB crosses, animals of the $RT1^{b/b}$ genotype having the highest incidence of thyroiditis and $RT1^{u/u}$ the lowest (Colle, Guttmann & Seemayer, 1985). Interestingly, the u haplotype is associated with diabetes. Selected F_2 mating pairs produced lines which still had variable incidences of thyroiditis, despite all animals being $RT1^{b/b}$, suggesting the influence of other unknown genes.

Environmental factors

OS chickens were originally developed from female birds with phenotypic signs of hypothyroidism, but both sexes now develop the condition equally; early treatment with testosterone reduces the severity of thyroiditis but has no effect after two to three weeks of age (Gause & Marsh, 1986). Although female Buf rats have a higher prevalence of thyroiditis than males in some studies (which may be related to multiple pregnancies and postpartum exacerbation of the autoimmune process), this is not always the case. In the BB rat both sexes are equally affected (Colle *et al.*, 1985).

An avian leukosis retrovirus produces a disease resembling Hashimoto's thyroiditis, but without Tg antibodies, when inoculated into white Leghorn chick embryos (Carter, Ow & Smith, 1983). Exogenous viruses have been observed in OS but not normal thyrocytes and preliminary investigations show particular endogenous retrovirus-like sequences in OS animals (Wick *et al.*, 1985; Ziemiecki *et al.*, 1988). However, much more work is clearly required in this area to establish an aetiological role for these viruses.

A major environmental determinant in all three models is dietary iodine (Bagchi *et al.*, 1985; Allen, Appel & Braverman, 1986a; Cohen & Weetman, 1988a). Excess iodine tends to enhance disease, whereas a low iodine diet ameliorates it. Several mechanisms might account for this, including direct thyroid cell toxicity with excess iodine, but in the OS chicken it is known that highly iodinated Tg is more immunogenic than poorly iodinated forms (Sundick *et al.*, 1987). It is not yet known whether abnormal iodine incorporation into Tg is one of the genetically determined target organ abnormalities in OS chickens. Although iodine may influence the immunogenicity of Tg, there is no evidence for any genetically determined abnormality in the OS chicken Tg molecule, the disease being dependent on exposure to Tg which can come from normal strains (Pontes de Carvalho *et al.*, 1982).

OS chickens require T4 supplementation to thrive, such is the severity of their thyroiditis, but the effect of T4 on the disease process has been assessed in BB rats which do not become overtly hypothyroid. Excessive exogenous T4, at concentrations sufficient to suppress serum TSH levels, reduces the severity of thyroiditis and suppresses Tg antibody formation, although this effect can be countered by giving iodine supplementation (Banovac *et al.*, 1988; Reinhardt *et al.*, 1988). Whether this amelioration is mediated through the high levels of T4 or suppressed TSH is unclear; similar findings, including a generalised immunological disturbance, were noted above in Tg-immunised rats.

A variety of chemicals enhance the development of thyroiditis in Buf rats. This discovery arose from the testing of compounds for carcinogenicity in this particular strain which has a propensity to develop spontaneous pituitary and adrenal neoplasms. Trypan blue, carbon tetrachloride and anthracene derivatives all cause thyroiditis but 3-methylcholanthrene has received the most attention (Glover, Reuber & Godfrey, 1969; Silverman & Rose, 1975). The disease appears similar to the truly spontaneous form and may be related to the immunosuppressive activity of this polycyclic aromatic hydrocarbon, which includes suppression of IL-2 and lymphotoxin production (Ghoneum, Wojdani & Alfred, 1987).

Thus, a wide variety of endogenous and exogenous factors can alter the induction and expression of thyroiditis in these genetically susceptible animals. The effect of iodine is particularly interesting, since there is accumulating evidence that this may also be important in human disease (see below). The observations on Buf rats also point to the possible involvement of unsuspected environmental pollutants in precipitating autoimmunity. No clear role for infection is suggested in these models. The same intestinal micro-organisms may be as necessary in Buf and BB rats as in thymectomy and irradiation-induced EAT but this has not been tested.

T cell responses

Thyroiditis in OS chickens is critically dependent on T cells: their complete removal within a day of hatching prevents disease (Pontes de Carvalho, Wick & Roitt, 1981). However, later thymectomy with less complete T cell depletion exacerbates thyroiditis (Wick, Kite & Witebsky, 1970). This is in keeping with the features noted previously in other forms of EAT and relates to further impairment of already incomplete centrally imposed tolerance and defective peripheral suppressor mechanisms. The importance of T cells in mediating OS thyroiditis is further shown by (i) the ability of T cells from bursectomised donors to transfer disease and (ii) the fact that a high proportion of the thyroid-infiltrating lymphocytes are activated T cells (Krömer et al., 1985). Dendritic cells are present in the thyroids of normal chickens and may be key APC; Ia$^+$ thyrocytes are only seen adjacent to areas of lymphocytic infiltration, indicating that Ia expression is a secondary event (Wick et al., 1984).

The effect of thymectomy on Buf rats has been discussed above. The importance of activated T cells in mediating this type of thyroiditis is shown by the complete prevention of disease if animals are given an IL-2 receptor blocking monoclonal antibody, together with a low dose of cyclosporin A (Cohen, Diamantstein & Weetman, 1990). Intrathyroidal dendritic cells are prominent early in the thyroiditis of BB rats, resembling the lesions in thymectomised Buf rats (Kabel et al., 1987). Depletion of macrophages with silica in the BB rat prevents the development of thyroiditis, again analogous to the Buf rat (Lee et al., 1988). Together these results suggest that macrophages and dendritic cells are the key APC, mediating spontaneous as well as induced animal thyroiditis.

B cell responses

A striking feature of OS chickens and BB rats is the development of polyendocrine autoimmunity, which obviously has parallels in some patients with autoimmune thyroid disease (Chapter 8). In OS chickens, this propensity is reflected by the production of antibodies to adrenal, exocrine pancreas and proventricular glands in the stomach, (the latter resembling the autoantibodies in pernicious anaemia) but non-organ-specific autoantibodies are detectable as well, suggesting a generalised hyper-responsiveness to autoantigens (Khoury et al., 1982). Thyroid microsomal as well as Tg antibodies are present and immune complex deposition in the basal lamina of thyroid follicles can be detected within three weeks of hatching (Katz, Kite & Albini, 1981).

In the Buf rat there is a rough correlation between Tg antibody levels and the severity of thyroiditis, although the serum levels decline with maximum lymphocytic infiltration (Noble et al., 1976). Immunofluorescence has revealed in vivo deposition of autoantibodies in these animals. Strain-related and interstrain recurrent idiotypes have been described on Tg antibodies from Buf rats, anti-idiotypic antibodies can be detected in animals with EAT and heterologous anti-idiotypes (raised in rabbits) can reduce the circulating level of Tg autoantibodies (Zanetti & Bigazzi, 1981; Zanetti, Barton & Bigazzi, 1983). However, effects of anti-idiotypic antibodies on thyroiditis were not assessed in these experiments.

Effector mechanisms

As in the other types of EAT, it seems likely that T cell-mediated cytotoxicity is important in thyroid injury. However, macrophages may also have an effector role, especially as these are the first cells to infiltrate the gland in Buf and BB rats. Antibodies seem more notable mediators of OS thyroiditis than the previously described forms of EAT: bursectomy (depleting B cells) suppresses disease (Wick et al., 1970) and thyroiditis can be precipitated by materno-embryonal transfer of antibodies, although full expression requires the development of the immune system (Katz, Albini & Kite, 1986). Besides complement fixation (mediated by microsomal antibodies), a pathogenic role for thyroid autoantibodies as mediators of ADCC has been suggested in OS thyroiditis (Wick et al., 1982).

Summary

All of these forms of thyroid autoimmunity have provided invaluable insights into aetiology and pathogenesis. In general, susceptibility to EAT is polygenic. Class II MHC genes make a major contribution, but other genes including those controlling T cells and the target organ also seem important, if currently ill-defined. A variety of endogenous and exogenous factors modulate this genetic susceptibility and of particular interest are the influence of dietary iodine and the possible role of cross-reacting microbial determinants. All models are T cell-dependent and incomplete tolerance to Tg is frequent. Autoreactivity is controlled by peripheral mechanisms which include suppressor cells, although these are not exclusively CD8$^+$. There is clear evidence for cytotoxic T cells as effectors of thyroid injury, whereas Tg antibodies appear to have little pathogenic role. However, there are important caveats in extrapolating the findings in EAT to human disease. Firstly, tolerance to an antigen which circulates, like Tg, may well be different from ostensibly fixed antigens like TPO. Secondly, EAT tends to remit, except in OS chickens in which disease occurs early in life; both features are unlike Hashimoto's thyroiditis. Finally, the non-spontaneous forms of EAT involve major perturbations produced by CFA, thymectomy or irradiation and the influence of these on general immune responsiveness must be considered in any analysis.

Autoimmune thyroid disease in man

The three main disorders, autoimmune hypothyroidism (Hashimoto's thyroiditis and primary myxoedema), Graves' disease (together with the associated ophthalmopathy and pretibial myxoedema) and postpartum thyroiditis, will be considered separately below. However, all share reactivity against the same thyroid components, albeit to varying extents and therefore the first part of this section will be devoted to a review of these autoantigens.

Autoantigens in thyroiditis

Thyroglobulin (Tg)

As described in the previous section, Tg was the first self antigen found to induce autoreactivity. The demonstration of Tg in the thyroid lymph and in the peripheral blood of normal animals effectively invalidated sequestration of this particular autoantigen as a mechanism for averting autoimmunity (Daniel et al., 1967). Tg is a homodimeric glycoprotein, each subunit being 330 kd, which is secreted by thyrocytes and stored in the follicular colloid. Tyrosine residues on the molecule are iodinated at the thyrocyte's apical surface and a subset of these iodotyrosyl residues are coupled to form T4 and triiodothyronine (T3). Release of these hormones depends on endocytosis and lysosomal hydrolysis of Tg. The gene encoding Tg occupies 200 kb on chromosome 8 and gives rise to an abundant mRNA after TSH activation of thyrocytes (Malthiery & Lissitzky, 1987). Tg from patients with Graves' disease cannot be distinguished immunologically from normal Tg (Chan et al., 1987).

Although many epitopes are recognised on xenogeneic Tg in immunisation experiments with animals, there is much greater restriction in the response to the autologous molecule. In man, each subunit possesses two major and one minor autoantigenic epitope recognised by autoantibodies from patients with thyroiditis (Nye, Pontes de Carvalho & Roitt, 1980). However, more recent epitope mapping with a large number of monoclonal antibodies revealed that the number of reacting determinants increases with rising titres of Tg autoantibody and that no epitopes are found with murine antibodies which are not also detectable with human sera (Bresler *et al.*, 1990). In contrast, natural Tg autoantibodies, of low affinity and titre from patients without biochemical evidence of thyroid disease, recognise only the hormonogenic regions, the most evolutionarily conserved portion of the molecule. Because the immunodominant epitopes are widely spaced on this large molecule, preventing IgG cross-linking, Tg antibodies do not fix complement (Adler *et al.*, 1984). T cell epitopes on Tg have not been defined so far.

Thyroid peroxidase (TPO)

Soon after the seminal discovery of Tg autoreactivity, antibodies against a second thyroid component were described which fixed complement (Trotter, Belyavin & Wadhams, 1957). Although these antibodies bound to the microsomal fraction, they also reacted with a cell surface antigen on the apical microvillar border and immunoglobulin deposited *in vivo* could be detected at this site in patients with thyroid autoimmunity (Khoury, Bottazzo & Roitt, 1984). Immunoprecipitation and immunoblotting revealed the microsomal antigen to be a poorly glycosylated protein of around 100–105 kd, which was defined as TPO from inhibition studies with TPO-specific monoclonal antibodies (Czarnocka *et al.*, 1985). Almost all of the microsomal antigenic determinants recognised by autoantibodies appear to be on TPO (Kotani *et al.*, 1986).

TPO is the haem-containing enzyme that is responsible for iodinating and coupling tyrosyl residues on Tg. It is encoded on chromosome 2 and gives rise to two coexisting proteins through alternate splicing of the gene (Kimura *et al.*, 1987). Antibodies against native TPO correspond to those detected by the standard haemagglutination assay, but a proportion of patients possess antibodies which react with denatured or reduced TPO (Hamada *et al.*, 1987). At least six B cell epitopes have been identified, including the catalytic sites for peroxidation, but it is unclear whether antibodies against these sites contribute to hypothyroidism by blocking normal T3 and T4 synthesis (Doble *et al.*, 1988). There is also an epitope which appears to be shared between Tg and TPO and autoantibodies which cross-react with these two are frequent in the sera of patients with thyroid autoimmunity, but not in normal subjects with naturally occurring Tg antibodies (Naito *et al.*, 1990). As yet little is known regarding T cell epitopes.

The TSH receptor

TSH stimulates thyroid cell function through a membrane receptor mainly utilising cyclic AMP (cAMP) as a second messenger. Adams & Purves (1956) discovered that a long-acting thyroid stimulator (LATS) occurred in Graves' disease and this led to the delineation of autoantibodies reacting with the TSH receptor as the cause of this disorder (Kriss, Pleshakov & Chien, 1964; Meek *et al.*, 1964). Subsequent work on TSH receptor antibodies is detailed below, but the central role of the receptor in thyroid physiology, and the almost unique stimulatory effects of autoantibodies to it, have made the further understanding of this molecule a major goal. A range of models has been proposed using biochemical techniques (reviewed by Rees Smith, McLachlan & Furmaniak, 1988), but molecular cloning has finally provided the answer. The TSH receptor shares many features with other receptors coupled to a G protein, the latter allowing adenylate cyclase stimulation. Indeed, this likelihood was used to isolate putative clones from a thyroid cDNA library, by selectively amplifying DNA segments with sequence similarity to genes for these already known receptors (Parmentier *et al.*, 1989).

The TSH receptor is 87 kd and comprises a large extracellular domain (398 amino acids), with five glycosylation sites, coupled to a carboxy terminal domain (346 residues) with seven transmembrane regions (Libert *et al.*, 1989; Nagayama *et al.*, 1989; Misrahi *et al.*, 1990). The amino terminal domain is probably the TSH binding site, sharing 45% sequence homology with the luteinising hormone receptor, while the transmembrane sequences show much greater homology, particularly the third intracellular loop which is the region interacting with the G protein. Dog and human TSH receptor sequences are more than 90% homologous. Interaction of the cloned and expressed TSH receptor with autoantibodies has already been reported and further analysis should soon permit a clearer understanding of TSH receptor–antibody interactions in autoimmune thyroid diseases.

Other antigens

Non-specific cyto-skeletal components, particularly tubulin, may be autoantigenic (Rousset *et al.*, 1983). A so-called second colloid antigen besides Tg has been known for a long time (Balfour *et al.*, 1961) but there is little information on its structure or function. Thyroid hormones themselves can give rise to autoantibodies, the main consequence being interference in thyroid hormone assays (Sakata, Nakamura & Miura, 1985). Other thyroid-specific autoantigens exist which can be revealed by molecular techniques. Screening of a thyroid cDNA with sera from patients with Hashimoto's thyroiditis has led to cloning of an antigen of unknown function, ATRA–1, which is recognised by about a third of sera (Hirayu *et al.*, 1987), and attempts to clone the TSH receptor revealed a cDNA encoding a 70 kd thyroid antigen which reacts with antibodies present in 65% of Graves' sera (Chan *et al.*, 1989). Further work will delineate the role of such molecules in thyroiditis, but it seems clear that the key thyroid autoantigens, Tg, TPO and the TSH receptor, have now been cloned and sequenced. The ability to produce pure, recombinant antigens will be invaluable not only in further understanding the autoimmune response, but also in producing diagnostic assays for autoantibodies.

Autoimmune hypothyroidism

This term encompasses several syndromes of autoimmune thyroid destruction but their nosological definition remains unclear. Broadly, goitrous autoimmune thyroiditis can be divided into three variants, oxyphil (the classical Hashimoto goitre), fibrous and lymphocytic (Doniach, Bottazzo & Russell, 1979), and these contrast with primary myxoedema, in which there is strikingly little evidence for any preceding goitre. The term Hashimoto's thyroiditis is often used in studies without clarifying whether the patients tested actually had goitrous hypothyroidism. The histology of primary myxoedema is similar to the fibrous variant of Hashimoto's thyroiditis, including lymphocytic infiltration (Katz & Vickery, 1974) and the severity of fibrosis is directly related to the development of hypothyroidism (Maagøe *et al.*, 1977), so that it is easy to imagine that these two entities might form a spectrum. However, the lymphocytic variant shows little change with time. A marked decrease in thyroid enlargement is observed in less than a third of patients receiving thyroid hormone replacement (which reduces TSH stimulation) and in even fewer not taking T4 (Hayashi *et al.*, 1985). There is also an overlap with Graves' disease, autoimmune hypothyroidism following thyrotoxicosis probably being part of the natural history of Graves' disease (Wood & Ingbar, 1979), while the reverse sequence of hypothyroidism followed by thyrotoxicosis is less common.

Autoimmune hypothyroidism is common. In an extensive survey of a village in North-East England, the prevalence was at least 1% in women but less than 0.1% in men (Tunbridge *et al.*, 1977). Thyroid autoreactivity, that is, the presence of thyroid autoantibodies without thyroid dysfunction, was even more common, being found in 10.3% of women and 2.7% of men, increasing with age in women only. This frequency is related to the prevalence of focal thyroiditis, found at routine autopsy in 6% of men and 22% of women; there is a close association between the presence of such lymphocytic infiltration and circulating thyroid antibodies (Williams & Doniach, 1962; Yoshida *et al.*, 1978). Thus, there is a high prevalence of thyroid autoreactivity in the community which progresses to overt disease in around 5–10% of cases. The emergence of gland dysfunction is a slow process. For instance, overt hypothyroidism developed at a rate of 5% per year in subjects who had thyroid antibodies and an elevated TSH (but normal T3 and T4) at presentation, while the presence of thyroid autoantibodies alone had no impact over a four year period (Tunbridge *et al.*, 1981). This is supported by follow-up studies on thyroid autoantibodies in middle-aged and elderly populations showing modest fluctuations in antibody levels but little progression to thyroid failure (Lazarus *et al.*, 1984; Aho *et al.*, 1985). These features suggest either the presence of protective mechanisms in the majority of such individuals which prevent autoreactivity becoming a frank, autoimmune disease or the existence of additional immunological responses (manifested by an elevated TSH as a marker of thyroid damage) in those subjects who become hypothyroid. These factors of course may be determined genetically or environmentally.

Immunogenetics

The importance of genetic factors in Hashimoto's thyroiditis was first established by the detection of thyroid autoantibodies in half the siblings of such patients (Hall, Owen & Smart, 1964). When MHC genes were first linked to many autoimmune disorders, it was somewhat surprising that no HLA associations with autoimmune hypothyroidism were immediately apparent. However, subdivision of Caucasian patients revealed that those without a goitre, i.e. primary myxoedema, had an increased frequency of HLA-B8, while those with a Hashimoto goitre did not (Irvine, 1978). These findings not only suggested the influence of MHC genes on susceptibility, but also provided support for the separability of the two types of thyroiditis.

HLA-B8 is in linkage disequilibrium with HLA-DR3 and an association of DR3, about as strong as for B8 (relative risk around 3.5), was found with atrophic thyroiditis (Moens & Farid, 1978). In contrast, Hashimoto's thyroiditis was associated with HLA-DR5, with a similar relative risk (Weissel *et al.*, 1980). This report on Austrian patients was apparently confirmed in those from Newfoundland and Denmark, although the DR5 association in the latter study was of only borderline significance and would not stand correction for the number of variables tested (Farid *et al.*, 1981; Thomsen *et al.*, 1983). However, using typing reagents distributed by the

Canadian Red Cross rather than locally available HLA antisera, one of these groups found subsequently that goitrous hypothyroidism was in fact associated with HLA-DR4 (Thompson & Farid, 1985). In this study, DR4 conferred a relative risk of 5.0, but there appears to have been no correction for the number of DR antigens tested on what was a small patient sample ($n = 21$). Further confusion is added by a Canadian study from Toronto in which HLA-DR5 was associated with Hashimoto's thyroiditis. The relative risk was 4.2 and the aetiological fraction 0.28 (Vargas et al., 1988). In addition, Hungarian patients actually showed an association with HLA-DR3, with a relative risk 3.3 and aetiological fraction of 0.29 (Stenszky et al., 1987). There was no linkage between DR3 and B8 in these patients, compatible with earlier findings since it suggests that the DR3-bearing haplotype in these Hashimoto patients does not include HLA-B8.

Clearly one variable which may explain these conflicting results is the use of different typing reagents. We have recently used RFLP to DR type English patients with Hashimoto's thyroiditis and found a significant association of the HLA-DR3 with autoimmune hypothyroidism irrespective of the presence of a goitre at presentation; DQw2, in strong linkage disequilibrium with DR3, was also increased in these patients (Tandon, Zhang & Weetman, 1991). The aetiological fraction was 0.35 for DR3 in Hashimoto's thyroiditis and 0.22 for primary myxoedema. Another reason for the differences between studies could be that intra-Caucasian ethnic differences in susceptibility exist, a possibility supported by the differing DR associations of Hashimoto's thyroiditis in non-Caucasian races. There is a strong association of HLA-DRw9 with Hashimoto's thyroiditis in Southern Chinese (Hawkins et al., 1987). Although in these patients primary myxoedema was not significantly associated with DRw9, this was due to the small number of patients studied: the frequency of this allele was the same in the goitrous and non-goitrous groups. In Japanese the DRw53 supertypic specificity (Gorski, Rollini & Mach, 1987) is dominantly associated with Hashimoto's thyroiditis (aetiological fraction 0.56), whereas the DR alleles 1 to 10 show no significant associations (Honda et al., 1989). Finally, it is possible that the disease and hence its genetic susceptibility are both changing with time. For instance, increasing iodine intake may influence the disorder (see below), and the more prosaic problem of ascertainment bias exists, particularly with the increasing application of accurate screening tests for hypothyroidism.

Thus, in Caucasians it seems that HLA-DR3 is associated with primary myxoedema and currently, at least in some regions, with Hashimoto's thyroiditis. About a third or less of the susceptibility to these diseases can be ascribed to DR3, clearly suggesting that other genes and/or environmental factors are also important. MHC immune response genes in linkage disequlibrium with DR3 are one possibility, but there is no obvious increase in risk with loci closer to either the DQ or the B regions. Three other sets of candidate genes have been investigated.

Study of IgG heavy chain allotypes in Japanese Hashimoto patients initially indicated that the G1m(1, 2); G3m(21) haplotype was increased (Nakao *et al.*, 1980), although two other studies, one from Japan and the other from Newfoundland, found no significant association with any Gm haplotype (Nakao *et al.*, 1982; Tamai *et al.*, 1985). However, a weak influence of allotypes was discerned in the Canadian subjects if only those with primary myxoedema were analysed. The other report (Tamai *et al.*, 1985) concerned families selected because two or more first degree relatives had Graves' disease, and the small percentage of remaining family members ($n = 14$) with Hashimoto's thyroiditis were studied. All of these shared the same HLA and Gm haplotypes, suggesting that genes linked to both sets of markers contributed to susceptibility but obviously this was a highly selected group, probably unrepresentative of the majority of patients. In Hungary, Gm allotype frequencies did not differ between Hashimoto and normal subjects, although a positive interaction between the G3m(21) phenotype and HLA-DR3 was found in these patients (Stenszky *et al.*, 1987). Finally, in selected families the inheritance of autoantibodies to Tg and TPO appears to be a dominant trait which is not linked to HLA markers, but linkage analysis for Gm markers unfortunately was not informative in this study (Phillips *et al.*, 1990).

A T cell receptor RFLP, located in the α chain V region, is associated with autoimmune hypothyroidism (Weetman *et al.*, 1987a), and in Japanese but not Caucasian patients, a T cell receptor β chain C region RFLP is associated with Hashimoto's thyroiditis (Ito *et al.*, 1989). Finally, a classical inherited common trait, the inability to taste phenylthiocarbamide (PTC), has been associated with hypothyroidism of unspecified cause, although a small study of 32 Hashimoto patients failed to find any difference from normal in taster status (Mourant, Kopeć & Domaniewska-Sobczak, 1978; Farid, Barnard & Bryant, 1977a). This may be worth further analysis, since PTC and other thiourea compounds block TPO and taster status may possibly be linked to the activity of this key enzyme (and autoantigen).

In summary, genetic susceptibility to autoimmune hypothyroidism is related to HLA-DR3, although other MHC susceptibility loci may be more closely associated, as appears to be the case for Japanese patients. There is incomplete agreement regarding the separate heritability of primary myxoedema and Hashimoto's thyroiditis based on DR alleles. T cell receptor and immunoglobulin genes may make an additional contribution to susceptibility, although, as previously described, the mere presence of thyroid autoantibodies does not necessarily lead to gland failure. The influence of other genes, including those governing PTC tasting, remains unclear.

Environmental factors

Woman have a greater chance of developing autoimmune hypothyroidism than men, presumably related to sex hormones, as in EAT. A somewhat conflicting finding is the excess of thyroid autoimmunity in Turner's but not Kleinfelter's syndrome (Doniach, Roitt & Polani, 1968). The severity of the autoimmune response is greater in mosaics (with abnormal sex chromosome structure) than pure XO ovarian dysgenesis; how this association arises is unknown. Trisomy 21 also appears to be a risk factor for thyroid auto-immunity, again of uncertain mechanism (Baxter *et al.*, 1975). There is no evidence implicating infections, subacute or viral thyroiditis very rarely leading to hypothyroidism. However, therapeutic irradiation to the head and neck is a risk factor, 30% of children so treated having Hashimoto's thyroiditis around 25 years later (Valdiserri & Borochovitz, 1980). This may relate to intensified antigen release from the damaged gland and a local inflammatory response.

As in EAT, iodine has received increasing attention. The increasing incidence of Hashimoto's thyroiditis in the mid-western states of the USA between 1920 and 1960 coincides with the introduction of iodine prophylaxis for endemic goitre (McConahey *et al.*, 1962; Weaver, Batsakis & Nishiyama, 1969) and a careful 20 year follow-up of thyroidectomy specimens revealed a much higher frequency of lymphocytic infiltration after the introduction of iodisation (Harach *et al.*, 1985). The introduction of iodised oil as prophylaxis on the island of Corfu resulted in the appearance of thyroid autoantibodies in 43% of subjects six months later (Boukis *et al.*, 1983). Iodine-containing drugs can also be responsible. Iodine in cough medicine was responsible for goitre in asthma patients, half of whom had thyroid autoantibodies (Hall, Turner-Warwick & Doniach, 1966). Amiodarone-induced hypothyroidism is commonly found in those with pre-existing thyroid autoimmunity and may act by potentiating the underlying thyroiditis (Martino *et al.*, 1987). This seems particularly so in iodine-deficient areas, since amiodarone has no such consistent effect in the UK where iodine intake is not only sufficient, but also rising (Weetman *et al.*, 1988a).

T cell responses

Studies on T cells in thyroiditis can be divided into those which characterise T cell phenotypes and those examining *in vitro* function. Many such analyses have perforce used circulating T cells which may reflect poorly (or not at all) the intrathyroidal pathology; one would not look at people driving to work in order to find out what they did on arrival. However, examination of the

Table 3.1. *T cell receptor phenotypes in Hashimoto's thyroiditis*

Author	Number of patients	CD4 : CD8 Ratio	Other comments
Circulating lymphocytes			
Thielemans et al., 1981	15	Increased	Due to low CD8[+] T cells; present in thyroiditis irrespective of T4 levels.
Canonica et al., 1982	11	Normal	Increased activated (Ia[+], 4F2[+]) T cells.
Bonnyns et al., 1983	58	Increased (on T4 replacement)	Ratio decreased in primary myxoedema when hypothyroid.
Fournier et al., 1983	23	Decreased	Due to low CD4[+] T cells.
Wall et al., 1983	53	Normal	Increased activated (Ia[+]) T cells.
Iwatani et al., 1983	23	Normal	No effect of high or low T4 levels.
Chan & Walfish, 1986	27	Normal	No effect of low T4 levels. Increased activated (Ia[+]) T cells.
Intrathyroidal lymphocytes[a]			
Jansson et al., 1984a	2	Mainly CD4[+]	Many Ia[+] T cells
Aichinger et al., 1985	7	Mainly CD4[+]	Some Leu 7[+] NK cells
Misaki et al., 1985	10	Mainly CD4[+]	Some Leu 7[+] NK cells

[a] By immunohistochemical analysis.

infiltrating T cells also has inherent problems, resulting from the slow evolution of disease which makes it almost impossible to separate primary and secondary changes.

Circulating T cell phenotypes have been analysed in some detail. Depending on the study, circulating CD8[+] T cell numbers may be normal or low, and 'activated' T cells, bearing MHC class II (or Ia) molecules, tend to be elevated (Table 3.1). However, these changes are found in many other autoimmune disorders. T cells comprise the bulk of the intrathyroidal lymphocytes and the CD4[+] phenotype predominates (Table 3.1). The T cells are often activated, and are found particularly in areas of glandular destruction. In one of two Hashimoto glands examined, an excess of $\gamma\delta$ receptor-bearing T cells has been observed compared to the peripheral blood. There was no obvious abnormality in the distribution of $V\beta$ gene family usage by $\alpha\beta$ receptor-bearing T cells in the thyroid or peripheral blood, although only a limited number of family-specific monoclonal anti-bodies were used to phenotype the cells (Teng et al., 1990a). This lack of restricted clonality is supported by Southern blot analysis of T cell receptor gene rearrangements. Only one of 11 Hashimoto's patients tested had a clonally restricted pattern in the infiltrating T cells (Kaulfersch et al., 1988; Katzin, Fishleder & Tubbs, 1989). However, it is possible that there is a pauciclonal T cell response early in disease which is impossible to detect later because non-specific T cells accumulate.

Lymphocytes binding Tg and thyroid microsomes can be detected in the circulation of healthy subjects (Bankhurst, Torrigiani & Allison, 1973; Roberts, Whittingham & McKay, 1973; Khalid, Hamilton & Cauchi, 1976). These are mainly B cells. T cells from normals which bind thyroid autoanti-gens may have only a low affinity and therefore little potential for causing autoimmune disease. Nonetheless such results suggest that B cell tolerance is normally incomplete. From the frequency of thyroiditis and thyroid autoantibodies in the population and the experimental results showing imperfect deletion of autoreactive T cells in other situations, it seems probable that thyroid-specific T cells are not totally deleted either. What holds them in check? T suppressor cells are obvious candidates for this and considerable efforts have been made to delineate a defect in T suppressor cell function as a cause for Hashimoto's thyroiditis. These experiments have usually assessed the same phenomena in Graves' disease simultaneously and can be divided broadly into those concerned with general suppressor effects and those which are thyroid-specific.

The generalised decrease in circulating $CD8^+$ cells has been equated with lowered suppressor function (Thielemans et al., 1981) but this seductive idea, based on the in vitro behaviour of T cells in mitogen-activated assays, is untenable, as CD8 simply indicates that the T cells are class I-restricted (Chapter 1). Such bracketing of phenotype with function has been a problem in this field, persisting latterly as a suppressor–inducer role was suggested for $CD45RA^+$ T cells. In any case, not all studies have found a lowered proportion of circulating $CD8^+$ T cells in Hashimoto's thyroiditis, which would account for the normal responses to the mitogen concanavalin A (which stimulates suppression in vitro), as well as normal autologous and allogeneic mixed lymphocyte reactions in these patients (Aoki, Pinnama-neni & DeGroot, 1979; Fournier et al., 1983). In contrast, others have found an increased $CD4^+ : CD8^+$ ratio in Hashimoto lymphocytes and exacerba-tion of this abnormality after culture for nine days; culture also led to a generalised enhancement of lymphocyte proliferation to a wide array of non-thyroidal autoantigens (Stern & Dau, 1987).

Antigen-specific T cells have been analysed by three main techniques: proliferative responses, migration inhibition assays and B cell co-culture experiments. The first of these relies on the proliferation (or blastogenesis) of sensitised T cells on contact with specific antigens *in vitro*, triggered by IL-2 production and IL-2 receptor expression. Weak proliferative responses to Tg and TPO are found in many patients with Hashimoto's thyroiditis and can be enhanced by selecting a population with putative helper properties or by removing $CD8^+$ T cells, which may be simply exerting a non-specific suppressor effect in such cultures (Aoki & DeGroot, 1979; Canonica *et al.*, 1984; Weetman, 1989). However, removal of $CD8^+$ T cells from normal individuals does not not lead to a stimulation of the remaining cells by Tg or TPO, suggesting either that thyroid-specific T cells cannot be detected in healthy subjects or that a non-$CD8^+$ T cell population suppresses their stimulation. Despite manipulations of the culture conditions, strong blasto-genic responses are never seen in Hashimoto's thyroiditis, although thyroid infiltrating T cells produce a slightly greater response than those in the circulation.

The migration inhibition assay utilises the production of a cytokine, migration inhibition factor (MIF), in response to an antigen as a marker of specific T cell sensitisation. There are many variants of the technique. In particular, the direct MIF test uses the same cells as both producers of the factor and responders in the assay of its concentration, whereas the indirect MIF test takes lymphocyte supernatants generated in response to the antigen and assays these on a separate cell population. The assay for MIF appears deceptively simple. Cells are packed into a capillary tube and their subsequent migration out of it measured by planimetry: the lower the area of migration, the greater the concentration of MIF. However, the assay is critically dependent on uniform cell packing in the capillary tube and an exactly similar tube length between replicates.

MIF production by Hashimoto T cells has been consistently observed in response to a crude thyroid extract, as well as to Tg and thyroid microsomal antigen (Brostoff, 1970; Calder *et al.*, 1973; Okita *et al.*, 1980; Vento *et al.*, 1984). A non-organ-specific response to mitochondria has also been detected in 34–55% of patients, compared to positive responses to thyroid extract in 63–100%. Few normal subjects produce a positive MIF test with thyroid antigens. These results are compatible with the frequent, albeit weak, blastogenic responses discussed above, but a striking anomaly is that this MIF production appears to be confined to circulating T cells; intra-thyroidal lymphocytes in Hashimoto's thyroiditis do not display sensitisa-tion in this assay (Tötterman, Andersson & Hayry, 1979).

Table 3.2. *Migration inhibition factor (MIF) assay for putative thyroid-specific T cells (Okita* et al., *1981)*

Source of responder lymphocytes	Thyroid Antigen[a]	Added Cells	Effect[b]
Normal	−	−	Normal migration
Normal	+	−	Normal migration
Hashimoto's thyroiditis	−	−	Normal migration
Hashimoto's thyroiditis	+	−	Reduced migration
Hashimoto's thyroiditis	+	Normal T cells (1 : 1–1 : 9)	Normal migration
Hashimoto's thyroiditis	+	Hashimoto T Cells (1 : 1)	Reduced migration
Hashimoto's thyroiditis	+	Mitomycin treated or irradiated normal T cells[c]	Reduced migration
Hashimoto's thyroiditis (Puromycin treated)[d]	+	−	Normal migration

[a] 800 g supernatant of a thyroid homogenate.
[b] Measured as the area of lymphocyte migration from a packed capillary tube; reduced migration implies production of MIF by sensitised T cells in response to antigen.
[c] Inhibits DNA synthesis.
[d] Inhibits protein synthesis.

Volpé and colleagues have utilised the direct MIF assay to test for the existence of thyroid-specific suppressor cells in thyroid autoimmunity. By adding allogeneic normal lymphocytes to Hashimoto lymphocytes, at a ratio of 1 : 9, the abnormal Hashimoto T cell migration was abolished (Table 3.2), implying that the normal T cells had prevented MIF production by the autoreactive T cells (Okita, Row & Volpé, 1980). Mixing allogeneic Hashimoto T cells had no such effect (in two tests) suggesting that this was not due to some effect of the mixed lymphocyte reaction. The allogeneic T cells which abolish MIF production are radiosensitive, a property regarded as a hallmark of suppressor cell function, but their phenotypic characterisation has not been performed (Topliss *et al.*, 1981). A similar correctable defect was also found in Graves' disease, yet cells from these patients were found to prevent MIF production by T cells from type 1 diabetic patients in response to an islet cell antigenic extract (Topliss *et al.*, 1983). This implies that the defect in Graves' disease and, by association Hashimoto's thyroiditis, is thyroid-specific.

Based on these findings, a cogent argument for a defect in antigen-specific suppressor cells causing autoimmune thyroiditis has been advanced (Volpé, 1988). The use of alloreactive T cells remains a problem, since it implies stimulation of the putative suppressor cells by autoantigen in a MHC-unrestricted fashion. Moreover, in view of the large number of epitopes in a crude tissue extract, the frequency of such suppressor cells in healthy individuals must be extremely high. Technical problems affecting the interpretation of these kinds of assay also exist (Chapter 1). The recent cloning of MIF should soon allow its distinction from other cytokines like IL-4 and γ-IFN with migration inhibiting properties, which may interfere in these assays, and allow a more accurate test to be developed for the further investigation of this aspect of immunoregulation (Weiser et al., 1989).

The third type of suppressor assay has used thyroid autoantibody-producing B cells as a readout of T cell function. Unfortunately, most methods have employed mitogens (usually pokeweed mitogen) to induce immunoglobulin production, which result in non-specific T cell activation and this makes interpretation of antigen specificity virtually impossible. The strategy of examining the differential production of autoantibody and total IgG is unhelpful, as this will generally reflect only the increased state of autoreactive B cell activation in these patients (see below) rather than T cell effects. Because B cells primarily rely on non-specific lymphokines for their activation, these assays may also be profoundly influenced by the pattern of T cell lymphokine release. This is of considerable interest but limited use as an index of specific suppression.

The initial culture techniques which permitted assay of thyroid autoanti-body production in vitro were achievements in themselves (see below) and were quickly applied to the analysis of T cell function. The addition of normal T cells to Hashimoto lymphocyte cultures had no effect on thyroid autoantibody production, taken to indicate an absence of activated suppressor cells in normals (McLachlan et al., 1980; Beall & Kruger, 1980a). In contrast, several studies have revealed an apparent defect in suppressor cell function, usually with Tg as the autoantigen under test. Using a plaque-forming cell assay which quantitates individual antibody-producing B cells, normal T cells or their antigen-stimulated supernatants were found to suppress Tg antibody production (in the absence of mitogens) by Hashimoto lymphocytes (Noma et al., 1982; Mori, Hamada & DeGroot, 1985; Row & Volpé, 1986). In apparent contrast to the MIF assay results in which the suppressor defect was universal, T cells from Hashimoto patients who did not have plaque-forming cells could also induce suppression and the defect appeared to be only partial even when present. Addition of autologous CD8$^+$ T cells to pokeweed mitogen-stimulated Hashimoto lymphocytes decreased thyroid autoantibody production, although there is little to support the contention that this is the result of an antigen-specific defect in CD4$^+$/CD8$^+$ T cell balance (Benveniste, Row & Volpé, 1985). Pokeweed mitogen or protein A (which cross-links B cell surface immunoglobulins) plus microsomal antigen as B cell stimulators have also been used to assess this; allogeneic CD8$^+$ T cells from normal individuals (or Hashimoto patients without circulating microsomal antibodies) are more efficient at suppressing microsomal antibody synthesis *in vitro* than CD8$^+$ T cells from Hashimoto patients with circulating antibodies (Iitaka *et al.*, 1988). However, the finding that total immunoglobulin as well as specific thyroid antibody production is reduced by allogeneic normal cells added to pokeweed mitogen-stimulated Hashimoto cultures certainly questions the specificity of any suppressor defect (Davies & Platzer, 1986).

Thus, there is evidence suggesting that, for Tg at least, suppressor cells may not be sufficiently effective in controlling the autoimmune response in Hashimoto's thyroiditis. There is also a good deal of data which does not completely support this, compatible instead with either a partial defect not universally found in this condition, or a generalised non-specific defect in suppressor cells. Whether these *in vitro* findings have counterparts *in vivo* is unknown, particularly since almost all experiments have relied on circulating T cells. From the lessons learnt with EAT, it would not be surprising if suppressor cells were important in preventing autoreactivity to Tg, but demonstrating that any defect in suppressor function detected in long-established disease represents a primary event in the aetiology is currently impossible. Finally, T cell regulation may be different for antigens like TPO and the TSH receptor which seem unlikely to be normal constituents of the circulation. The completeness of tolerance to these antigens can be assessed only when sufficient pure material is available.

At least it seems clear that autoantigen-responsive T cells exist in Hashimoto's thyroiditis: how are these stimulated? As expected, conventional APC (macrophages and dendritic cells) are capable of this as Tg presentation has been observed *in vitro* (Weetman, McGregor & Hall, 1983b; Farrant *et al.*, 1986). Morphological evidence certainly suggests that Tg may be presented *in vivo* by intrathyroidal follicular dendritic cells (Kasajima, Yamakawa & Imai, 1987). However, considerable attention has focussed on the possibility that thyrocytes themselves may act as APC. This hypothesis developed from the finding of MHC class II$^+$ thyrocytes in thyroidectomy specimens from patients with Hashimoto's thyroiditis and Graves' disease but not in normal tissue (Hanafusa *et al.*, 1983). Furthermore, thyrocytes in culture were found to express class II molecules after treatment with lectins, an action at first thought to be independent of their lymphocyte-stimulating properties (Pujol-Borrell *et al.*, 1983). The concept developed of such aberrant class II expression being the initiating event in autoimmune thyroiditis, possibly working in concert with an antigen-specific T suppressor cell defect (Bottazzo *et al.*, 1983).

Although no correlation between class II expression and the lymphocytic infiltrate was observed in the original report, subsequent studies have found a consistent close relationship (Jansson, Karlsson & Forsum, 1984a; Aichinger, Fill & Wick, 1985). It has also become clear that lectins exert their effect by stimulating T cells which inevitably contaminate thyrocyte cultures, and that the key lymphokine inducing the class II expression is γ-IFN (Todd *et al.*, 1985; Weetman *et al.*, 1985a). Normal thyrocytes and those from patients with autoimmune thyroid disease respond to γ-IFN in an identical fashion. Other cytokines have no effect on class II induction, although the effect of γ-IFN is enhanced by TNF, probably by increasing the binding of γ-IFN (Weetman & Rees, 1988; Bucsema *et al.*, 1989). Both γ-IFN and TNF are known to be produced by the thyroidal infiltrate in thyroiditis (Margolick, Weetman & Burman, 1988; Turner, Londei & Feldmann, 1987). Another factor increasing thyrocyte class II expression is TSH, which appears to act by stimulating progress through the cell cycle (Todd *et al.*,1987; Weetman, Green & Borysiewicz, 1987b). The raised TSH in autoimmune hypothyroidism could therefore enhance the class II-inducing effect of γ-IFN.

Thus it seems far more likely that thyrocyte class II expression arises secondary to the gland infiltration, and is therefore unlikely to initiate autoreactivity. This is borne out by the observations discussed in EAT. However, the phenomenon could still be important as a means of perpetuating the autoimmune response. Primary cultures of class II-expressing thyroid cells have been shown to present influenza peptides, but not whole virus, to histocompatible peptide-specific T cell clones and to stimulate T cells in the autologous mixed lymphocyte reaction (Londei *et al.*, 1984; Davies, 1985). Moreover, T cell lines or clones, expanded from the intra-thyroidal lymphocytes by culture with IL-2, proliferate in response to autologous class II$^+$ thyrocytes but not conventional APC, which indicates presentation of a thyrocyte component to specific autoreactive T cells, rather than merely an autologous mixed lymphocyte reaction (Londei, Bottazzo & Feldmann, 1985; Weetman, *et al.*; 1986a; Iwatani *et al.*, 1986). Thyrocytes may also synthesise IL-1 (Grubeck-Loebenstein *et al.*, 1989), but this appears to be a variable property and mRNA for IL-1 has not been detected in Graves' thyrocytes by *in situ* hybridisation, although capillary endothelial cells are positive (Miyazaki *et al.*, 1989). Together, these results provide reasonable evidence for thyrocytes serving as APC. However, just as T cells inevitably contaminate primary thyrocyte cultures, so do dendritic cells and macrophages. The potency of dendritic cells in particular could be sufficient to allow small numbers to produce such effects and this is especially possible because these cells are increased in Graves' and Hashimoto glands (Kabel et al., 1988).

In contradistinction, class II expression by thyrocytes might confer tolerising rather than antigen presenting properties, resulting from the inability of these cells to provide a necessary second signal for T cell stimulation (Fig. 1.3). This possibility has so far not been tested with thyrocytes, although it was raised early in these investigations (Iwatani et al., 1986). Considerably greater evidence supports the hypothesis in type 1 diabetes, as discussed in Chapters 1 and 4, and it seems unlikely that the thyroid will behave differently from the islets of Langerhans in this regard. Such tolerising properties of class II^+ thyrocytes would certainly explain why it has been so difficult to establish long-term autoreactive T cell lines and clones from intrathyroidal lymphocytes and why the conventional assays for T cell sensitisation show such weak responses by what should be a population enriched for thyroid specificity.

Moreover, class II expression by thyrocytes is a widespread phenomenon, occurring in subacute thyroiditis and neoplasia (Lloyd et al., 1985; Karlsson, Tötterman & Jansson, 1986). Thyrocyte class II expression alone is therefore insufficient to trigger the initiation of autoimmune thyroiditis, and the accompanying lymphocytic infiltrate in these conditions may be prevented from expanding by the Ia^+ thyroid cells, which is why permanent thyroid dysfunction so rarely ensues. Thus, in addition to active suppression, a second mechanism to back up thymically imposed tolerance may exist in autoimmune thyroid diseases. This gives rise to new hypotheses for their aetiology. In particular, could this peripheral tolerance be defective in subjects who develop thyroiditis? It is also possible that prolonged exposure to class II^+ thyrocytes could alter lymphocyte function tested subsequently in vitro and that anergy in particular T cell subsets imposed by this means could explain some of the differences between patients and controls apparent in co-culture experiments.

B cell responses

Evidence cited at the beginning of the last section suggests that thyroid-reactive B cells are incompletely tolerised in normal subjects. One consequence of this is the frequent appearance of Tg autoantibodies after viral infections and in old age (Fong et al., 1981). These antibodies are generally of low affinity and are often IgM isotype, characteristics of natural autoantibodies with limited pathological significance. In patients with thyroiditis, the concentrations and affinities of Tg and TPO antibodies are much higher, and they are mainly IgG. The IgG subclass distribution of antibody reactivity has been investigated since this is an important functional determinant. IgG_1

and IgG_4 make up the majority of both antibodies, although the IgG_2 and IgG_3 subclasses are also present; the raised proportion of IgG_4 does not account for the inability of Tg antibodies to fix complement (Parkes et al., 1984). These studies indicate a polyclonal B cell response which is borne out by the lack of light chain restriction. Furthermore the sera from 30 of 31 Hashimoto patients gave a Tg antibody spectrotype on isoelectric focussing characteristic of a polyclonal response (Nye, Pontes de Carvalho & Roitt, 1981). The spectrotypes differed between patients but the individual patterns remained constant over several years (Delves & Roitt, 1988).

Thus a monoclonal origin for these thyroid autoantibodies seems to be a rare event. The thyroid is a major site of synthesis although bone marrow and lymph nodes are also important sources (Weetman et al., 1984b). The infiltrating B cells in Hashimoto's thyroiditis form follicles which are strikingly similar to gut-associated lymphoid tissue and all isotypes are represented, although light chain restriction may be found in occasional patients, compatible with a diagnosis of low-grade lymphoma (Wilkin & Casey, 1984; Hyjek & Isaacson, 1988). It seems likely that the infiltrate can further change with the emergence of a single dominant clone in some patients, so that parafollicular B cells give rise to high-grade non-Hodgkin's lymphoma, a recognised but rare complication of Hashimoto's thyroiditis. Immunoglobulin heavy and light chain gene rearrangements have also been studied with similar results: restricted clonality is only observed with the emergence of lymphoma in Hashimoto's thyroiditis (Kaulfersch et al., 1988; Katzin, Fishleder & Tubbs, 1989).

The detection of Tg and TPO autoantibody production in vitro was alluded to in the previous section and many studies have been performed on the regulation of this. A variety of non-specific B cell stimulators, particularly pokeweed mitogen, have been used together with techniques for detecting antibodies secreted into the culture supernatants (by haemagglutination, ELISA or radioimmunoassay) or for detecting individual antibody-producing cells by their formation of plaques or ELISA-spots. Spontaneous autoantibody secretion by circulating Hashimoto B cells is generally only detectable with very sensitive methods, in contrast to the easily measured production by thyroidal lymphocytes (McGregor et al., 1979a; Beall & Kruger, 1980b; McLachlan et al., 1981; Weetman et al., 1984b).

Although thyroid autoantibody synthesis by lymphocytes from healthy subjects was not detected in these studies, Tg and TPO antibody production by mitogen-stimulated normal lymphocytes has been described (Tao, Leu & Kriss, 1985; Iitaka et al., 1988). Such results are compatible with the notion that B cell tolerance is less complete than that for T cells and powerful stimuli in vitro can induce synthesis which is much less likely to occur in vivo. However, a problem of antibody specificity remains; most natural autoantibodies have low affinity and react with multiple epitopes. This would appear to be the case in one study in which around 7000 Tg antibody-producing cells were detected per million mononuclear cells in healthy subjects (Tao *et al.*, 1985). Assuming that as many as 20% of the circulating lymphocytes are B cells, this means that 3.5% of normal blood-borne B cells are Tg-reactive, clearly too high a number for these to be truly Tg-specific.

Attempts to stimulate antibody production with autoantigen alone have met with limited success. Only a variable proportion of peripheral blood lymphocyte cultures respond (usually from selected patients with high circulating antibody levels) and special manipulations of APC and antigen are required for optimum production (Beall, 1982; McLachlan *et al.*, 1983; Weetman *et al.*,1983b; Benveniste *et al.*, 1984; Logtenberg *et al.*, 1986; Sekino *et al.*, 1988). In one of these studies (Logtenberg *et al.*, 1986) the response appeared to be T cell-independent. This was possibly because the Tg was coupled to beads, although *a priori* some additional source of lymphokines would appear to be necessary. In contrast to circulating cells, thyroid lymphocytes often show enhanced Tg antibody production after stimulation with Tg, but decreased production after mitogen stimulation (McLachlan *et al.*, 1983; Atherton *et al.*, 1985). It is interesting to note that intrathyroidal B cells are heterogeneous in this regard, those near the follicles making the most thyroid antibodies (McLachlan *et al.*, 1986a).

These differences and indeed some of the variability between reports seem due at least in part to the diverse states of B cell activation in Hashimoto's thyroiditis: some differentiated cells need little triggering, while less completely activated B cells require more. Circulating B cells from different patients with Hashimoto's thyroiditis give unique responses to a diverse panel of stimulators, consistent with individual subjects having differing proportions of autoreactive B cells at the various stages of evolution into plasma cells (Weetman *et al.*, 1985b; Sekino *et al.*, 1988). This heterogeneity in B cell activation may affect results in experiments on T cell interactions (see above), also making analysis of B cell function difficult. It is unclear how the activation state of these circulating lymphocytes relates to intrathyroidal, lymph node or bone marrow lymphocytes making autoantibodies, although correlation between circulating B cell autoantibody production and serum titres has been observed for TPO and, inconsistently, for Tg antibodies (Benveniste *et al.*, 1984; Sekino *et al.*, 1988).

The lymph nodes and bone marrow are obvious sites for antibody formation and the accumulation of APC and T cells at the site of autoantigen production suggests a simple explanation for the localisation of thyroid antibody-producing B cells in the gland. Whilst it is highly likely that the intrathyroidal T cells are capable of producing the lymphokines necessary to stimulate B cell activation through to differentiation, an additional source of a key cytokine in this progression, namely IL-6, turns out to be the thyrocyte itself (Grubeck-Loebenstein *et al.*, 1989). Thyrocyte production of IL-6 *in vitro* is enhanced by other cytokines known to be produced by infiltrating mononuclear cells, in particular γ-IFN, IL-1 and TNF, as well as by TSH which is elevated in autoimmune hypothyroidism (Weetman, Bright-Thomas & Freeman, 1990a). Thus, the thyroid may contribute to its own destruction by release of IL–6 which stimulates intrathyroidal B (and T) cell proliferation and differentiation.

Effector mechanisms

Several mechanisms probably contribute to tissue injury and hypo-thyroidism (Fig. 3.2). TPO antibodies are found in about 90% of patients with Hashimoto's thyroiditis or primary myxoedema by haemagglutination assay (Pinchera *et al.*, 1980). It is not yet clear whether more sensitive assays with recombinant TPO (Kaufman *et al.*, 1990), including the use of reduced or denatured antigen (Hamada *et al.*, 1987), will increase the frequency of positive patients still further. It is also possible that patients negative for circulating TPO antibodies could have sufficient intrathyroidal synthesis to mediate pathogenic effects, as suggested by a recent case report (Baker *et al.*, 1988).

TPO antibodies are important in tissue injury: they bind to thyrocytes *in vivo* and are cytotoxic in the presence of complement *in vitro* (Khoury *et al.*,

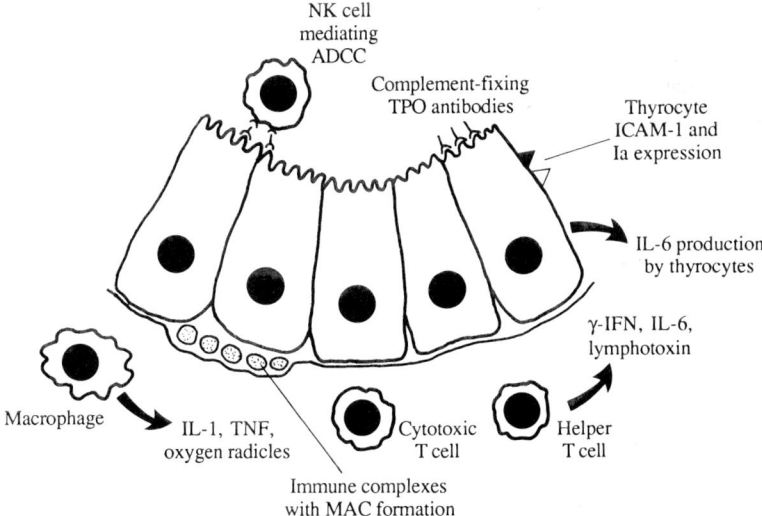

Fig. 3.2 Possible effector mechanisms in thyroiditis. The thyrocyte itself may contribute to the process by secretion of IL-6 and expression of ICAM-1 and Ia (see text). These phenomena are stimulated by T cell- and macrophage-derived cytokines.

1981; Khoury, Bottazzo & Roitt, 1984). However, in common with many nucleated cells, thyrocytes are relatively resistant to homologous complement. Sublethal membrane attack complex formation impairs thyroid cell function *in vitro*; sustained attack may well exhaust the cell metabolically and lead to lysis (Weetman, Freeman & Morgan, 1990b). There is considerable evidence for immune complex formation in Hashimoto's thyroiditis. Elevated levels of terminal complement complexes are present in the circulation and these are also localised around the thyroid follicles (Kappelgaard *et al.*, 1983; Pfaltz & Hediger, 1986; Weetman *et al.*, 1989a). In addition to this strong evidence for complement-mediated injury, a proportion of TPO antibodies can inhibit the function of this key enzyme, which could also lead to thyroid dysfunction (Kohno *et al.*, 1986; Doble *et al.*, 1988).

TSH receptor-blocking antibodies may contribute separately to hypothyroidism in some patients. Thyroid-stimulating antibodies, the cause of Graves' disease, will be considered in detail below. However, it was clear at an early stage that TSH receptor-binding antibodies occurred in up to 14% of patients with autoimmune hypothyroidism if assays measuring inhibition of radiolabelled TSH binding to thyroid membranes were used (Mukhtar *et al.*, 1975). The functional significance of such antibodies could only be appreciated with the development of sensitive bioassays as some TSH receptor antibodies may neither stimulate nor block the receptor *in vivo*. IgG-mediated inhibition of TSH-stimulated cAMP production by thyrocytes was reported initially in a patient with autoimmune hypothyroidism (Endo *et al.*, 1978) and then in two siblings with neonatal hypothyroidism (Matsuura *et al.*, 1980). Subsequent studies have found that blocking antibodies are present in both Hashimoto's thyroiditis and primary myxoedema (Steel *et al.*, 1984; Kraiem *et al.*, 1987a), although in Japanese patients the phenomenon may be confined to primary myxoedema (Konishi *et al.*, 1983; Arikawa *et al.*, 1985). In a series of 50 Israeli patients with autoimmune hypothyroidism, 16% had TSH receptor-blocking antibodies (Kraiem *et al.*, 1987a). The presence of such antibodies is often first detected because their transplacental passage causes transient neonatal hypothyroidism. This may occur in patients with Graves' disease who also possess thyroid-stimulating antibodies with insufficient potency to overcome the blocking antibodies (Matsuura *et al.*, 1988). Meticulous analysis of such blocking antibodies suggests that they may be of restricted clonality and can arise long after the autoimmune process has been established (Zakarija, McKenzie & Eidson, 1990).

The existence of a separate set of growth-stimulating and blocking antibodies has been suggested: those which stimulate growth were only detected in a small subgroup of Hashimoto patients whose goitres regrew after surgery, while growth-blocking antibodies were proposed as key mediators of thyroid atrophy in primary myxoedema (Drexhage *et al.*, 1980, 1981; Doniach, 1981). These findings have aroused considerable controversy, particularly since they employed the Feulgen cytochemical bioassay which is a difficult method to reproduce. Compelling evidence has been adduced that thyroid growth-stimulating antibodies are inseparable from TSH receptor-stimulating antibodies, at least in Graves' disease (Zakarija, Jin & McKenzie, 1988), suggesting that growth-blocking antibodies could well overlap with TSH receptor-blocking antibodies. These contrasting views have been extended to congenital hypothyroidism and endemic cretinism, in which certain studies have suggested a major role for growth-blocking antibodies (Van der Gaag, Drexhage & Dussault, 1985; Boyages *et al.*, 1989). However, alternative assays to the Feulgen method have shown that TSH receptor-blocking antibodies are indistinguishable from putative growth-inhibiting antibodies and only rarely (one of 24 cases) account for congenital hypothyroidism (Brown, Keating & Mitchell, 1990). Thus, the role of a separate group of growth-blocking antibodies causing primary myxoedema and congenital hypothyroidism is currently far from certain.

Although cytotoxic T cells are important in EAT, only one truly thyroid-specific, cytotoxic T cell clone has been identified so far in man. This CD8$^+$ clone was derived from a patient with Hashimoto's thyroiditis (MacKenzie *et al.*, 1987). Unfortunately the thyroid cell surface autoantigen recognised by these T cells was not identified. The expression of class II MHC molecules by thyrocytes may make them susceptible to attack by CD4$^+$ cytotoxic T cells, but this has not been demonstrated so far. $\gamma\delta$ receptor-bearing T cells may be a third type of effector. Besides class II, thyrocytes also express ICAM–1 in response to various cytokines and this increases T lymphocyte binding to the thyroid cell surface (Weetman *et al.*, 1990c). While this could be involved in a variety of T cell interactions, it is certainly important in establishing the necessary binding of T cells for cytotoxicity to occur *in vitro*. Other thyrocyte adhesion molecules may also be important in binding effector T cells, since blocking ICAM–1 in these experiments only partially inhibited thyroid cell killing.

In general, expansion of thyroidal lymphocytes from Hashimoto patients has produced CD8$^+$ T cells which are indiscriminately cytotoxic, killing cells typically used as NK cell targets (Canonica *et al.*, 1985; Del Prete *et al.*, 1986; MacKenzie *et al.*, 1987). These features almost certainly reflect the conditions used to expand the cells (especially exogenous IL-2) The relevance of such cytotoxicity to disease pathogenesis is unclear, although the potential for T cell-mediated cytotoxicity is obvious. Such lymphokine-activated T cells merge functionally with NK cells and there have been many studies of NK cells in autoimmune hypothyroidism but so far a clear consensus has not emerged. Of course, rather than indiscriminate killing, NK cells could produce specific thyroid injury via ADCC, demonstrated for both Tg and

TPO antigen-coated model targets *in vitro* (Calder *et al.*, 1973). An increase in circulating NK cells in Hashimoto's thyroiditis has been suggested in some studies (Calder *et al.*, 1976; Amino *et al.*, 1982a; Bogner, Schleusener & Wall, 1984) but not others (Endo *et al.*, 1983; Sack *et al.*, 1986) using functional assays including ADCC. The reasons for these discrepancies are unclear, but probably relate in part to differences in the assays used: what relevance modest changes in circulating NK cell numbers may have to tissue injury is unknown. Perhaps the most compelling evidence that NK cells may have a pathogenic role comes from the development of autoimmune hypothyroidism after administering IL-2, alone or with lymphokine-activated killer cells, to patients with malignancy (Atkins *et al.*, 1988; Van Liessum *et al.*, 1989). Although enormous concentrations of IL-2 were involved, these observations at least show that non-specific activation of NK and T cells may influence what seems likely to have been underlying thyroid autoreactivity.

The intrathyroidal production of cytokines and other soluble mediators is a final effector mechanism mediating gland dysfunction. TNF and γ-IFN together are cytostatic for the $FRTL_5$ rat thyroid cell line (Weetman & Rees, 1988), although such clear results are not found when these cytokines are added to primary human thyrocytes in culture (McLachlan *et al.*, 1990). However, γ-IFN alone does inhibit T3 and Tg release by thyrocytes in response to TSH (Nagayama *et al.*, 1987). TNF, IL-1 and IL-6 also reduce the effect of TSH on thyroid function, including adenylate cyclase stimulation and thyroid hormone release (Sato *et al.*, 1990; Weetman *et al.*, 1990a). The activities of many other cytokines, alone or in combination, have not yet been assessed. Additional molecules with pro-inflammatory effects are likely to play an effector role, including reactive oxygen metabolites, prostaglandins and leukotrienes, which will be released locally by lymphocytes and macrophages in response to a variety of stimuli including membrane attack complexes.

In summary, thyroid injury in autoimmune hypothyroidism is likely to result from a combination of humoral and cell-mediated effector mechanisms. TPO antibodies fix complement and will participate in ADCC: thyrocyte-specific cytotoxic T cells, and possibly non-specific NK cells, are probably also involved. In addition, thyroid function is impaired by TSH receptor-blocking antibodies and possibly some TPO antibodies in a small percentage of patients, while cytokines and other soluble mediators may have similar effects on a wider scale.

Treatment

The only treatment necessary is thyroid hormone replacement. Any goitre usually shrinks somewhat but often does not disappear (Doniach *et al.*,

Table 3.3. *Major clinical features of postpartum thyroiditis.*

(i)	Definition: Transient thyroid dysfunction within the year after delivery.
(ii)	Thyrotoxicosis typically 3–4 months after delivery; hypothyroidism typically 1–2 months later (in some patients only one phase is apparent).
(iii)	Moderate goitre which decreases in size within a year.
(iv)	TPO antibodies often detectable in early pregnancy; significant increase 3–6 months postpartum, and then decrease.
(v)	Normal thyroid biochemistry one year after delivery; tends to recur after subsequent pregnancies.

1979). This effect is the result of decreased TSH stimulation. Antibody levels usually decline but can fluctuate or remain high. An increased $CD4^+ : CD8^+$ ratio in circulating T cells has been ascribed to thyroxine supplementation (Bonnyns *et al.*, 1983). Very rarely a Hashimoto goitre may be painful: while raising the suspicion of lymphoma, this can be due to the uncomplicated disease (Shigemasa *et al.*, 1990). Prednisone (with or without azathioprine) is often successful in controlling such symptoms, but thyroidectomy may be necessary in some patients because of unacceptable steroid side effects.

Postpartum thyroiditis

Pregnancy has profound effects on the immune system, the changes being necessary to prevent rejection of paternal alloantigens borne by the fetus. The immunosuppressive effect of pregnancy is mediated by local placental mechanisms as well as by more generalised changes in T and B lymphocyte numbers and function produced by hormones and pregnancy-associated plasma proteins. Following delivery there is a rebound in immune reactivity. This sequence explains why immunologically mediated disorders, like asthma or SLE, improve during pregnancy but worsen postpartum. This certainly applies to thyroid autoimmunity, both Hashimoto's thyroiditis and Graves' disease often remitting in the last trimester but returning thereafter accompanied by rising autoantibody levels (Amino & Miyai, 1983).

These observations suggested that the common subclinical form of thyroiditis could develop into overt disease after delivery and indeed transient hypothyroidism or thyrotoxicosis was discovered in 5.5% of otherwise healthy Japanese women postpartum (Amino *et al.*, 1982b). This condition of postpartum thyroiditis has been reviewed extensively (Amino & Miyai, 1983; Jansson, Dahlberg & Karlsson, 1988). The major clinical features of the condition are now well established (Table 3.3). It is common, surveys in the year after delivery showing a prevalence of 3.9–6.7% in Japan, Sweden, USA and Denmark (Amino *et al.*, 1982b; Jansson *et al.*, 1984b; Nikolai, Turney & Roberts, 1987; Lervang, Pryds & Østergaard Kristensen, 1987). An apparently higher prevalence of 16.7% in Wales was the result of patient selection and the true figure would almost certainly be in keeping with the other studies (Fung *et al.*, 1988), but the prevalence in Thailand is only 1.1%, presumably related to unidentified genetic or environmental influences (Rajatanavin *et al.*, 1990).

The important underlying pathological events are painless destruction of the thyroid accompanied by a lymphocytic infiltrate, which explain the typical features of a small goitre, low radioiodine uptake and the alternation from thyrotoxicosis to hypothyroidism as stored hormones are initially released from the damaged gland and then function becomes impaired. Recovery within the year after delivery is a *sine qua non* for the diagnosis: permanent hypothyroidism or thyrotoxicosis reflects the postpartum development of autoimmune hypothyroidism or Graves' disease. Long-term follow-up suggests that some patients with postpartum thyroiditis will go on to develop either of these two conditions subsequently, but the exact risk has not yet been established because any follow-up period has been relatively short (Tachi *et al.*, 1988; Jansson *et al.*, 1988; Othman *et al.*, 1990). However, recurrence of transient thyroiditis during subsequent pregnancies occurs in at least two-thirds of patients.

The condition needs to be separated from subacute or de Quervain's thyroiditis and painless or 'silent' thyroiditis, although this is rarely difficult clinically. Considerable debate has centred around the syndrome of painless thyroiditis in the absence of a preceding pregnancy. Some of these cases may represent unusual forms of the more common autoimmune thyroid disorders, but it is now obvious that many outbreaks of silent thyroiditis have been due to the inadvertent ingestion of animal thyroid tissue (Kinney *et al.*, 1988). Despite previous speculation that it may represent a separate autoimmune disorder (Farid, Hawe & Walfish, 1983), this condition will not be considered further.

Immunogenetics

A family history of other autoimmune thyroid disorders is frequently reported by these patients and a familial aggregation of postpartum thyroiditis itself has been documented (Singer & Gorsky 1985). The disease has been associated with HLA-DR4 in Denmark, Sweden and Newfoundland, with an aetiological fraction of 0.37 in Sweden (Lervang *et al.*, 1984; Jansson, Säfwenberg & Dahlberg, 1985; Thompson & Farid, 1985), whereas in the USA and Wales the association appears to be with HLA-DR3 (Fein *et al.*,

1985; Kologlu *et al.*, 1987). Although the American study did not match for local controls and the significance of the Welsh data did not survive correction, the results are very suggestive of a true association since HLA-B8 was also increased. A second study from Denmark revealed an association with HLA-DR5 (relative risk 4.4) but not DR4, when considered singly (Pryds *et al.*, 1987). However, the phenotype DR4/5 conferred an increased relative risk (16.2) compared to DR5 in combination with any other allele. A weak association with HLA-DR3 was found in Japanese patients, but there is a much stronger effect of HLA-DRw8 and -DRw9 (Tachi *et al.*, 1988). No influence of HLA haplotype was found in a small group of Caucasian women who developed permanent hypothyroidism two to four years after postpartum thyroiditis (Othman *et al.*, 1990), whereas HLA-B51 and -DRw9 were associated with this outcome in Japanese patients (Tachi *et al.*, 1988). Other genetic markers have not been assessed.

Environmental factors

Age, parity and breast-feeding do not have an effect (Jansson *et al.*, 1984b; Fung *et al.*, 1988). Initial reports that giving birth to a girl or smoking increased the risk of developing postpartum thyroiditis (Amino *et al.*, 1982b; Fung *et al.*, 1988) have not been confirmed (Jansson *et al.*, 1984b). The postpartum effects of T4 (100 μg daily) or iodide supplementation (150 μg daily) have been tested on women with TPO antibodies antepartum; T4 had a clinical benefit but did not alter the course of postpartum thyroiditis, while the increase in dietary iodide worsened the thyroid dysfunction (Kämpe, Jansson & Karlsson, 1990). Whether this effect of iodide was due to a biochemical or immunological action is unknown.

T cell responses

Functional analysis of T cells in postpartum thyroiditis has not been performed. No consistent changes in circulating T cell phenotypes have been found after delivery in these women, although activated (Ia$^+$) T cells are increased (as in many autoimmune conditions) and a rise in the ratio of CD4$^+$ to CD8$^+$ cells has been reported (Jansson *et al.*, 1984c; Chan & Walfish, 1986). In the thyroid, B and T cells accumulate, with more CD4$^+$ than CD8$^+$ T cells (ratio 3 : 1) (Jansson *et al.*, 1984b).

B cell responses

Antibodies to TPO are detectable postpartum in 75–95% of women with hypothyroidism and prospective studies show that low levels of TPO

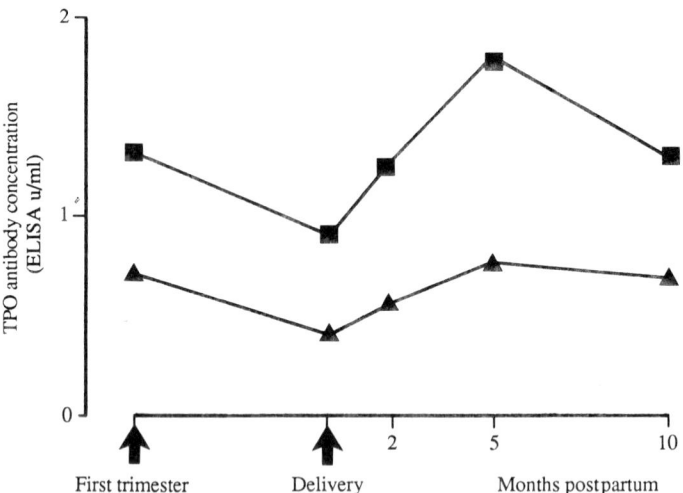

Fig. 3.3   Changes in TPO autoantibodies during and after pregnancy.
Values in women ($n = 23$) who had postpartum thyroiditis are shown as
squares. Antibody levels in women ($n = 49$) who were TPO antibody-
positive in the first trimester, yet did not develop postpartum thyroiditis,
are shown as triangles. Mean TPO antibody levels were significantly
higher, and had a greater increase postpartum, in the patients with
thyroid dysfunction.

antibodies are present in many women in the antenatal period (Amino *et al.*,
1982b; Jansson *et al.*, 1984b; Nikolai *et al.*, 1987; Fung *et al.*, 1988; Vargas *et
al.*, 1988). More sensitive tests, like ELISA, detect a higher proportion of
women with antibodies who do not actually develop biochemical dysfunction than the conventional haemagglutination assay because low levels of
TPO antibodies reflect only subclinical damage in the postpartum period.
TPO antibody levels change in a characteristic fashion during and after
pregnancy, with a slight fall in the last trimester and a considerable rise six
months after delivery, before returning to antepartum levels (Fig. 3.3). The
rise is directly proportional to the maximum elevation in TSH postpartum.
Although a specific increase in TPO antibodies of the IgG_1 subclass has been
associated with the development of postpartum hypothyroidism (Jansson *et
al.*, 1986), more sensitive assays show a symmetrical change in all four IgG
subclasses irrespective of clinical outcome (Weetman *et al.*, 1990d). Tg
antibodies have a lower prevalence than TPO antibodies in this condition.
TSH receptor-stimulating antibodies may appear during the postpartum
period, but then the diagnosis is Graves' disease; these antibodies show a
similar pattern of change to TPO antibodies in pregnancy and the postpartum period (Jansson *et al.*, 1988).

Effector mechanisms

Little is known of the effector mechanisms in postpartum thyroiditis, how these are controlled and why remission ensues. However, it seems highly likely that the same processes occur as in Hashimoto's thyroiditis. TPO antibodies probably play a major role, but may be undetectable in the serum of up to a quarter of patients (Fung *et al.*, 1988). Circulating NK cell activity is identical to healthy postpartum controls, although there is a general decrease in NK cell function in all women after delivery (Hayslip *et al.*, 1988). Since NK cells can suppress immunoglobulin synthesis *in vitro* (Mason *et al.*, 1988), this decrease may contribute to the rise in all autoantibodies after delivery.

Treatment

If symptomatic, treatment with beta-blockers for thyrotoxicosis or thyroxine for hypothyroidism is indicated, but should be stopped one year after delivery, as recovery is expected. Anticipatory treatment with thyroxine does not affect the immunological events, although it may arrest development of symptoms (Kämpe *et al.*, 1990). Excess dietary iodine (e.g. kelp tablets) should be avoided. There is no need for any immunomodulatory treatment.

Graves' disease

Graves' disease is caused by thyroid-stimulating antibodies (TSAb) which bind to the TSH receptor and activate adenylate cyclase, resulting in thyrotoxicosis. As already discussed, there are many features shared with autoimmune hypothyroidism, including the presence of Tg and TPO antibodies, thyroid lymphocytic infiltration and the behaviour of T cells in assays of function *in vitro*. This section will concentrate on immunological features unique to Graves' thyroid disease: Graves' ophthalmopathy and pretibial myxoedema will be reviewed separately.

Hyperthyroidism is common, affecting at least 1.9% of women and 0.16% of men surveyed in the North-East of England (Tunbridge *et al.*, 1977). The majority of these patients have Graves' disease but exact diagnostic criteria have been variable. Whilst it is assumed that all patients with Graves' disease have TSAb (see below), the detection of these antibodies depends on assay sensitivity and availability. Often the diagnosis is made on clinical grounds, usually supplemented by tests for other thyroid antibodies. In 850 European patients with hyperthyroidism, the condition was defined by the

Table 3.4. *Main HLA associations with Graves' disease.*

Study	Country	Number of Patients	Antigen	Relative Risk	Aetiological Fraction
Caucasians					
Bech *et al.*, 1977	Denmark	86	B8	2.80	0.30
			Dw3	3.94	0.38
Farid, Stone & Johnson, 1980	Canada	175	B8	3.05	0.34
		83	DR3	5.67	0.53
McGregor *et al.*, 1980a	England	65	DR3	3.20	0.31
Dahlberg *et al.*, 1981	Sweden	78	B8	4.43	0.41
			DR3	3.89	0.41
McKenna *et al.*, 1982	Ireland	86	B8	2.51	0.31
			DR3	2.62	0.33
Allannic *et al.*, 1983	France	94	B8	3.40	0.34
			DR3	4.21	0.41
Stenszky *et al.*, 1985	Hungary	256	B8	3.48	0.32
			DR3	4.80	0.40
Frecker *et al.*, 1986	Hungary	117	B8	3.19	0.29
			DR3	5.09	0.42
Weetman *et al.*, 1986b	Wales	65	DR3	2.89	0.34
De Bruin *et al.*, 1988	Holland	58	DR3	2.70	0.28
Frecker *et al.*, 1988	Canada	133	B8	2.43	0.27
			DR3	3.12	0.38
Kendall-Taylor *et al.*, 1988	England	127	B8	2.77	0.32
			DR3	2.13	0.25
Weetman *et al.*, 1988b	England	101	DR3	1.10[a]	0.04
Schleusener *et al.*, 1989	Germany	253	DR3	2.52[b]	0.24
Non-Caucasians					
Sasazuki *et al.*, 1983	Japan	30	DR5	8.14	0.26
			DRw8	3.07	0.25
Cho *et al.*, 1987	Korea	128	B13	3.8	0.11
			DR5	4.4	0.13
			DRw8	2.3	0.17
Hawkins *et al.*, 1985	Southern Chinese	132	Bw46[c]	4.8	0.44
Sridama *et al.*, 1987	USA Blacks	73	No DR association[d]		
Omar *et al.*, 1990	South African Blacks	103	DR1	3.48	0.10
			DR3	2.35	0.33
Tandon *et al.*, 1990	Asian Indian	57	B8	4.1[e]	0.23
			DQw2	5.5	0.50

presence of TSH receptor-binding antibodies and/or Graves' ophthalmopathy; 59.5% had Graves' disease while 31.3% remained unclassified (Reinwein *et al.*, 1986). It is probable that some of the latter also had Graves' disease, although not fulfilling these criteria. Regional variations in prevalence exist in Europe and within the UK (Barker & Phillips, 1984). The peak age for developing Graves' disease is between 40 and 49.

Immunogenetics

Family studies by Bartels demonstrated a genetic susceptibility in Graves' disease as long ago as 1941, and retrospective studies have shown that 50–60% of monozygotic twins share thyrotoxicosis, in contrast to 3–9% of dizygotic twins (reviewed by Farid, 1981). This high concordance may be inflated by ascertainment bias, however. Many studies have examined HLA associations (Table 3.4). HLA-DR3 is more strongly associated than B8 in Caucasians, but the relative risks and aetiological fractions are modest. There is also a trend towards a weaker association over the time these studies have been conducted. Non-Caucasians display a variety of different associations and in North American Blacks no overall susceptibility could be linked to any DR allele, although subdivision of the patients revealed that DRw6 was associated with thyroid antibody formation. Other subdivisions of Caucasian patients have suggested that HLA-B8 is more prevalent in those with severe disease, a large goitre and frequent disease in relatives (Stenszky *et al.*, 1983). No associations with genes in the DQ or DP regions have been found in Caucasians with Graves' disease (Weetman *et al.*, 1990e). The DR3 association, in linkage disequilibrium with B8, is common in many autoimmune disorders and may be related to a non-specific effect of this haplotype on immune function (Chapter 2). Another possibility is that DR3 could be in linkage disequilibrium with polymorphisms of the TNF gene and a weak association of a RFLP with Graves' disease has been identified (Badenhoop *et al.*, unpublished data).

Family studies in over 500 index cases show a low penetrance of disease-related genotypes and that the risk to HLA-identical siblings is only 7%, even lower than the concordance for monozygotic twins (Stenszky *et al.*,

---

Notes to Table 3.4

[a] By RFLP analysis.
[b] Extrapolated from previous control data.
[c] Weak association with DRw9, not surviving correction, with smaller numbers of patients (Bw46 is in linkage disequilibrium with DRw9 in Chinese).
[d] DRw6 was associated with the presence of TPO and/or Tg antibodies.
[e] Weak association with DR3, not surviving correction; HLA-A10 also associated.

1985). Even allowing for bias in the twin studies, these facts suggest that other genetic (as well as environmental) factors may be involved in disease susceptibility. Associations of Graves' disease with immunoglobulin allotypes have been examined in population surveys. In Canadian and Hungarian patients the fb haplotype was more frequent than controls, but this was insignificant in one study and did not survive correction in another (Farid *et al.*, 1977b; Kozma *et al.*, 1985). No association was found in a repeat study in Hungary or in Welsh patients (Frecker *et al.*, 1986; Weetman & Brazier, 1988). There is also disagreement in Japanese populations (Nakao *et al.*, 1980; Tamai *et al.*, 1985). However, a selected family study showed a strong effect of both HLA and Gm allotypes on susceptibility (Uno *et al.*, 1981). Because no particular allotype was delineated in the affected patients, the Gm-associated disease-susceptibility gene could not have been in significant linkage disequilibrium with Gm. Immunoglobulin switch region RFLP patterns are normal in Graves' disease, but a weak association with a lambda light chain C region RFLP has been observed (Weetman *et al.*, 1988b; Williams *et al.*, 1988).

T cell receptor RFLP analysis initially suggested an association of a β chain C region polymorphism with Graves' disease in Caucasians, although it is unclear whether both patients and controls came from the same geographical area (Demaine *et al.*, 1987). Repeat analyses on English patients by the same group and by others have failed to confirm this (Weetman *et al.*, 1988b; Demaine *et al.*, 1989). However, this latter study reported an association between Tg antibodies and a particular $C\beta$ genotype. This suggests a T cell-mediated genetic influence on Tg antibody production but it is perhaps surprising that Hashimoto patients, who frequently have these antibodies, do not differ from controls in their $C\beta$ genotypes (Weetman *et al.*, 1987a). In Japanese patients, the $C\beta$ RFLP pattern in Graves' disease differs from controls (Ito *et al.*, 1989), so geographical diversity may well operate. A small study of 10 American patients found abnormal distributions of both a $C\alpha$ and a $V\alpha$ T cell receptor RFLP (Oksenberg *et al.*, 1989). The data together at least hint at possible T cell receptor gene involvement in susceptibility. Finally, the ability to taste phenylthiocarbamide is much more frequent in patients with Graves' disease than controls, with a relative risk of 2.1 and aetiological fraction of 0.44 (Kitchin *et al.*, 1959). As discussed in the section on autoimmune hypothyroidism, the gene involved and the reasons for this association are unknown, but certainly warrant further study.

Environmental factors

Although some of the incomplete concordance in twin studies may be due to differing T cell receptor and immunoglobulin repertoires, it also suggests the involvement of environmental factors as susceptibility determinants. Being female obviously predisposes to Graves' disease and pregnancy may be an added risk factor: excluding nulliparous women, two-thirds of women aged 20–35 had a postpartum onset of the disorder (Jansson et al., 1987). Stress has often been discussed as a precipitant and certainly a vast literature has blossomed on the interactions between neuroendocrine and immunological responses, indicating possible mechanisms for this. However, no causal relationship has so far been proved (Gray & Hoffenberg, 1985), although this is a difficult hypothesis to test. Mantle irradiation for haematological malignancy is a more clearly defined precipitant, possibly related to thyroidal damage and release of autoantigens (Mortimer et al., 1986).

Iodine, as discussed in previous sections, may be of considerable importance in some areas. Iodisation programmes always precipitate thyrotoxicosis in some predisposed individuals, including patients with Graves' disease, but it is difficult to disassociate an immunological from a biochemical effect as the cause of this (Adams et al., 1975). The prevalence of thyroid antibodies in Graves' disease is higher in iodine-sufficient areas compared to iodine-deficient areas in Europe (although exceptions exist) which suggests that there is some effect of iodine on the autoimmune response (Reinwein et al., 1986).

The role of infectious agents as precipitants is unclear. Analysis of 857 British cases of Graves' disease over a 10 year period revealed no clustering of cases in time or space, indicating that infections behaving in an epidemic fashion are unlikely precipitating factors (Cox, Phillips & Osmond, 1989). Antibodies to Yersinia enterocolitica are found with increased frequency in Graves' disease (Shenkman & Bottone, 1976) and a saturable binding site for TSH was discovered in lysozyme-treated extracts of this organism (Weiss et al., 1983). Such a TSH receptor-like molecule could provoke the formation of cross-reactive TSAb. Further investigations have suggested that antibodies against a plasmid-encoded protein in enteropathogenic strains of Yersinia are strongly associated with various forms of thyroid autoimmunity, although how this can be reconciled with the specific induction of Graves' disease is unclear (Wenzel et al., 1988). Similar TSH receptor-binding material has been found in mycoplasma (Sack et al., 1989). An exogenous retrovirus has also been implicated, based on hybridisation of an HIV-I gag probe with thyroidal DNA from Graves' but not control subjects, although it is unclear where the virus is located and what it is (Ciampolillo et al., 1989). Further work is obviously required in this area.

Finally, the hyperthyroidism of the disease itself may modify the immune response. For instance, chronic supranormal concentrations of T4 may depress NK cell activity (Papic et al., 1987), although this has recently been disputed (Pedersen et al., 1989). Such effects in man have been difficult to disentangle from the immunological factors producing disease. Further examples are considered in detail below, in the context of antithyroid drugs.

T cell responses

As in autoimmune hypothyroidism and indeed often in simultaneous studies, T cells have been analysed by phenotyping and by *in vitro* functional assays. There is some disagreement regarding the distribution of T cell subsets in untreated Graves' disease and the results of a large number of studies are reviewed elsewhere (Burman & Baker, 1985; DeGroot *et al.*, 1985). Subsequent reports have tended to confirm the impression that there is a generalised reduction in circulating CD8$^+$ T cells (Ludgate *et al.*, 1984; Di Mario *et al.*, 1986; Gerstein *et al.*, 1987), although these were normal in another study from Japan (Ueki *et al.*, 1988). Circulating T cells are activated, expressing Ia and 4F2. For reasons which are not clear, LFA-1 expression by circulating lymphocytes is decreased in Graves' disease; the functional consequence of this is unknown (Guerin *et al.*, 1989). Attempts have been made to subdivide the CD8$^+$ subset phenotypically into suppressor and cytotoxic cells with monoclonal antibodies (CD11b and Leu 15) but, as discussed in Chapter 1, no such clear partition exists functionally (Gerstein *et al.*, 1987; Ueki *et al.*, 1988). The distribution of CD29$^+$ and CD45RA$^+$ T cells in the blood is normal (Ueki *et al.*, 1988).

Variable proportions of intrathyroidal CD4$^+$ and CD8$^+$ T cells have been found by immunohistochemistry (Table 3.5), possibly related to differences in counting techniques and pretreatment of patients prior to thyroidectomy. Intraepithelial lymphocytes are greatly increased compared to the small number present normally. These cells are CD3$^-$CD8$^+$. Their function is unknown but they have an obvious potential for interaction with otherwise inaccessible thyroid antigens. A large percentage of the intrathyroidal T cells are activated (expressing Ia and the IL-2 and transferrin receptors) and production of γ-IFN has been shown by *in situ* staining (Table 3.5). The proportion of CD4$^+$CD29$^+$ cells (staining with the monoclonal reagent 4B4) is higher than in the peripheral blood, whereas intrathyroidal CD4$^+$CD45RA$^+$ cells are decreased with respect to the circulation (Ueki *et al.*, 1988). Although taken to indicate an excess of helper-inducers and a dearth of suppressor-inducers, this seems far more likely to reflect the increased numbers of activated and memory T cells in the gland. No obviously abnormal distribution of T cell receptor Vβ gene family usage has been identified, although there is a slight excess of intrathyroidal T cells bearing the $\gamma\delta$ receptor (Teng *et al.*, 1990a). Southern blot analysis of T cell receptor genes confirms the polyclonal T (and B) cell response within the thyroid (Kaulfersch *et al.*, 1988). However, this does not exclude the possibility of a monoclonal or pauciclonal origin for the autoimmune process in the early stages of the disease.

In functional assays, Graves' T cells behave in a similar fashion to those from Hashimoto patients, but effects on autoantibody production have not

Table 3.5. *Intrathyroidal T cell phenotypes in Graves' disease identified by immunohistochemical staining. In almost all cases patients had been pretreated with antithyroid drugs which may have altered the infiltrate*

Author	Number of Patients	CD4 : CD8 Ratio	Other markers
Bene *et al.*, 1983	15	Mainly CD8	–
Margolick *et al.*, 1984	4	2 : 1	Intraepithelial lymphocytes $CD3^-$, $CD8^+$
Warford *et al.*, 1984	16	1 : 2	Some $OKT6^+$ (Langerhans) cells
Jansson *et al.*, 1984a	11	2 : 1–4 : 1	Many Ia^+ T cells
Misaki *et al.*, 1985	11	2 : 1 in follicle 1 : 2 in interstitium	Some IL-2 receptor-positive cells; some NK cells
Margolick *et al.*, 1988	5	Mainly CD4	Mainly $CD45RA^+$; some IL-2 receptor-positive cells; some γ-interferon-producing T cells
Cohen & Weetman, 1988c	5	Mainly CD8	Mainly $CD45R0^+$, few $CD45RA^+$; some transferrin receptor-positive cells; some NK cells

been tested because the measurement of TSAb secreted *in vitro* is difficult. General impairment of suppressor cell activity has been found, particularly in responsiveness to the mitogen concanavalin A (Aoki *et al.*, 1979; Pacini & DeGroot, 1983). Although likely to be due to the reduction in circulating $CD8^+$ cells which are stimulated by the mitogen, this defect was confined to the thyroid in one study (Ueki *et al.*, 1988). Another non-specific T cell functional abnormality is an impaired autologous mixed lymphocyte reaction which may be caused by some unidentified inhibitory factor in Graves' serum (Fournier *et al.*, 1983; Bagnasco *et al.*, 1985).

Antigen-specific T cell responses have been tested using Tg and TPO, or crude thyroid extracts in which the low abundance of TSH receptors must be swamped by these two antigens, although partially purified TSH receptor stimulates blastogenesis in Graves' lymphocytes (Wenzel *et al.*, 1981). The recent cloning of this antigen will now allow localisation of T cell epitopes. The proliferative response of T cells to Tg and TPO seems the same as in Hashimoto's thyroiditis (although the prevalence of positive responders is lower), confirming the existence of circulating and intrathyroidal sensitised T cells. The MIF assay has been employed to demonstrate a universal antigen-specific T suppressor cell defect in Graves' disease, exactly as in Hashimoto's thyroiditis (reviewed by Volpé, 1988). Particularly compelling is the demonstration that an islet cell antigen preparation will not stimulate MIF production by Graves' T cells but does so in patients with diabetes mellitus; Graves' T cells suppress this response and diabetic T cells suppress the response of Graves' T cells to a thyroid extract (Topliss et al., 1983). Although MIF production by circulating and intrathyroidal T cells cultured with a thyroid extract has been found in most Graves' patients in a separate study (Tötterman et al., 1979), this assay has been completely normal in other laboratories (Brostoff, 1970; Ludgate et al., 1985). Such conflicting results could be related to antigenic and technical differences; clearly more robust assays with defined, pure antigens are required to address the question of T cell function in vitro. The cloning of antigen-specific T cells would also be useful in this regard. Tg- and TPO-reactive helper T cell lines and clones have been produced from one patient with Graves' disease using fibroblasts as APC, but even so the proliferative responses to antigen were weak (Fisfalen et al., 1988).

Thyrocyte Ia expression and its potential role in T cell stimulation or peripheral tolerisation generally mirrors that found in Hashimoto's thyroiditis. The functional assays described previously have often used Graves' thyrocytes, as these are readily available at thyroidectomy. The addition of monocytes enhances the ability of thyrocytes to stimulate the response of autologous T cells to the antigen PPD (Eguchi et al., 1988). This could be taken as evidence for the capacity of thyrocytes to present antigen, albeit suboptimally, or alternatively for insufficient conventional APC contaminating the thyrocyte cultures to sustain a maximal response. In the first case, the thyrocytes must have the ability to process the antigen, which a previous study was unable to demonstrate (Londei et al., 1984). Intrathyroidal dendritic cells are abundant in Graves' disease and appear to form clusters with T cells (Kabel et al., 1988). Contamination of thyrocyte cultures by these and other APC could explain the weak antigen presentation observed in these experiments.

B cell responses

A variety of assays have been established for TSH receptor antibodies (Table 3.6). TSAb, which cause the disease, require bioassay for their detection (reviewed by Marshall & Ealey, 1986) and the most frequently employed technique measures cAMP production by human thyrocytes or by the FRTL$_5$ rat thyroid cell line in response to added immunoglobulin preparations. TSH receptor binding antibody (TBII) production *in vitro* has been detected using mitogen stimulation (McLachlan *et al.*, 1977) but further analysis of regulation has been precluded by assay insensitivity. Thyroidal lymphocytes are one source of these autoantibodies (McLachlan *et al.*, 1986b), although the effects of thyroidectomy in some patients suggest that the lymph nodes and bone marrow are more important sites (De Bruin *et al.*, 1988).

There is some evidence that TSAb, unlike Tg and TPO antibodies, may have a pauciclonal or even monoclonal origin, an idea expressed eloquently by Adams (1978). Isoelectric focussing showed that TSAb and LATS activity were present in only one or two fractions of separated sera (Lonergan, Babiarz & Burke, 1973; Zakarija & McKenzie, 1978). Of seven Gm heterozygote Graves' patients, five had TSH receptor antibodies expressing only one Gm haplotype (Pepper, Noel & Farid, 1981). There is usually light chain restriction, with 22 of 30 patients so far examined using exclusively lambda light chains in their TSAb, four using kappa and only four being unrestricted (Zakarija, 1983; Knight *et al.*, 1986; Williams *et al.*, 1988). This is unexpected, not only since restricted clonality is implied, but also because kappa light chains are preponderant in a normal antibody response (2 : 1 ratio with lambda). Finally, in all 14 patients so far tested, TSAb activity is restricted to the IgG$_1$ subclass (Zakarija, 1983; Weetman *et al.*, 1990f).

Thus it is possible that TSAb may arise from only one or a few B cells. This could be due to inadequate deletion or antigen-driven selection of these autoreactive clones or even to the presence of appropriate V region genes only in a group of subjects therefore predisposed to Graves' disease. However, it is probable that all of these patients were selected for study because their TSAb levels were very high, making assay of fractions possible; the methods themselves are not sensitive enough to detect minor components and it is unclear whether similar restriction applies to all Graves' patients. Furthermore, patients obviously may have multiple TSH receptor antibodies, some binding, some stimulating and some blocking. Because these can be transferred across the placenta, their effects can best be seen in certain babies whose circulation contains maternal antibodies with varying biological effects depending on the different rates of breakdown of the individual antibody species (Zakarija, McKenzie & Hoffman, 1986). Heterogeneity in TSH receptor antibody binding and subsequent biological activity (Carayon *et al.*, 1983) are not necessarily evidence against the pauciclonal origin of TSAb, as somatic mutation upon exposure to antigen is the usual mechanism for increasing the affinity of antibodies during the evolution of an immune response. Thus there is evidence that potent TSAb at least may have a mono- or oligoclonal origin, but their

Table 3.6. *Assays for TSH receptor antibodies*[a]

Assay system	Species	Response	Name of stimulator	Reference
Non-functional	Human	Inhibition of LATS[b] binding by thyroid membranes *in vitro*; LATS subsequently tested by *in vivo* bioassay	LATS-P[c]	Adams & Kennedy, 1967; Munro, 1984
	Human	Inhibition of radio-labelled TSH binding to thyroid membranes	TBII[d]	Smith & Hall, 1974
	Guinea pig	Binding to guinea pig membranes detected by ELISA[f]	–	Baker *et al.*, 1983
	Guinea pig	Inhibition of radio-labelled TSH binding to fat cell membranes	FBI[e]	Shinozawa, Villadolid & Ingbar, 1986
In vivo bioassay	Guinea pig or mouse	Release of ^{125}I from preloaded thyroid	LATS	Adams & Purves, 1956; McKenzie, 1964

In vitro bioassay	Pig or man	Stimulation of cAMP, iodide trapping or thyroid hormone release by thyroid membranes, cells or slices	TSAb[g], HTS[h], HTACS[i]	Zakarija, McKenzie & Banovac, 1980; Atkinson & Kendall-Taylor, 1981; Rapoport et al., 1984
	Rat FRTL$_5$ cells	Stimulation of cAMP production or iodine uptake, ESTA[j]	—	Marcocci et al., 1983; Ealey et al., 1988
	Guinea pig	Cytochemical bioassay measuring alteration in thyroid cell lysosomal permeability	—	Ealey, Marshall & Ekins, 1981

[a] An almost overwhelming amount of information has accumulated on the assay of TSH receptor antibodies; key methods only are given here and assays for growth are given in the text.

[b] LATS: long-acting thyroid stimulator.

[c] LATS-P: long-acting thyroid stimulator-protector.

[d] TBII: TSH binding-inhibiting immunoglobulins.

[e] FBI: fat cell-binding IgG (fat cells have TSH receptors but preparations of them are not contaminated by TPO, Tg and other thyroid antigens).

[f] ELISA: enzyme-linked immunosorbent assay.

[g] TSAb: thyroid stimulating antibodies.

[h] HTS: human thyroid stimulator.

[i] HTACS: human thyroid adenylate cyclase stimulator.

[j] ESTA: eluted stain assay; microculture application of the cytochemical bioassay.

pathological effect will be influenced, among other things, by affinity maturation and by competition with other TSH receptor antibodies without a stimulatory action.

Another potential modulator of TSAb activity is the generation of an anti-idiotypic antibody response. Indeed, it has even been suggested that formation of antibodies against TSH could create an idiotype looking like the TSH receptor and that anti-idiotypic antibodies made in response would act as TSAb, because they would bind to the TSH receptor-like idiotype on the anti-TSH antibody (Islam *et al.*, 1983; Beall *et al.*, 1986). However, TSH-binding antibodies have been found in less than half of Graves' patients, suggesting that this is an unlikely general mechanism for TSAb formation (Raines *et al.*, 1985). Instead, such TSH receptor antibodies could have been generated in response to TSAb and would act as anti-idiotypes to modify TSAb action. At odds with this view is a recent study which found a very low prevalence of anti-TSH antibodies in Graves' disease (0.32% of 2500 cases) and, even when present, there was no evidence that they interfered with the activity of TSAb or TSH receptor-binding antibodies (Ochi *et al.*, 1989).

Finally, a consistent two-fold increase in circulating $CD5^+$ B cells has been found in untreated Graves' disease, conventional $CD5^-$ B cells being present at normal concentrations (Iwatani *et al.*, 1989). In destructive thyrotoxicosis, the level of $CD5^+$ B cells was unaltered, leading the authors to propose that prolonged (rather than transient) hyperthyroidism may be responsible. However, the increase in $CD5^+$ B cells found with other autoimmune conditions suggests that the abnormality is part of the aberrant immune response. Whether these B cells make thyroid antibodies is unknown.

Effector mechanisms

A long-term outcome in Graves' disease is hypothyroidism (Wood & Ingbar, 1979) and occasionally patients may fluctuate rapidly from thyrotoxicosis to hypothyroidism, or vice versa (Doniach *et al.*, 1979). The clinical picture of Graves' disease is therefore probably a balance between stimulation mediated by TSAb and inhibition of gland function by humoral and cellular mechanisms. Circulating TPO antibodies are found in about 80% of Graves' patients (Pinchera *et al.*, 1980) and presumably cause the same mechanisms of tissue injury in both Graves' disease and Hashimoto's thyroiditis: certainly, complement membrane attack complexes are deposited around the thyroid follicles in both conditions (Weetman *et al.*, 1989a). Non-specific cytotoxic T cells, produced by expansion with IL-2 *in vitro*, are not elicited from Graves' thyroids, in contrast to those from Hashimoto patients (MacKenzie *et al.*, 1987; Bagnasco *et al.*, 1988). This dichotomy is of considerable interest, although the pathological role of these unrestricted cells in Hashimoto's thyroiditis is unclear. Thyroid-specific cytotoxic T cells have not been demonstrated in Graves' disease. Thyrotoxicosis may actually reduce NK function (Papic *et al.*, 1987). Although NK cells are present in the thyroid (Table 3.5), their distribution in the untreated stage of disease is unknown.

Of course, the key clinical features of Graves' disease are the result of TSAb formation. These antibodies are detectable in virtually all patients provided a suitably sensitive assay is used (Zakarija, McKenzie & Banovac, 1980; Rapoport *et al.*, 1984). They may also occur in ophthalmic Graves' disease (see below) or, rarely, in Hashimoto's thyroiditis; in these two settings their clinical effect is presumably limited by concentration or concurrent thyroid destruction. The lack of correlation between the severity of thyrotoxicosis and the serum concentration of TSAb could have many causes (Takata *et al.*, 1980) but for reasons just discussed, the effect of tissue injury produced by TPO antibodies seems particularly likely to have a major role.

The possible involvement of a separate set of antibodies mediating thyroid growth was mentioned above. Using tritiated thymidine incorporation by the FRTL$_5$ rat thyroid cell line as a measure of growth stimulation (rather than a cytochemical bioassay), such antibodies were found in about 90% of newly diagnosed Graves' patients (Valente *et al.*, 1983). Because there was no correlation between this activity and the stimulation of thyroid cAMP release, it was believed that growth-stimulating antibodies were a distinct and separate population. Although this has been supported by an assay using primary cultures of rat follicles, with 68% of newly diagnosed Graves' patients positive (Chiovato *et al.*, 1983), the use of thymidine incorporation alone as a measure of growth has been criticised. Experiments assessing growth by directly measuring DNA concentration, the proportion of cells in S phase or the number of cells in metaphase, all indicate that the stimulation of growth is mediated by cAMP (Ealey *et al.*, 1985; Jin *et al.*, 1986). It is difficult to explain these discrepancies, although so far the evidence favours a single group of TSAb which stimulates both adenylate cyclase and growth. Contamination of Graves' IgG preparations with variable concentrations of cytokines (like γ-IFN, IL-1 and IL-6) might explain some of the differences, since these could modify long-term assays like growth yet have no effect on short-term cAMP production.

Treatment

Most patients in the UK are treated initially with the antithyroid drugs carbimazole (active metabolite: methimazole) or propylthiouracil, generally for 6–18 months. About 50% of patients will relapse in the subsequent year and these are then offered radioiodine or partial thyroidectomy. All three forms of therapy are accompanied by immunological phenomena which may influence the outcome. Understanding the basis for these changes may shed light on the autoimmune response.

Currently it is unclear why half the patients treated with antithyroid drugs enter remission after a suitable period of treatment. Other reviews have considered this in depth (Weetman, McGregor & Hall, 1984c; Ratana-chaiyavong & McGregor, 1985; Volpé et al., 1986). There seems little doubt that these agents have a direct effect on the disease process as the alternative explanation, that a suitable period of biochemical normality allows spontaneous remission to occur, is not borne out by the evidence. In particular, the remission rate is substantially higher with antithyroid drugs (considering all patient categories) than propranolol (used only to treat the mildest cases), and all patients treated with long-term sodium iodate promptly relapsed on stopping this inhibitor of thyroid hormone release (Weetman et al., 1984c; Shen et al., 1985). Moreover, if patients are treated with high doses of antithyroid drugs supplemented by T4 to prevent hypothyroidism, remission rates are much better than if euthyroidism is achieved by titrating the dose of drugs (Romaldini et al., 1983). Unless they were having a direct effect, it is difficult to see why the amount of antithyroid drugs given should influence outcome.

The basis for remission seems to be the decrease in TSAb which occurs during treatment (Pinchera et al., 1969; McGregor et al., 1980b). Tg and TPO antibody levels also decline, as do incidentally occurring DNA antibodies (Murakami et al., 1988), whereas gastric parietal cell antibodies do not (McGregor et al., 1982). These results are explicable if thyroid (and DNA) antibody synthesis is occurring in the gland where, by concentrating the drug, an immunological effect is produced; B cells making parietal cell antibodies, probably in the stomach, would not be exposed to an adequate concentration of drug. Methimazole and propylthiouracil are immunologically active in vitro, decreasing pokeweed mitogen and antigen-stimulated autoantibody and total IgG production (McGregor et al. 1980b; Weiss & Davies, 1981; Weetman, McGregor & Hall, 1983b; McLachlan et al., 1985). They also enhance T cell proliferation and alter subset distributions in mitogen-stimulated cultures, at least in part by increasing IL-2 synthesis (Hallengren, Forsgren & Melander, 1980; Weetman, 1986; Wilson et al., 1988, 1990). One way such effects might be mediated is by the action of these drugs as oxygen radical scavengers (Weetman et al., 1984d; Balázs et al., 1986). By removing reactive oxygen metabolites generated in cultures by monocytes, T cell behaviour may be modified, with subsequent effects on B cells.

It is unknown whether antithyroid drugs have similar effects in vivo. However, other immunological changes occur with treatment, including shrinkage of the thymus, which is often enlarged in Graves' disease, and diminution in the thyroid lymphocytic infiltrate (Michie *et al.*, 1967; Nilsson, 1972; Young *et al.*, 1976). Although the abnormal responses in the MIF test are present after remission has been induced by antithyroid drugs (How *et al.*, 1983), another test of circulating T cell sensitisation, procoagulant activity production in response to thyroid antigen, is normalised (Iitaka *et al.*, 1987). Non-specific suppressor cell abnormalities also return to normal, as do the reduced number of $CD8^+$ and increased number of Ia^+ T cells (reviewed by Volpé *et al.*, 1986).

These changes could be a direct result of antithyroid drugs acting on the intrathyroidal lymphocytes, as suggested by the *in vitro* observations described above, but there are other possibilities. Volpé (1985) has argued that the hyperthyroidism of untreated Graves' disease may influence the autoimmune response adversely and that the restoration of euthyroidism by antithyroid drugs reverses these changes. There is little categorical evidence to support this possibility because it is difficult to dissociate the effects of hyperthyroidism from the underlying immune process. At least the T cell subset alterations corrected by antithyroid drugs seem to be independent of thyroid hormone status, as no abnormality in circulating T cell subsets was found in patients with thyrotoxicosis caused by an adenoma (Bagnasco *et al.*, 1983), while the low $CD8^+$ T cell number in patients with toxic multinodular goitre seems related more to a concurrent autoimmune response than hyperthyroidism, as discussed below (Grubeck-Loebenstein *et al.*, 1985). The most compelling proof that antithyroid drugs have immunological effects which are independent of changes in thyroid hormones comes from experiments on EAT. In all three major models, immunisation-induced, thymectomy-induced and spontaneous, the severity of thyroiditis is greatly reduced by antithyroid drugs (Rennie *et al.*, 1983; Davies, Weiss & Gerber, 1984; Allen *et al.*, 1986b; Cohen & Weetman, 1988b). This effect occurs despite maintenance of euthyroidism. Variable effects on Tg antibody formation have been found but, unlike man, the thyroid is not a major source of thyroid antibodies in EAT.

A second possibility is that the drugs impair antigen presentation by the thyrocytes (Volpé *et al.*, 1986; Tötterman *et al.*, 1987). There is no evidence so far to support this. Antithyroid drugs have no effect on thyrocyte autoantigen or MHC class II molecule expression (Cohen & Weetman, 1988b; Aguayo *et al.*, 1988) and, as discussed previously, it is unclear currently whether thyrocytes actually present antigen. However, alternative immunological actions on thyrocytes are possible. These cells release reactive oxygen metabolites in response to complement membrane attack complexes *in vitro*, which might have pro-inflammatory effects (Weetman *et al.*, 1990b). By their oxygen radical scavenging activity, antithyroid drugs could reduce this phlogistic response. Thyrocyte IL-6 production, in response to cytokine stimulation *in vitro*, is also inhibited by antithyroid drugs (Weetman *et al.*, 1990a).

There have been many attempts to define patient characteristics which would predict remission after antithyroid drug treatment. The levels of TSAb or other TSH receptor antibodies at the end of treatment have some predictive value but are of low sensitivity and specificity (reviewed in Schleusener *et al.*, 1989; Edan *et al.*, 1989). Pretreatment values are not related to outcome. In initial studies HLA-DR3 was associated with an increased risk of relapse (Bech *et al.*, 1977; McGregor *et al.*, 1980a), but several groups subsequently have found no link with any DR antigen (Dahlberg *et al.*, 1981; McKenna *et al.*, 1982; Allannic *et al.*, 1983; Weetman *et al.*, 1986b; Schleusener *et al.*, 1989).

In summary, antithyroid drugs have a direct effect in Graves' disease leading to remission. This may be the result of their immunomodulatory activity, which includes suppression of thyrocyte IL-6 and oxygen radical production. At least some of these immunological actions are independent of the restoration of euthyroidism, as thyroiditis in EAT is ameliorated by antithyroid drugs. There are no reliable predictors of outcome.

After partial thyroidectomy, circulating LATS-P and TSAb levels show a transient increase, followed by a slow and progressive decline (Hardisty, Talbot & Munro, 1981; Bech *et al.*, 1982). Tg antibodies follow the same trend although the period of initial elevation may be somewhat longer (Feldt-Rasmussen *et al.*, 1982). The decrease in antibody levels could be due to loss of intrathyroidal synthesis, removal of the bulk of autoantigen or stimulation of suppressor cells by a bolus of antigen from the damaged thyroid. A more recent study found no consistent change in TBII and TPO antibody levels in the months after thyroidectomy, although the initial transient rise was observed and ascribed to leakage of TSH receptor antibodies from the manipulated gland (De Bruin *et al.*, 1988). These observations demonstrate the importance of extrathyroidal sites of autoantibody synthesis in at least some Graves' patients.

To circumvent the interference from preoperative antithyroid drugs, 26 patients were followed who had been pretreated with propranolol alone. TSAb fell in 19 (73%) by six weeks after surgery, whereas TBII fell in only two (15%) of 11 patients in whom they were detectable (Steel *et al.*, 1987). Substantial falls in TPO antibodies were seen in about half of these patients. It is unclear why TSAb and TBII did not change in parallel, although, as previously stressed, the two assays measure only partially overlapping sets of antibodies. In those patients whose TSAb persisted, relapse was infrequent (although the disappearances of TSAb and TBII probably predicts that relapse is highly unlikely). It is also surprising that in one study the size of remnant left was not related to subsequent thyroid status (Tweedle *et al.*,

1977). One important determinant of outcome is the accompanying destructive autoimmune response; high titres of complement-fixing TPO antibodies are associated with early postoperative hypothyroidism (Irvine, McGregor & Stuart, 1962; Van Welsum *et al.*, 1974). TSAb may therefore be unable to induce relapse because there is insufficient thyroid and because autoimmune tissue injury prevents regrowth. If an underlying destructive process is in part responsible for hypothyroidism, this would explain the fact that remnant size is unimportant. Whether thyroidectomy somehow tips the balance in favour of injury rather than stimulation is unclear.

Radioiodine results in a rise in TSAb, LATS-P and TBII around three to six months after therapy, followed by a fall to pretreatment levels by two years (McGregor *et al.*, 1979b; Bech & Madsen, 1980; Hardisty, Fowles & Munro, 1984a). Two possible explanations have been advanced for this phenomenon. Firstly, suppressor cells are more radiosensitive than helper cells, at least *in vitro*, and their intrathyroidal irradiation may tip the balance in favour of increased T cell help, stimulating autoantibody production within the gland (McGregor *et al.* 1979c). Although the thyroid is generally depleted of all lymphocytes after ^{131}I treatment (Kennedy & Thomson, 1974), circulating T cells may be affected by their passage through the gland in the days after treatment (Blomgren *et al.*, 1987) which could have extrathyroidal consequences. Secondly, radiation damage to the gland could release autoantigen and stimulate the autoimmune response, including antibody synthesis in the bone marrow and lymph nodes.

As a result of either mechanism, circulating T cell subsets change after ^{131}I, in particular there being a rise in activated (Ia$^+$, CDw26$^+$, CD45R0$^+$) T cells which is not related to thyroid hormone levels (Teng *et al.*, 1990b). Another study found gradual restoration to normal of circulating CD8$^+$ T cell levels in Graves' disease after radioiodine, which was ascribed to the amelioration of hyperthyroidism, based on the uncertain premise that radioiodine has no direct immunological effects (Volpé *et al.*, 1986; Gerstein *et al.*, 1987). In fact, the changes in CD8$^+$ cells occurred over a much longer period than it took to restore euthyroidism. The rise in autoantibodies after radioiodine is also completely independent of fluctuations in thyroid hormone levels (Bech & Madsen, 1980) as are the circulating T and B cell changes which result from irradiation (Blomgren *et al.*, 1987). Finally, methimazole prevents the rise of TBII after ^{131}I, once again unrelated to circulating thyroid hormone concentrations, providing strong evidence that both agents induce autoantibody changes independent of thyroid status (Gamstedt, Wadman & Karlsson, 1986). As with thyroidectomy, the presence of complement-fixing TPO antibodies (which presumably increase in parallel to TSH receptor antibodies after ^{131}I) may be a minor risk factor for the subsequent development of hypothyroidism (Lundell *et al.*, 1981).

Table 3.7. *Classification of eye signs in Graves' ophthalmopathy (Van Dyk, 1981)*

Class or Grade[a]	Signs and symptoms
0	No physical signs or symptoms
1	Upper eye lid retraction, stare and lid lag; no symptoms
2	Signs and symptoms of soft tissue involvement, especially periorbital oedema
3	Proptosis (or exophthalmos)
4	Restriction of extraocular movement
5	Corneal exposure or ulceration
6	Visual field defect due to optic nerve compression

[a] Although patients with a particular grade of eye involvement often have the preceding grades as well, this is not inevitable. Grades can be subdivided into mild (a), moderate (b) or severe (c).

This is even the case when TPO antibodies accompany a toxic adenoma (Mariotti *et al.*, 1986).

In summary, partial thyroidectomy and radioiodine both have a major impact on the autoimmune response in Graves' disease. Several explanations have been advanced for these changes; it seems unlikely that the restoration of euthyroidism alone is responsible. With both treatments, autoantigen is released but at a different tempo and concentration. Since EAT can be made better or worse by injecting varying concentrations of autoantigen (Kong, 1986), it is possible that the differences in autoantibody response after the two therapies could relate in part to this phenomenon. Immunosuppressive treatment for Graves' disease is not warranted, although prednisone will induce remission (Werner & Platman, 1965). However, if the disease can be shown to have an oligoclonal T or B cell origin, then specific immunotherapy might be feasible.

Graves' ophthalmopathy

Graves' thyrotoxicosis is frequently associated with the signs or symptoms of Graves' ophthalmopathy, caused by an autoimmune process principally affecting the extraocular muscles (Trokel & Jakobiec, 1981). A grading system is generally used to classify the signs but does not necessarily reflect progressive changes (Table 3.7). Even in Graves' patients without clinically obvious eye muscle involvement, the condition can be detected in up to 90%

by ultrasonography, computerised tomographic scanning, exophthalmo-
metry or evaluation of saccadic eye movement fatigue (Werner, Coleman &
Frantzen, 1974; Enzmann, Donaldson & Kriss, 1979; Amino et al., 1980;
Mauri et al., 1984). Although it is therefore a very frequent disorder in
Graves' disease, it is not yet clear if all such patients have ophthalmopathy,
with minimal disease escaping detection even by these sensitive (but
indirect) techniques. Moreover, the same ophthalmopathy can occur in
patients with Hashimoto's thyroiditis or in the absence of any overt biochemical disturbance of thyroid function, this being termed ophthalmic
Graves' disease. Yet even in the ostensibly euthyroid patients with ophthalmic Graves' disease, a variety of thyroid abnormalities can frequently be
found, including suppressed TSH, thyroid lymphocytic infiltration and
detectable TPO and TSH receptor autoantibodies, as well as antibodies
mediating ADCC against thyrocytes (Teng & Yeo, 1977; Salvi et al., 1990).

Graves' ophthalmopathy is therefore a disorder associated closely with
Graves' disease and less frequently with Hashimoto's thyroiditis or subclinical thyroid autoimmunity (about 10% of cases). Whether the eye disease
ever occurs in the absence of any thyroid abnormality is debatable; the
relative insensitivity of tests for thyroiditis is a major problem in addressing
this. In most patients there is a close temporal relationship between the
onset of thyroid and eye disease, strengthening their association (Wiersinga
et al., 1988). At present it seems most likely that Graves' ophthalmopathy
and autoimmune thyroid disease are associated because there is antigenic
cross reactivity in the two target tissues which is identified by the autoimmune response. The nature of this is unknown and it is also unclear why so
few patients with Hashimoto's thyroiditis have any eye signs and why the
clinically evident range of eye involvement in Graves' disease is so great.
These last two features suggest that there are unique genetic or environmental influences which may operate in ophthalmopathy through different
immunopathogenic mechanisms to those in thyroid autoimmunity. Extensive reviews of earlier work on ophthalmopathy have been published
(Jacobson & Gorman, 1984; Pope, Ludgate & McGregor, 1986). Like
Graves' disease, there is no satisfactory animal model and investigation has
also been hampered by the inaccessibility of the retrobulbar tissue.

Immunogenetics

An immunogenetic predisposition to develop Graves' ophthalmopathy has
long been sought but so far there is no consistent evidence for this. The lack
of consensus may reflect differences in classifying the disorder. If, as seems
likely, virtually all patients with Graves' disease have eye involvement then
one is looking for an added genetic susceptibility to develop significantly
worse ophthalmopathy. The question is, what is significant? An early

association of Graves' ophthalmopathy with HLA-Cw3 was suggested but the patients were not graded for the severity of their eye signs (Mayr *et al.*, 1976). This association has not been confirmed in subsequent studies (Farid, Stone & Johnson, 1980). Nine of 14 patients with grade 4–5 ophthalmopathy were HLA-Bw35 in another study, compared to 12.1% of controls, giving a relative risk of 13.1 (Sergott *et al.*, 1983). Although an impressive result, seven of 30 patients with grade 0 ophthalmopathy were also Bw35, an insignificant difference from those with severe eye involvement, when corrected for the number of variables tested.

An increased frequency of the HLA-B8,-DR3 haplotype in Caucasians with ophthalmopathy (above that of Graves' disease alone) has been found in some studies (Farid *et al.*, 1980; Schleusener *et al.*; 1983). In addition to the DR3 effect, DR7 enhanced susceptibility in Hungarian patients in the presence of B8, but was protective in its absence (Frecker *et al.*, 1986). This has been confirmed in a separate study from Newfoundland (Frecker *et al.*, 1988). By contrast, others in Denmark, France and England have found no differences in DR types between Graves' patients with and without ophthal-mopathy (Bech *et al.*, 1977; Allannic *et al.*, 1983; Kendall-Taylor *et al.*, 1988; Weetman *et al.*, 1988b). HLA-DR4 and DRw6 were significantly associated with eye disease in American Blacks with Graves' disease when frequencies were compared to normal controls (Sridama *et al.*, 1987). Once again, however, there was no significant difference (after correction) in these distributions compared to a group of concurrently studied Graves' disease patients without ophthalmopathy. HLA-DPB2.1 appears to protect against ophthalmopathy in Caucasian patients with Graves' disease; the distribution of HLA-DQ alleles is unaltered (Weetman *et al.*, 1990e).

The distribution of Gm allotypes is not abnormal in patients with ophthalmopathy, nor are any of the T cell receptor RFLP genotypes so far examined, although it is possible that certain Gm allotypes may interact with HLA-B8 to enhance susceptibility (Frecker *et al.*, 1986; Weetman *et al.*, 1988b). A wide variety of other polymorphisms have been tested without further associations being turned up: an increased frequency of the blood group P^+ phenotype in ophthalmopathy patients was insignificant after correction (Kendall-Taylor *et al.*, 1988).

Environmental factors

The female preponderance found in autoimmune thyroid disease is less obvious in Graves' ophthalmopathy. One possible reason for this is the association of ophthalmopathy with smoking (Hägg & Asplund, 1987; Shine *et al.*, 1990). The presence and severity of the eye disease both appear to be associated with increasing tobacco consumption. The reasons for this are unknown but cigarette smoking is known to be goitrogenic and to increase the release of Tg (Borup Christensen *et al.*, 1984). Thus a potentially cross-reactive thyroid autoantigen might reach circulatory levels sufficient to cause a retrobulbar autoimmune response more readily in smokers. Alternatively smoking could have a deleterious non-specific effect on the immune system, for instance by enhancing IL-1 release (Francus *et al.*, 1989).

T cell responses

The earliest pathological feature of Graves' ophthalmopathy is the appearance of T and B lymphocytes in the extraocular muscles. In three of four patients examined with an extensive infiltrate, activated/memory T cells (CD45R0$^+$) predominated (Tallstedt & Norberg, 1988; Weetman *et al.*, 1989b). The retrobulbar muscle fibroblasts express Ia molecules as do some of the T cells, but the muscle cells are Ia$^-$. Macrophages were prominent in one patient who had received steroid treatment prior to biopsy. The percentages of circulating CD4$^+$ and CD8$^+$ T cells appear normal in ophthalmic Graves' disease (Pedersen *et al.*, 1989).

For obvious reasons, functional T cell studies have been confined to the peripheral blood. Blastogenic responses to a lacrimal gland extract were observed in nine of 22 patients with ophthalmopathy (Wall *et al.*, 1978). Lacrimal gland infiltration can occur in this condition but no correlation with evidence of such involvement was given in these patients, as determining this is difficult. T cells also proliferate in response to eye muscle membranes, but this is not specific as patients with Hashimoto's thyroiditis and Graves' disease without overt ophthalmopathy respond equally well and skeletal and extraocular muscle induce the same proliferative responses (Weetman, Fells & Shine, 1989c). Since skeletal muscle lymphocytic infiltrates are found in biopsies from some patients with Graves' disease (Ramsay, 1966), the selective nature of the disease may be relative, perhaps relating to enhanced susceptibility of the highly specialised extraocular muscles.

MIF production in response to crude retrobulbar antigen extracts provides further evidence of circulating T cell sensitisation to this tissue in ophthalmopathy (Mahieu & Winand, 1972; Munro *et al.*, 1973). Partial purification suggested that Tg, or some component of it, was responsible for these results (Mullin *et al.*, 1977). It has been proposed that Tg travels from the thyroid to the retrobulbar space by lymphatic channels, binds to the muscles and thus provokes an autoimmune response (Kriss, 1970; Konishi, Herman & Kriss, 1974). There are several problems with this hypothesis, including the fact that Tg is a normal circulating antigen anyway. More particularly, the autoimmune response against Tg is much stronger in Hashimoto's thyroiditis than Graves' disease, whereas ophthalmopathy has the opposite predilection. There are also studies which have failed to find

significant MIF production by T cells from these patients in response to
retrobulbar or lacrimal gland antigen preparations (Wall *et al.*, 1978, 1979).
As previously discussed, the MIF test for T cell sensitisation in Graves'
disease has also proven erratic in reproducibility. Leucocyte procoagulant
production has been used as a potentially more robust assay for T cell
sensitisation and two-thirds of ophthalmopathy patients gave positive responses (Wall, 1986).

Allowing for patient and assay variability, it seems that a proportion of
patients, generally selected for overt ophthalmopathy, have peripheral
blood T cells sensitised to retrobulbar antigens. However, a wide variety of
potential targets are included in these antigen preparations. T cell reactivity
may be against several antigens or against epitopes shared with (at a
minimum) skeletal muscle and lacrimal gland.

B cell responses

The search for autoantibodies against retrobulbar tissues has become a
Grail-like quest recently, despite the lack of any evidence that humoral
mechanisms cause ophthalmopathy (indeed oversight of this fact has caused
some confusion in antibody terminology). On the other hand, the difficulty
of studying ophthalmopathy is so great that the availability of a sensitive and
specific antibody test would have considerable diagnostic and research
utility, even if only indirectly related to the disease process. Certainly, the
conventional thyroid antibodies against Tg, TPO and the TSH receptor do
not seem to play a significant role in the development and course of
ophthalmopathy, although TSH receptor antibody levels tend to be higher
in these Graves' patients than in those without eye signs (Bech, 1989).

Several approaches have been adopted to identify retrobulbar antibodies.
A gel-purified soluble antigen derived from human eye muscle cytosol
reacted with sera from 74% of ophthalmopathy patients by ELISA but with
none of 16 sera from Graves' disease patients without eye signs (Kodama *et
al.*, 1982). The gel fractionation removed human IgG which interfered with
the assay. Porcine eye muscle has also been used to circumvent this problem.
In an ELISA using ultracentrifuged membranes, antibody binding was
found in 64% of ophthalmopathy patients but in none of 11 patients with
Graves' thyroid disease alone (Atkinson, Holcombe & Kendall-Taylor,
1984). The assay was initially thought to be eye muscle-specific and these
results were supported by apparently similar reactivity using human eye
muscle membranes and radiolabelled protein A to measure antibody binding (Farnya, Nauman & Gardas, 1985).

However, subsequent studies have found far less clear distinction between patient groups (Sikorska & Wall, 1985; Kadlubowski, Irvine &
Rowland, 1986; Ahmann *et al.*, 1987; Weetman *et al.*, 1989c). Moreover,

these studies and further investigation by the original group (Kendall-Taylor, Jones & Atkinson, 1987) have confirmed that there is little evidence for eye muscle specificity, as these antibodies generally bind equally well to skeletal or thyroid membranes. At least some of the autoantigens have been characterised, namely actin, tubulin and acetylcholine receptor (Kadlubowski, Irvine & Rowland, 1987). One group has detected, by immunoblotting, high frequency of antibodies against a 64 kd human eye muscle protein in patients with ophthalmopathy (Salvi, Miller & Wall, 1988). Less frequently, antibodies were detected against 55 and 95 kd proteins; the 55 kd antigen appears to be eye muscle-specific whereas the 64 and 95 kd antigens are shared with thyroid membranes (Zhang et al., 1989). Recently a cDNA encoding a 64 kd protein of unknown function has been cloned which may explain these results (Dong, Ludgate & Vassart, 1991). The antigen is widespread in canine tissue but apparently confined to human eye muscle and thyroid. However, no obvious relationship between antibodies to this antigen and the presence of ophthalmopathy has yet emerged, particularly as some normal sera bind to it.

The interest in Tg as a possible cross-reactive antigen in ophthalmopathy has been revived by the demonstration of Tg sequence homology with acetylcholinesterase, particularly as hydropathy profiles also indicate the two proteins may share antigenic determinants (Swillens et al., 1986). This suggests that antibodies to Tg could bind to eye muscle membrane acetylcholinesterase and cause ophthalmopathy. A shared epitope has been defined which reacted with all eight Graves' ophthalmopathy sera tested but with only one of 10 Hashimoto sera, even though these contained high levels of Tg antibodies (Ludgate et al., 1989). This antigen is not related to the 64 kd antigen. Since acetylcholinesterase is widely distributed, it is difficult to see why the extraocular muscles should be singled out for immunological attack on this basis. The fact that many patients with ophthalmopathy do not have Tg antibodies also does not accord with this hypothesis.

Most attempts to delineate antibodies in ophthalmopathy have used extraocular muscle membranes as a source of antigen, but many other cells besides muscle cells contribute to the proteins present in these preparations. The evidence for muscle cell injury in Graves' ophthalmopathy is slender and it has been argued that the retrobulbar fibroblast may be the key target of the autoimmune response (Bahn, Smith & Gorman, 1989a). Certain monoclonal TSH receptor antibodies stimulate collagen synthesis by normal skin fibroblasts and circulating antibodies with this activity have been found in Graves' patients, their levels correlating closely with the severity of ophthalmopathy (Rotella et al., 1986). Others have found that sera from nine of 39 Graves' ophthalmopathy patients bound to cultured retrobulbar but not skin fibroblasts, suggesting site specificity in the antigens expressed by these cells (Bahn et al., 1987). Somewhat at odds with this is the recent demonstration of a 23 kd protein in fibroblasts from diverse sites, which reacts with antibodies in 56% of Graves' sera compared to 15% of controls (Bahn et al., 1989b). However, there was no relationship between the occurrence of these antibodies and eye signs in the Graves' group and, in contrast to the experience of Wall and colleagues, antibodies to a 64 kd protein were universally present in both normal and autoimmune subjects.

In summary, a considerable effort has been made in recent years to identify circulating autoantibodies against retrobulbar tissues in ophthalmopathy. No consensus has yet been reached. Hypotheses suggesting cross reactivity of Tg or TSH receptor antibodies with shared epitopes present in extraocular muscle must explain why serum levels of these common antibodies do not correlate with disease and why eye muscle is specifically involved. The existence of a novel 64 kd protein shared between thyroid and eye muscle may explain these paradoxes but further characterisation is required. So far there is no antibody against retrobulbar tissue which is a sensitive and specific marker for ophthalmopathy: given the sophistication of the methodology recently applied, it may be that this is the ultimate truth.

Effector mechanisms

Although the extraocular muscles are infiltrated by lymphocytes, the target organ reaction is oedema (probably due to increased production of mucopolysaccharides by fibroblasts), fibrosis and, occasionally, fat cell infiltration (Campbell, 1984). Stimulation of retrobulbar fibroblasts by autoantibodies or, probably more likely, cytokines from the T cell infiltrate could well induce these pathological features (Sisson & Vanderburg, 1972). Only rarely are lymphocytes seen cuffing degenerating muscle fibres, suggesting that muscle cell destruction is not of importance to the disease. Nonetheless, cytotoxicity against cultured extraocular muscle cells has been shown by two groups. In a single patient with ophthalmopathy, circulating lymphocytes killed allogeneic extraocular but not skeletal muscle cells (Blau et al., 1983). The exact effector cells responsible for this unusual MHC-unrestricted but target-specific effect were not established. In another study, sera from five of 13 patients with ophthalmopathy contained antibodies which mediated ADCC against cultured extraocular but not skeletal muscle cells (Wang et al., 1986). These antibodies did not fix complement nor correlate closely with those reacting with the 64 kd antigen previously identified by the same group (Zhang et al., 1989). Antibodies producing this type of ADCC were found in eight of 14 Graves' patients without clinical evidence of eye disease but not in controls and their concentration was directly related to the severity of the ophthalmopathy (Hiromatsu et al., 1990). However, besides the already mentioned lack of histological evidence for muscle cell destruction, circulating NK cell activity is depressed in Graves' ophthalmopathy

(Wang *et al.*, 1986; Pedersen *et al.*, 1989), which makes ADCC seem a less likely pathogenic mechanism.

In essence, the pathogenesis of this disorder is unclear. It is possible that the localised inflammatory cells produce cytokines which act directly on fibroblasts and mast cells to induce oedema and ultimately fibrosis. A role for humoral or cell-mediated cytotoxicity remains to be confirmed. Any postulate for an effector mechanism must take into account the localisation of the disorder to the extraocular muscles and the frequent asymmetry of the changes.

Treatment

The therapy of mild to moderate ophthalmopathy is often merely symptomatic, as the condition usually remains stable until fibrosis ensues and further progression is prevented. However, severe or congestive ophthalmopathy requires prompt treatment to prevent or reverse visual failure. Non-specific immunosuppression using steroids, cyclophosphamide, azathioprine, cyclosporin A, plasma exchange and orbital irradiation have all been used with varying degrees of success (Gorman, 1986). Cyclosporin A may be a useful steroid-sparing agent in extended treatment regimens (Kahaly *et al.*, 1986; Prummel *et al.*, 1989). When rapid action is necessary, orbital decompression is probably the treatment of choice if an initial trial of high-dose steroids fails. Part of the apparent variability in response seen with all treatment modalities lies in the imprecise definition of disease severity and duration. Once fibrosis has intervened, then little short of corrective surgery will produce benefit.

From the immunological point of view, the effect of therapy for concurrent Graves' disease on ophthalmopathy is intriguing. One might expect some relationship if a cross-reactive antigen is involved, given the autoimmune sequelae of such treatment discussed previously. In one study, progression of the eye disease was slightly slower after partial thyroidectomy or radioiodine, but enhanced by antithyroid drugs (Gwinup, Elias & Ascher, 1982). More recently it has become apparent that radioiodine worsens pre-existing ophthalmopathy, although it does not initiate clinical disease in Graves' patients without eye signs before treatment (Bartalena *et al.*, 1989). This deterioration could be prevented by prednisone and may have been due to enhanced release of a cross-reactive antigen or to effects on T cell activation. Regardless of the mode of antithyroid treatment, two recent retrospective studies have suggested that persistently abnormal thyroid function is related to more severe eye disease (Karlsson *et al.*, 1989; Prummel *et al.*, 1990). However, it is impossible to conclude that these effects are caused directly by the abnormal thyroid hormone levels, which could simply reflect a more powerful autoimmune response in turn associated with worse eye disease. Problems of grading eye signs and the statistical assessment used also make these findings somewhat difficult to evaluate (Feldon, 1990).

Pretibial myxoedema

The dermopathy of Graves' disease affects about 1% of patients, who are almost always those with severe ophthalmopathy. It is not necessarily confined to the pretibial region; similar but less pronounced changes may be found on the feet and forearms and it may appear elsewhere in response to trauma (Wortsman et al., 1981; Noppakun, Bancheum & Chandraprasert, 1986). The histology and relationship of this condition to thyroid autoimmunity have been reviewed extensively (Smith, Bahn & Gorman, 1989). The dermis of affected skin contains a great increase of glycosaminoglycans, particularly hyaluronic acid, without any evidence of lymphocytic infiltration. The fibroblast is thought to be the source of these changes, but the effector mechanism is unknown. One striking feature is that LATS and LATS-P are found in 90–100% of patients with pretibial myxoedema yet occur in only 15–25% of Graves' patients without it (Schermer et al., 1970; Hardisty, Fowles & Munro, 1984b). However, the levels of LATS and LATS-P do not correlate with the severity of the dermopathy or its clinical course, and LATS is not deposited in affected skin. In vitro experiments have also failed to show that LATS or other TSAb can stimulate fibroblasts.

Mitogen-stimulated normal lymphocytes increase glycosaminoglycan production by retrobulbar fibroblasts, suggesting a role for cytokines as mediators in ophthalmopathy and, by analogy, dermopathy (Sisson & Vanderburg, 1972). Serum from patients with pretibial myxoedema contains a similar activity which enhances hyaluronic acid synthesis by pretibial fibroblasts from healthy subjects and patients with dermopathy (Cheung et al., 1978). Others have also found an uncharacterised activity in dermopathy serum which will stimulate normal fibroblasts (Jolliffe et al., 1979). In neither case was this effect mediated by IgG. In contrast, immunoglobulins from dermopathy patients were found to stimulate glycosaminoglycan production by the $FRTL_5$ rat thyroid cell line (Rotella et al., 1987). This has been confirmed recently, although it was also noted that generalised enhancement of thyroid cell growth and protein synthesis occurred and, more importantly, the antibodies did not stimulate syngeneic pretibial fibroblasts in vitro (Tao, Leu & Kriss, 1989). These studies suggest that there may be a subgroup of TSH receptor antibodies, possibly LATS or LATS-P, which are unusually potent at stimulating thyroid cell growth and protein synthesis (via cAMP). Such dermopathy-associated TSAb are closely linked to pretibial myxoedema, but how disease is induced remains unknown, although a direct effect of dermopathy-associated TSAb on skin fibroblasts seems unlikely. Treatment is usually with potent topical steroids such as triamcinolone or betamethasone. The possible benefits of other treatments such as plasma exchange described in single case reports have not been evaluated further (T. J. Smith *et al.*, 1989).

Multinodular goitre

The hypothesis that growth-stimulating antibodies may be responsible for non-toxic simple goitre has already been discussed. In addition, it is worth mentioning that toxic and non-toxic multinodular goitre may be associated with immunological features which suggest that a subset of these patients may have a variant of autoimmune thyroid disease. Some individuals give positive MIF responses to thyroid antigens (Kiy *et al.*, 1981) and the thyrocytes in a multinodular gland may express class II antigens, although they appear to be incapable of stimulating the T cells which also infiltrate the gland (Grubeck-Loebenstein *et al.*, 1988). About half of a group of Israeli patients with toxic multinodular goitre had circulating TSAb, with a distinct scintiscan appearance and concurrent thyroid antibodies, indicative of underlying Graves' disease (Kraiem *et al.*, 1987b).

Summary

Autoimmune thyroid disease has been the paradigm of organ-specific autoimmunity for over 30 years. Reproducible animal models of thyroiditis, ready access to thyroidal lymphocytes and the frequency of these disorders have sustained the growth in understanding their aetiology and pathogenesis. Genetic susceptibility is in part related to HLA-DR3 in Caucasians, possibly due to non-specific, heightened immune reactivity seen in such individuals. Non-MHC genes encoding T cell receptors or immunoglobulins may also play a role. Few environmental factors contributing to the aetiology of thyroiditis have been clearly defined but dietary iodine, pregnancy and infections have all been implicated. Tissue injury in hypothyroidism seems likely to be the result of complement-fixing TPO antibodies and cell-mediated effector mechanisms; hyperthyroidism in Graves' disease is produced by TSAb, which may be clonally restricted. All forms of treatment for Graves' disease influence the autoimmune response and several hypotheses have been advanced to account for this, but none is totally proven. Far less is known about Graves' ophthalmopathy, although it seems possible that a cross-reactive antigen in the thyroi i a٠d the extraocular muscles explains the observed associations. The fibroblast rather than the muscle cells may be the target in this disorder. The recent cloning of TPO, the TSH receptor and other previously unsuspected thyroid antigens should allow clarification of many of the uncertainties which remain.

References

Adams, D.D. (1978). The V gene theory of inherited autoimmune disease. *Journal of Clinical and Laboratory Immunology*, **1**, 17–24.

Adams, D.D. & Purves, H.D. (1956). Abnormal responses in the assay of thyrotrophin. *Proceedings of the University of Otago Medical School*, **34**, 11–12.

Adams, D.D. & Kennedy, T.H. (1967). Occurrence in thyrotoxicosis of a gamma globulin which protects LATS from neutralisation by an extract of thyroid gland. *Journal of Clinical Endocrinology and Metabolism*, **27**, 173–7.

Adams, D.D., Kennedy, T.H., Stewart, J.C., Utiger, R.D. & Vidor, G.I. (1975). Hyperthyroidism in Tasmania following iodide supplementation: measurements of thyroid stimulating autoantibodies and thyrotropin. *Journal of Clinical Endocrinology and Metabolism*, **41**, 221–8.

Adler, T.R., Beall, G.N., Curd, J.G., Heiner, D.C. & Sabharwal, U.K. (1984). Studies of complement fixation and IgG subclass restriction of anti-thyroglobulin. *Clinical and Experimental Immunology*, **56**, 383–9.

Aguayo, J., Iitaka, M., Row, V.V. & Volpé, R. (1988). Studies of HLA-DR expression on cultured human thyrocytes: effect of antithyroid drugs and other agents on interferon-gamma-induced HLA-DR expression. *Journal of Clinical Endocrinology and Metabolism*, **66**, 903–8.

Ahmann, A., Baker, J.R., Weetman, A.P., Wartofsky, L., Nutman, T.B. & Burman, K.D. (1987). Antibodies to porcine eye muscle in patients with Graves' ophthalmopathy; identification of serum immunoglobulins directed against unique determinants by immunoblotting and enzyme-linked immunosorbent assay. *Journal of Clinical Endocrinology and Metabolism*, **64**, 454–60.

Aho, K., Gordin, A., Palosuo, T. & Takala, J. (1985). Development of thyroid autoimmunity. *Acta Endocrinologica*, **108**, 61–4.

Aichinger, G., Fill, H. & Wick, G. (1985). *In situ* immune complexes, lymphocyte subpopulations, and HLA-DR positive epithelial cells in Hashimoto's thyroiditis. *Laboratory Investigation*, **52**, 132–40.

Allannic, H., Fauchet, R., Lorcy, Y., Gueguen, M., Le Guerrier, A.-M. & Genetet, B. (1983). A prospective study of the relationship between relapse of hyperthyroid Graves' disease after antithyroid drugs and HLA haplotype. *Journal of Clinical Endocrinology and Metabolism*, **57**, 719–22.

Allen, E.M., Appel, M.C. & Braverman, L.E. (1986a). The effect of iodine ingestion on the development of spontaneous lymphocytic thyroiditis in the diabetes prone BB/W rat. *Endocrinology*, **118**, 1977–81.

Allen, E.M., Rajatanavin, R., Nogimori, T., Cushing, G., Ingbar, S.H. & Braverman, L.E. (1986b). The effect of methimazole on the development of spontaneous lymphocytic thyroiditis in the diabetes-prone BB/W rat. *American Journal of the Medical Sciences*, **29**, 267–71.

Amino, N., Yuasa, T., Yabu, Y. & Miyai, K. (1980). Exophthalmos in autoimmune thyroid disease. *Journal of Clinical Endocrinology and Metabolism*, **51**, 1232–4.

Amino, N., Mori, H., Iwatani, Y., Asari, S., Izumiguchi, Y. & Miyai, K. (1982a). Peripheral K lymphocytes in autoimmune thyroid disease: decrease in Graves' disease and increase in Hashimoto's disease. *Journal of Clinical Endocrinology and Metabolism*, **54**, 587–91.

Amino, N., Mori, H., Iwatani, Y., Tanizawa, O., Kawashima, M., Tsuge, I., Ibaragi, K., Kumahara, Y. & Miyai, K. (1982b). High prevalence of transient post-partum thyrotoxicosis and hypothyroidism. *New England Journal of Medicine*, **306**, 849–52.

Amino, N., & Miyai, K. (1983). Postpartum autoimmune endocrine syndromes. In *Auto-immune Endocrine Disease*, ed. T.F. Davies, pp. 247–72, New York: John Wiley.

Ansar Ahmed, S., Young, P.R. & Penhale, W.J. (1983). The effects of female sex steroids on the development of autoimmune thyroiditis in thymectomized and irradiated rats. *Clinical and Experimental Immunology*, **54**, 351–8.

Aoki, N. & DeGroot, J. (1979). Lymphocyte blastogenic response to human thyroglobulin in Graves' disease, Hashimoto's thyroiditis, and metastatic thyroid cancer. *Clinical and Experimental Immunology*, **38**, 523–30.

Aoki, N., Pinnamaneni, K.M. & DeGroot, L.J. (1979). Studies on suppressor cell function in thyroid diseases. *Journal of Clinical Endocrinology and Metabolism*, **48**, 803–10.

Arikawa, K., Ichikawa, Y., Yoshida, T., Shinozawa, T., Homma, M., Momotani, N. & Itoh, K. (1985). Blocking type antithyrotropin receptor antibody in patients with nongoitrous hypothyroidism: its incidence and characteristics of action. *Journal of Clinical Endocrinology and Metabolism*, **60**, 953–9.

Atherton, M.C., McLachlan, S.M., Pegg, C.A.S., Dickinson, A., Baylis, P., Young, E.T., Proctor, S.J. & Rees Smith, B. (1985). Thyroid autoantibody synthesis by lymphocytes from different lymphoid organs: fractionation of B cells on density gradients. *Immunology*, **55**, 271–9.

Atkins, M.B., Mier, J.W., Parkinson, D.R., Gould, J.A., Berkman, E.A. & Kaplan, M.M. (1988). Hypothyroidism after treatment with interleukin–2 and lymphokine-activated killer cells. *New England Journal of Medicine*, **318**, 1557–63.

Atkinson, S. & Kendall-Taylor, P. (1981). The stimulation of thyroid hormone secretion in vitro by thyroid-stimulating antibodies. *Journal of Clinical Endocrinology and Metabolism*, **53**, 1263–66.

Atkinson, S., Holcombe, M. & Kendall-Taylor, P. (1984). Ophthalmopathic immunoglobulin in patients with Graves' ophthalmopathy. *Lancet*, **ii**, 374–6.

Bagchi, N., Brown, T.R., Urdanivia, E. & Sundick, R.S. (1985). Induction of autoimmune thyroiditis in chickens by dietary iodine. *Science*, **230**, 325–7.

Bagnasco, M., Canonica, G.W., Ferrini, S., Biassoni, P., Melioli, G., Ferrini, O. & Giordano, G. (1983). T lymphocyte subpopulations in Graves' disease: relationship with clinical conditions. *Acta Endocrinologica*, **102**, 213–19.

Bagnasco, M., Ciprandi, G., Orlandi, A., Torre, G., Canonica, G.W. & Giordano, G. (1985). Autologous mixed lymphocyte reaction in Graves' disease: relationship to clinical status. *Acta Endocrinologica*, **110**, 366–72.

Bagnasco, M., Venuti, D., Prigione, I., Torre, G.C., Ferrini, S. & Canonica, G.W. (1988). Graves' disease: phenotypic and functional analysis at the clonal level of the T-cell repertoire in peripheral blood and in thyroid. *Clinical Immunology and Immunopathology*, **47**, 230–9.

Bahn, R.S., Gorman, C.A., Woloschak, G.E., David, C.S., Johnson, P.M. & Johnson, C.M. (1987). Human retroocular fibroblasts *in vitro*: a model for the study of Graves' ophthalmo-pathy. *Journal of Clinical Endocrinology and Metabolism*, **65**, 665–70.

Bahn, R.S., Smith, T.J. & Gorman, C.A. (1989a). The central role of the fibroblast in the pathogenesis of extrathyroidal manifestations of Graves' disease. *Acta Endocrinologica*, **121** (Suppl. 2), 75–81.

Bahn, R.S., Gorman, C.A., Johnson, C.M. & Smith, T.J. (1989b). Presence of antibodies in the sera of patients with Graves' disease recognizing a 23 kilodalton fibroblast protein. *Journal of Clinical Endocrinology and Metabolism*, **69**, 622–8.

Baker, J.R., Lukes, Y.G., Smallridge, R.C., Berger, M. & Burman, K.D. (1983). Partial characterization and clinical correlation of circulating human immunoglobulins directed against thyrotrophin binding sites in guinea pig fat cell membranes. *Journal of Clinical Investigation*, **72**, 1487–97.

Baker, J.R., Saunders, N.B., Tseng, Y.C., Wartofsky, L. & Burman, K.D. (1988). Seronegative Hashimoto thyroiditis with thyroid autoantibody production localized to the thyroid. *Annals of Internal Medicine*, **108**, 26–30.

Balázs, C., Kiss, E., Leovey, E. & Farid, N.R. (1986). The immunosuppressive effect of methimazole on cell-mediated immunity is mediated by its capacity to inhibit peroxidase and scavenge free radicals. *Clinical Endocrinology*, **25**, 7–16.

Balfour, B.M., Doniach, D., Roitt, I.M. & Couchman, K.G. (1961). Fluorescent antibody studies in human thyroiditis: autoantibodies to an antigen of the thyroid colloid distinct from thyroglobulin. *British Journal of Experimental Pathology*, **42**, 307–16.

Bankhurst, A.D., Torrigiani, G. & Allison, A.C. (1973). Lymphocytes binding human thyroglobulin in healthy people and its relevance to tolerance for autoantigens. *Lancet*, **i**, 226–30.

Banovac, K., Ghandur-Mnaymneh, L., Zakarija, M., Rabinovich, A. & McKenzie, J.M. (1988). The effect of thyroxine on spontaneous thyroiditis in BB/W rats. *International Achives of Allergy and Applied Immunology*, **87**, 301–5.

Barker, D.J.P. & Phillips, D.I.W. (1984). Current incidence of thyrotoxicosis and past prevalence of goitre in 12 British towns. *Lancet*, **ii**, 567–70.

Bartalena, L., Marcocci, C., Bogazzi, F., Panicucci, M., Lepri, A. & Pinchera, A. (1989). Use of corticosteroids to prevent progression of Graves' ophthalmopathy after radioiodine therapy for hyperthyroidism. *New England Journal of Medicine*, **321**, 1349–52.

Bartels, E.D. (1941). *Heredity in Graves' Disease*. Copenhagen: Munksgaard.

Baxter, R.G., Martin, F.I.R., Myles, K., Larkins, R.G., Heyma, P. & Ryan, L. (1975). Down syndrome and thyroid function in adults. *Lancet*, **ii**, 794–5.

Beall, G.N. (1982). Production of human antithyroglobulin in vitro. IV. Specific stimulation by antigen. *Journal of Clinical Endocrinology and Metabolism*, **54**, 1–5.

Beall, G.N. & Kruger, S.R. (1980a). Production of human antithyroglobulin in vitro. II Regulation by T cells. *Clinical Immunology and Immunopathology*, **16**, 498–503.

Beall, G.N. & Kruger, S.R. (1980b). Production of human antithyroglobulin in vitro. I Stimulation by mitogens. *Clinical Immunology and Immunopathology*, **16**, 485–90.

Beall, G.N., Rapoport, B., Chopra, I.J. & Kruger, S.R. (1986). Studies on auto-anti-idiotypic thyroid-stimulating antibodies. *International Archives of Allergy and Applied Immunology*, **81**, 351–6.

Bech, K. (1989). Thyroid antibodies in endocrine ophthalmopathy. A review. *Acta Endocrinologica*, **121** (Suppl. 2), 117–22.

Bech, K., Lumholz, B., Nerup, J., Thomson, M., Platz, P., Ryder, L.P., Svejgaard, A., Siersbock-Nielsen, K., Mølholm-Hansen, J. & Larsen, J.H. (1977). HLA antigens in Graves' disease. *Acta Endocrinologica*, **86**, 510–15.

Bech, K. & Madsen, S.N. (1980). Influence of treatment with radioiodine and propylthiouracil on thyroid stimulating immunoglobulins in Graves' disease. *Clinical Endocrinology*, **13**, 417–24.

Bech, K., Feldt-Rasmussen, U., Bliddal, H., Date, J. & Blichert-Toft, M. (1982). The acute changes in thyroid stimulating immunoglobulins, thyroglobulin and thyroglobulin antibodies following subtotal thyroidectomy. *Clinical Endocrinology*, **16**, 235–42.

Ben-Nun, A., Maron, R., Ron, Y. & Cohen, I.R (1980). H-2 gene products influence susceptibility of target thyroid gland to damage in experimental autoimmune thyroiditis. *European Journal of Immunology*, **10**, 156–9.

Bene, M.-C., Derennes, V., Faure, G., Thomas, J.L., Duheille, J. & Leclere, J. (1983). Graves' disease: *in situ* localization of lymphoid T cell subpopulations. *Clinical and Experimental Immunology*, **52**, 311–16.

Benveniste, P., Wenzel, B.E., Khalil, A., Row, V.V. & Volpé, R. (1984). Spontaneous secretion of thyroid autoantibodies by cultured peripheral blood lymphocytes from patients with Hashimoto's thyroiditis detected by micro-ELISA techniques. *Clinical and Experimental Immunology*, **58**, 273–82.

Benveniste, P., Row, V.V. & Volpé, R. (1985). Studies on the immunoregulation of thyroid autoantibody production *in vitro*. *Clinical and Experimental Immunology*, **61**, 274–82.

Blau, H.M., Kaplan, I., Tao, T.W. & Kriss, J.P. (1983). Thyroglobuin-independent cell-mediated cytotoxicity of human eye muscle cells in tissue culture by lymphocytes of a patient with Graves' disease. *Life Sciences*, **32**, 45–53.

Blomgren, H., Petrini, B., Wasserman, J., Schnell, P-O. & Lundell, G. (1987). Changes in blood lymphocyte population following 131-I treatment for nodular goitre. *International Journal of Radiation Oncology, Biology, Physics*, **13**, 209–15.

Bogner, U., Schleusener, H. & Wall, J.R. (1984). Antibody-dependent cell mediated cytotoxicity against human thyroid cells in Hashimoto's thyroiditis but not Graves' disease. *Journal of Clinical Endocrinology and Metabolism*, **54**, 734–8.

Bonnyns, M., Bentin, J., Devetter, G. & Duchateau, J. (1983). Heterogeneity of immunoregulatory T cells in human thyroid autoimmunity: influence of thyroid status. *Clinical and Experimental Immunology*, **56**, 251–4.

Borup Christensen, S., Ericsson, U.B., Janzon, L., Tibblin, S. & Melander, A. (1984). Influence of cigarette smoking on goiter formation, thyroglobulin, and thyroid hormone levels in women. *Journal of Clinical Endocrinology and Metabolism*, **58**, 615–18.

Bottazzo, G.F., Pujol-Borrell, R., Hanafusa, T. & Feldmann, M. (1983). Role of aberrant HLA-DR expression and antigen presentation in induction of endocrine autoimmunity. *Lancet*, **ii**, 1115–19.

Boukis, I.A., Koutras, D.A., Souvantzoglou, A., Evangelopolou, A., Vrontakis, A. & Moulopoulos, S.D. (1983). Thyroid hormone and immunological studies in endemic goitre. *Journal of Clinical Endocrinology and Metabolism*, **57**, 859–62.

Boyages, S.C., Halpern, J.P., Maberly, G.F., Eastman, C.J., Chen, J., Zhen-Hua, W., Van der Gaag, R.D. & Drexhage, H.A. (1989). Endemic cretinism: possible role for thyroid autoimmunity. *Lancet*, **ii**, 529–32.

Braley-Mullen, H., Tompson, J.G., Sharp, G.C. & Kyriakos, M. (1980). Suppression of experimental autoimmune thyroiditis in guinea pigs by pretreatment with thyroglobulin-coupled spleen cells. *Cellular Immunology*, **51**, 408–13.

Bresler, H.S., Burek, C.L., Hoffman, W.H. & Rose, N.R. (1990). Autoantigenic determinants on human thyroglobulin. II Determinants recognised by autoantibodies from patients with chronic autoimmune thyroiditis compared to autoantibodies from healthy subjects. *Clinical Immunology and Immunopathology*, **54**, 76–86.

Brostoff, J. (1970). Migration inhibition studies in human disease. *Journal of the Royal Society of Medicine*, **63**, 905–6.

Brown, R.S., Keating, P. & Mitchell, E. (1990). Maternal thyroid-blocking immunoglobulins in congenital hypothyroidism. *Journal of Clinical Endocrinology and Metabolism*, **70**, 1341–6.

Bucsema, M., Todd, I., Deuss, U., Hammond, L., Mirakian, R., Pujol-Borrell, R. & Bottazzo, G.F. (1989). Influence of tumor necrosis factor-α on the modulation by interferon-γ of HLA class II molecules in human thyroid cells and its effect on interferon-γ binding. *Journal of Clinical Endocrinology and Metabolism*, **69**, 433–9.

Burman, K.D. & Baker, J.R. (1985). Immune mechanisms in Graves' disease. *Endocrine Reviews*, **6**, 183–232.

Calder, E.A., Penhale, W.J., McLeman, D., Barnes, E.W. & Irvine, W.J. (1973). Lymphocyte-dependent antibody-mediated cytotoxicity in Hashimoto's thyroiditis. *Clinical and Experimental Immunology*, **14**, 153–8.

Calder, E.A., Irvine, W.J., Davidson, N.M. & Wu, F. (1976). T, B and K cells in autoimmune thyroid disease. *Clinical and Experimental Immunology*, **25**, 17–22.

Campbell, R.J. (1984). Pathology of Graves' ophthalmopathy. In *The Eye and Orbit in Thyroid Disease*, ed. C.A. Gorman, R.A. Waller & J.A. Dyer, pp. 25–31. New York: Raven Press.

Canonica, G.W., Bagnasco, M., Corte, G., Ferrini, S., Ferrini, O. & Giordano, G. (1982). Circulating T lymphocytes in Hashimoto's disease: imbalance of subsets and presence of activated cells. *Clinical Immunology and Immunopathology*, **23**, 616–25.

Canonica, G.W., Cosulich, M.E., Croci, R., Ferrini, S., Bagnasco, M., Dirienzo, W., Ferrini, O., Bargellesi, A. & Giordano, G. (1984). Thyroglobulin-induced T-cell *in vitro* proliferation in Hashimoto's thyroiditis: identification of the responsive subset and effect of monoclonal antibodies directed to Ia antigens. *Clinical Immunology and Immunopathology*, **32**, 132–41.

Canonica, G.W., Caria, M., Bagnasco, M., Cosulich, M.E., Giordana, G. & Moretta, L. (1985). Proliferation of T8-positive cytolytic T lymphocytes in response to thyroglobulin in human autoimmune thyroiditis: analysis of cell interactions and culture requirements. *Clinical Immunology and Immunopathology*, **36**, 40–8.

Carayon, P., Adler, G., Roulier, R. & Lissitzky, S. (1983). Heterogeneity of the Graves' immunoglobulins directed toward the thyrotropin receptor-adenylate cyclase system. *Journal of Clinical Endocrinology and Metabolism*, **56**, 1202–8.

Carter, J.K., Ow, C.L. & Smith, R.E. (1983). Rous-associated virus type 7 induces a syndrome in chickens characterized by stunting and obesity. *Infection and Immunity*, **39**, 410–21.

Champion, B.R., Varey, A.M., Katz, D., Cooke, A. & Roitt, I.M. (1985). Autoreactive T-cell lines specific for mouse thyroglobulin. *Immunology*, **54**, 513–19.

Chan, C.T.J., Byfield, P.G.H., Himsworth, R.I. & Shepherd, P. (1987). Human antibodies to thyroglobulin are directed towards a restricted number of human specific epitopes. *Clinical and Experimental Immunology*, **70**, 516–23.

Chan, J.Y., Lerman, M.I., Prabhakar, B.S., Isozaki, O., Santisteban, P., Kuppers, R.C., Oates, E.L., Notkins, A.L. & Kohn, L.D. (1989). Cloning and characterization of a cDNA that encodes a 70-kDa novel human thyroid autoantigen. *Journal of Biological Chemistry*, **264**, 3651–4.

Chan, J.Y.C. & Walfish, P.G. (1986). Activated (Ia) T-lymphocytes and their subsets in autoimmune thyroid diseases: analysis by dual laser flow microfluorocytometry. *Journal of Clinical Endocrinology and Metabolism*, **62**, 403–9.

Cheung, H.S., Nicoloff, J.T., Kamiel, M.B., Spolter, L. & Nimni, M.E. (1978). Stimulation of fibroblast biosynthetic activity by serum of patients with pretibial myxedema. *Journal of Investigative Dermatology*, **71**, 12–17.

Chiovato, L., Hammond, L.J., Hanafusa, T., Pujol-Borrell, R., Doniach, D. & Bottazzo, G.F. (1983). Detection of thyroid growth immunoglobulins (TGI) by [³H]-thymidine incorporation in cultured rat thyroid follicles. *Clinical Endocrinology*, **19**, 581–90.

Cho, B.Y., Rhee, B.D., Lee, D.S., Lee, M.S., Kim, G.Y., Lee, H.K., Koh, C.-S., Min, H.K. & Lee, M. (1987). HLA and Graves' disease in Koreans. *Tissue Antigens*, **31**, 119–21.

Ciampolillo, A., Marini, V., Mirakian, R., Bucsema, M., Schulz, T., Pujol-Borrell, R. & Bottazzo, G.F. (1989). Retrovirus-like sequences in Graves' disease: implications for human autoimmunity. *Lancet*, **i**, 1096–100.

Cohen, S.B. & Weetman, A.P. (1987). Characterization of different types of experimental autoimmune thyroiditis in the Buffalo strain rat. *Clinical and Experimental Immunology*, **69**, 25–32.

Cohen, S.B. & Weetman, A.P. (1988a). The effect of iodine depletion and supplementation in the Buffalo strain rat. *Journal of Endocrinological Investigation*, **11**, 625–7.

Cohen, S.B. & Weetman, A.P. (1988b). Antithyroid drugs ameliorate thymectomy-induced experimental autoimmune thyroiditis. *Autoimmunity*, **1**, 51–8.

Cohen, S.B. & Weetman, A.P. (1988c). Activated interstitial and interepithelial lymphocytes in autoimmune thyroid disease. *Acta Endocrinologica*, **119**, 161–6.

Cohen, S.B., Dijkstra, C.D. & Weetman, A.P. (1988). Sequential analysis of experimental autoimmune thyroiditis induced by neonatal thymectomy in the Buffalo strain rat. *Cellular Immunology*, **114**, 126–36.

Cohen, S.B. & Weetman, A.P. (1990). Serological analysis of experimental autoimmune thyroiditis in the Buffalo strain rat. *International Archives of Allergy and Applied Immunology*, **91**, 47–53.

Cohen, S.B., Diamantstein, T. & Weetman, A.P. (1990). The effect of T cell subset depletion on experimental autoimmune thyroiditis in the Buffalo strain rat. *Immunology Letters*, **23**, 263–8.

Colle, E., Guttman, R.D. & Seemayer, T.A. (1985). Association of spontaneous thyroiditis with the major histocompatibility complex of the rat. *Endocrinology*, **116**, 1243–7.

Cox, S.P., Phillips, D.I.W. & Osmond, C. (1989). Does infection initiate Graves' disease? A population based 10 year study. *Autoimmunity*, **4**, 43–9.

Creemers, P., Rose, N.R. & Kong, Y-C. (1983). Experimental autoimmune thyroiditis: *in vitro* cytotoxic effects of T lymphocytes on thyroid monolayers. *Journal of Experimental Medicine*, **157**, 559–71.

Czarnocka, B., Ruf, J., Ferrand, M., Carayon, P. & Lissitzy, S. (1985). Purification of the human thyroid peroxidase and its identification as the microsomal antigen involved in autoimmune thyroid diseases. *FEBS Letters*, **190**, 147–51.

Dahlberg, P.A., Holmlund, G., Karlsson, F.A. & Säfwenberg, J. (1981). HLA-A, -B, -C and -DR antigens in patients with Graves' disease and their correlation with signs and clinical course. *Acta Endocrinologica*, **97**, 42–7.

Daniel, P.M., Pratt, O.E., Roitt, I.M. & Torrigiani, G. (1967). Thyroglobulin in the lymph draining from the thyroid gland and in the peripheral blood of rats. *Quarterly Journal of Experimental Physiology*, **52**, 184–99.

Davies, T.F. (1985). Co-cultures of human thyroid monolayer cells and autologous T cells – impact of HLA class II antigen expression. *Journal of Clinical Endocrinology and Metabolism*, **61**, 418.

Davies, T.F., Weiss, I. & Gerber, M.A. (1984). Influence of methimazole on murine thyroiditis. Evidence for immunosuppression. *Journal of Clinical Investigation*, **73**, 397–404.

Davies, T.F. & Platzer, M. (1986). The T cell suppressor defect in autoimmune thyroiditis: evidence for a high set 'autoimmunostat'. *Clinical and Experimental Immunology*, **63**, 73–9.

De Bruin, T.W.A., Patawardhan, N.A., Brown, R.S. & Braverman, L.E. (1988). Graves' disease: changes in TSH receptor and anti-microsomal antibodies after thyroidectomy. *Clinical and Experimental Immunology*, **72**, 481–5.

DeGroot, L.J., Sridama, V., Hara, Y., Mori, H., Hamada, N. & Ryan, M. (1985). Quantitative and qualitative abnormalities in circulating lymphocytes in autoimmune thyroid disease. In *Autoimmunity and the Thyroid*, ed. P.G. Walfish, J.R. Wall & R. Volpé, pp. 67–74. Orlando: Academic Press.

Del Prete, G.F., Vercelli, D., Tiri, A., Maggi, E., Mariotti, S., Pinchera, A., Ricci, M. & Romagnani, S. (1986). *In vivo* activated cytotoxic T cells in the thyroid infiltrate of patients with Hashimoto's thyroiditis. *Clinical and Experimental Immunology*, **65**, 140–7.

Delves, P.J. & Roitt, I.M. (1988). Long term spectrotypic and idiotypic stability of thyroglobu-lin autoantibodies in patients with Hashimoto's thyroiditis. *Clinical and Experimental Immunology*, **71**, 459–63.

Demaine, A., Welsh, K.I., Hawe, B.S. & Farid, N.R. (1987). Polymorphism of the T cell receptor β-chain in Graves' disease. *Journal of Clinical Endocrinology and Metabolism*, **65**, 643–6.

Demaine, A.G., Ratanachaiyavong, S., Pope, R., Ewins, D., Millward, B.A. & McGregor, A.M. (1989). Thyroglobulin antibodies in Graves' disease are associated with T-cell receptor beta chain and major histocompatibility complex loci. *Clinical and Experimental Immunology*, **77**, 21–4.

Di Mario, U., Scardellato, A., Irvine, W.J., Kennedy, L., Kadlubowski, M., Kennedy, R., Cavatorta, F.P. & Andreani, D. (1986). Immunity in Graves' disease at diagnosis: corre-lation between activated T cells and humoral immune factors. *Acta Endocrinologica*, **113**, 493–9.

Doble, N.D., Banga, J.P., Pope, R., Lalor, E., Kilduff, P. & McGregor, A.M. (1988). Autoantibodies to the thyroid microsomal/thyroid peroxidase antigen are polyclonal and directed to several distinct antigenic sites. *Immunology*, **64**, 23–9.

Dong, Q., Ludgate, M. & Vassart, G. (1991). Cloning and sequencing of a 64kd autoantigen expressed in the thyroid and extra-ocular muscle. *Journal of Clinical Endocrinology and Metabolism*, (in press).

Doniach, D. (1981). Hashimoto's thyroiditis and primary myxoedema viewed as separate entities. *European Journal of Clinical Investigation*, **11**, 245–7.

Doniach, D., Roitt, I.M. & Polani, P.E. (1968). Thyroid antibodies and sex-chromosome anomalies. *Proceedings of the Royal Society of Medicine*, **61**, 278–80.

Doniach, D., Bottazzo, G.F. & Russell, R.C.G. (1979). Goitrous autoimmune thyroiditis. *Clinics in Endocrinology and Metabolism*, **8**, 63–80.

Drexhage, H.A., Bottazzo, G.F., Doniach, D., Bitensky, L. & Chayen, J. (1980). Evidence for thyroid growth-stimulating immunoglobulins in some goitrous thyroid diseases. *Lancet*, **ii**, 287–92.

Drexhage, H.A., Bottazzo, G.F., Bitensky, L., Chayen, J. & Doniach, D. (1981). Thyroid growth-blocking antibodies in primary myxoedema. *Nature*, **289**, 594–6.

Ealey, P.A., Marshall, N.J. & Ekins, R.P. (1981). Time-related thyroid stimulation by thyrotropin and thyroid-stimulating antibodies, as measured by the cytochemical section bioassay. *Journal of Clinical Endocrinology and Metabolism*, **52**, 483–7.

Ealey, P.A., Emmerson, J.M., Bidey, S.P. & Marshall, N.J. (1985). Thyrotrophin stimulation of mitogenesis of the rat thyroid cell strain FRTL–5: a metaphase index assay for the detection of thyroid growth stimulation. *Journal of Endocrinology*, **106**, 203–10.

Ealey, P.A., Yateman, M.E., Holt, S.J. & Marshall, N.J. (1988). ESTA:A bioassay system for the determination of the potencies of hormones and antibodies which mimic their action. *Journal of Molecular Endocrinology*, **1**, R1–R4.

Ebner, S.A., Stein, M.E., Minami, M., Dorf, M.E. & Stadecker, M.J. (1987). Murine thyroid follicular epithelial cells can be induced to express class II (Ia) gene products but fail to present antigen *in vivo*. *Cellular Immunology*, **104**, 154–68.

Edan, G., Massart, C., Hody, B., Poirer, J.Y., Reun, M.L., Hespel, J.P., Leclech, G. & Simon, M. (1989). Optimum duration of antithyroid drug treatment determined by assay of thyroid stimulating antibody in patients with Graves' disease. *British Medical Journal*, **298**, 359–61.

Eguchi, K., Otsubo, T., Kawabe, Y., Shimomura, C., Ueki, Y., Nakao, H., Tezuka, H., Matsunaga, M., Fukuda, T., Ishikawa, N., Ito, K. & Nagataki, S. (1988). Synergy in antigen presentation by thyroid epithelial cells and monocytes from patients with Graves' disease. *Clinical and Experimental Immunology*, **72**, 84–90.

Eishi, Y. & McCullagh, P. (1988). The relative contributions of the immune system and target organ variation in susceptibility of rats to experimental allergic thyroiditis. *European Journal of Immunology*, **18**, 657–60.

ElRehewy, M., Kong, Y.M., Giraldo, A.A. & Rose, N.R. (1981). Syngeneic thyroglobulin is immunogenic in good responder mice. *European Journal of Immunology*, **11**, 146–51.

Endo, K., Kasagi, K., Konishi, J., Ikekubo, K., Okuno, T., Takeda, Y., Mori, T. & Torizuka, K. (1978). Detection and properties of TSH-binding inhibitor immunoglobulins in patients with Graves' disease and Hashimoto's thyroiditis. *Journal of Clinical Endocrinology and Metabolism*, **46**, 734.

Endo, Y., Aratake, Y., Yamamoto, I., Nakagawa, H., Kuribayashi, T. & Ohtaki, S. (1983). Peripheral K cells in Graves' disease and Hashimoto's thyroiditis in relationship to circulating immune complexes. *Clinical Endocrinology*, **18**, 187–94.

Enzmann, D.R., Donaldson, S.S. & Kriss, J.P. (1979). Appearance of Graves' eye disease on orbital computed tomography. *Journal of Computer Assisted Tomography*, **3**, 815–19.

Farid, N.R. (1981). Graves' disease. In *HLA in Endocrine and Metabolic Disorders*, ed. N.R. Farid, pp. 85–143. New York: Academic Press.

Farid, N.R., Barnard, J.M. & Bryant, D.G. (1977a). HLA and phenylthiocarbamide (PTC) tasting in autoimmune thyroid disease. *Tissue Antigens*, **10**, 414–16.

Farid, N.R., Newton, R.M., Noel, E.P. & Marshall, W.H. (1977b). Gm phenotypes in autoimmune thyroid disease. *Journal of Immunogenetics*, **4**, 429–32.

Farid, N.R., Stone, E. & Johnson, G. (1980). Graves' disease and HLA – clinical and epidemiological associations. *Clinical Endocrinology*, **13**, 535–44.

Farid, N.R., Sampson, L., Moens, H. & Barnard, J.M. (1981). The association of goitrous autoimmune thyroiditis with HLA-DR5. *Tissue Antigens*, **17**, 265–8.

Farid, N.R., Hawe, B.S. & Walfish, P.G. (1983). Increased frequency of HLA-DR3 and 5 in the syndrome of painless thyroiditis with transient thyrotoxicosis: evidence for an autoimmune aetiology. *Clinical Endocrinology*, **19**, 699–704.

Farnya, M., Nauman, J. & Gardas, A. (1985). Measurement of autoantibodies against human eye muscle plasma membranes in Graves' ophthalmopathy. *British Medical Journal*, **290**, 191–3.

Farrant, J., Bryant, A., Chan, J. & Himsworth, R.L. (1986). Thyroglobulin-treated blood dendritic cells induce IgG anti-thyroglobulin antibody in vitro in Hashimoto's thyroiditis. *Clinical Immunology and Immunopathology*, **41**, 433–42.

Fein, H.G., Metz, S., Nikolai, T.F., Johnson, A.H. & Smallridge, R.C. (1985). HLA antigens in thyroiditis: differences between silent and postpartum lymphocytic forms, and comparison with subacute and goitrous autoimmune thyroiditis. In *Autoimmunity and the Thyroid*, ed. P.G. Walfish, J.R. Wall & R. Volpé, pp. 373–5. Orlando: Academic Press

Feldon, S.E. (1990). Graves' ophthalmopathy. Is it really thyroid disease? *Archives of Internal Medicine*, **150**, 948–50.

Feldt-Rasmussen, U., Blichert-Toft, M., Christiansen, C. & Date, J. (1982). Serum thyroglobulin and its autoantibody following subtotal thyroid resection of Graves' disease. *European Journal of Clinical Investigation*, **12**, 203–8.

Fisfalen, M.E., DeGroot, L.J., Quintans, J., Franklin, W.A. & Soltani, K. (1988). Microsomal antigen-reactive lymphocyte lines and clones derived from thyroid tissue of patients with Graves' disease. *Journal of Clinical Endocrinology and Metabolism*, **66**, 776–84.

Flynn, J.C., Conaway, D.H., Cobbold, S., Waldmann, H. & Kong, Y.-C.M. (1989). Depletion of L3T4$^+$ and Lyt-2$^+$ cells by rat monoclonal antibodies alters the development of adoptively transferred experimental autoimmune thyroiditis. *Cellular Immunology*, **122**, 377–90.

Fong, S., Tsoukas, C.D., Frincke, L.A., Lawrence, S.K., Holbrook, T.L., Vaughan, J.H. & Carson, D.A. (1981). Age associated changes in Epstein–Barr virus induced human lymphocyte autoantibody production. *Journal of Immunology*, **126**, 910–14.

Fournier, C., Chen, H., Leger, A. & Charreire, J. (1983). Immunological studies of auto-immune thyroid disorders: abnormalities in the inducer T cell subset and proliferative responses to autologous and allogeneic stimulation. *Clinical and Experimental Immunology*, **54**, 539–46.

Francus, T., Manzo, G., Canki, M., Thompson, L.C. & Szabo, P. (1989). Two peaks of interleukin 1 expression in human leukocyte cultures with tobacco glycoprotein. *Journal of Experimental Medicine*, **170**, 327–32.

Frecker, M., Stenszky, V., Balázs, C., Kozma, L., Kraszits, E. & Farid, N.R. (1986). Genetic factors in Graves' ophthalmopathy. *Clinical Endocrinology*, **25**, 479–85.

Frecker, M., Mercer, G., Skanes, V.M. & Farid, N.R. (1988). Major histocompatibility complex (MHC) factors predisposing to and protecting against Graves' eye disease. *Autoimmunity*, **1**, 307–15.

Fung, H.Y.M., Kologlu, M., Collison, K., John, R., Richards, C.J., Hall, R. & McGregor, A.M. (1988). Postpartum thyroid dysfunction in Mid Glamorgan. *British Medical Journal*, **296**, 241–4.

Gamstedt, A., Wadman, B. & Karlsson, A. (1986). Methimazole, but not betamethasone, prevents ^{131}I treatment-induced rises in thyrotropin receptor autoantibodies in hyperthyroid Graves' disease. *Journal of Clinical Endocrinology and Metabolism*, **62**, 773–7.

Gause, W.C. & Marsh, J.A. (1986). Effect of testosterone treatments for varying periods on autoimmune development and on specific infiltrating leukocyte populations in the thyroid gland of obese strain chickens. *Clinical Immunology and Immunopathology*, **39**, 464–78.

Gerstein, H.C., Rastogi, B., Iwatani, Y., Iitaka, M., Row, V.V. & Volpé, R. (1987). The decrease in non-specific suppressor T lymphocytes in female hyperthyroid Graves' disease is secondary to the hyperthyroidism. *Clinical and Investigative Medicine*, **10**, 337–44.

Ghoneum, M., Wojdani, A. & Alfred, L. (1987). Effect of methylcholanthrene on human natural killer cell cytotoxicity and lymphokine production in vitro. *Immunopharmacology*, **14**, 27–33.

Glover, E.L., Reuber, M.D. & Godfrey, E.F. (1969). Methylcholanthrene-induced thyroidi-tis: susceptibility of Buffalo strain rats. *Archives of Environmental Health*, **18**, 901–3.

Gorman, C.A. (1986). Extrathyroid manifestations of Graves' disease. In *The Thyroid*, ed. S.H. Ingbar & L.E. Braverman, pp. 1015–38. Philadelphia: J.B.Lippincott Company.

Gorski, J., Rollini, P. & Mach, B. (1987). Structural comparison of the genes of two HLA-DR supertypic groups: the loci encoding DRw52 and DRw53 are not truly allelic. *Immunogenetics*, **25**, 397–402.

Gray, J. & Hoffenberg, R. (1985). Thyrotoxicosis and stress. *Quarterly Journal of Medicine*, **54**, 153–60.

Grubeck-Loebenstein, B., Derfler, K., Kassal, H., Knapp, W., Krisch, K., Liszka, K., Smyth, P.P.A. & Waldhäusl, W. (1985). Immunological features of nonimmunogenic hyperthy-roidism. *Journal of Clinical Endocrinology and Metabolism*, **60**, 150–5.

Grubeck-Loebenstein, B., Londei, M., Greenall, C., Pirich, K., Kassal, H., Waldhäusl, W. & Feldmann, M. (1988). Pathogenetic relevance of HLA class II expressing thyroid follicular cells in nontoxic goiter and in Graves' disease. *Journal of Clinical Investigation*, **81**, 1608–14.

Grubeck-Loebenstein, B., Buchan, B., Chantry, D., Kassal, H., Londei, M., Pirich, K., Barrett, K., Turner, M., Waldhäusl, W. & Feldmann, M. (1989). Analysis of intrathyroidal cytokine production in thyroid autoimmune disease: thyroid follicular cells produce interleukin–1α and interleukin–6. *Clinical and Experimental Immunology*, **77**, 324–30.

Guerin, V., Bene, M.C., Amiel, C., Hartemann, P., Leclere, J. & Faure, G. (1989). Decreased lymphocyte function-associated antigen–1 molecule expression on peripheral blood lymphocytes from patients with Graves' disease. *Journal of Clinical Endocrinology and Metabolism*, **69**, 648–53.

Gwinup, G., Elias, A.N. & Ascher, M.S. (1982). Effect on exophthalmos of various methods of treatment of Graves' disease. *Journal of the American Medical Association*, **247**, 2135–8.

Hägg, E. & Asplund, K. (1987). Is endocrine ophthalmopathy related to smoking? *British Medical Journal*, **295**, 634–5.

Hála, K. (1988). Hypothesis: immunogenetic analysis of spontaneous autoimmune thyroiditis in obese strain (OS) chickens: a two-gene family model. *Immunobiology*, **177**, 354–73.

Hall, R., Owen, S.G. & Smart, G.S. (1964). Evidence for genetic predisposition to formation of thyroid autoantibodies. *Lancet*, **ii**, 187–8.

Hall, R., Turner-Warwick, H. & Doniach, D. (1966). Autoantibodies in iodide goitre and asthma. *Clinical and Experimental Immunology*, **1**, 285–96.

Hallengren, B., Forsgren, A. & Melander, A. (1980). Effect of antithyroid drugs on lymphocyte function *in vitro*. *Journal of Clinical Endocrinology and Metabolism*, **51**, 298–301.

Hamada, N., Jaeduck, N., Portman, L., Ito, K. & DeGroot, L. J. (1987). Antibodies against denatured and reduced thyroid microsomal antigen in autoimmune thyroid disease. *Journal of Clinical Endocrinology and Metabolism*, **64**, 230–8.

Hanafusa, T., Pujol-Borrell, R., Chiovato, L., Russell, R.C.G., Doniach, D. & Bottazzo, G.F. (1983). Aberrant expression of HLA-DR antigen on thyrocytes in Graves' disease: relevance for autoimmunity. *Lancet*, **ii**, 1111–15.

Harach, H.R., Escalante, D.A., Oñativia, A., Lederer Outes, J., Saravia Day, E. & Williams, E.D. (1985). Thyroid carcinoma and thyroiditis in an endemic goitre region before and after iodine prophylaxis. *Acta Endocrinologica*, **108**, 55–60.

Hardisty, C.A., Talbot, C.H. & Munro, D.S. (1981). The effect of partial thyroidectomy for Graves' disease on serum long-acting thyroid stimulator protector (LATS-P). *Clinical Endocrinology*, **14**, 181–8.

Hardisty, C.A., Fowles, A. & Munro, D.S. (1984a). The effect of radioiodine and antithyroid drugs on serum long-acting thyroid stimulator protector (LATS-P). A three year prospective study. *Clinical Endocrinology*, **20**, 597–605.

Hardisty, C.A., Fowles, A. & Munro, D.S. (1984b). Serum long-acting thyroid stimulator (LATS) and LATS-protector in Graves' disease associated with localized myxoedema. *Journal of Endocrinological Investigation*, **7**, 151–5.

Hassman, R., Weetman, A.P., Gunn, C., Stringer, B.M., Wynford-Thomas, D., Hall, R. & McGregor, A.M. (1985). The effects of hyperthyroidism on experimental autoimmune thyroiditis in the rat. *Endocrinology*, **116**, 1253–8.

Hawkins, B.R., Ma, J.T.C., Lam, K.S.L., Wang, C.C.L. & Yeung, R.T.T. (1985). Association of HLA antigens with thyrotoxic Graves' disease and periodic paralysis in Hong Kong Chinese. *Clinical Endocrinology*, **23**, 245–52.

Hawkins, B.R., Lam, K.S.L., Ma, J.T.C., Wang, C. & Yeung, R.T.T. (1987). Strong association between HLA-DRw9 and Hashimoto's thyroiditis in Southern Chinese. *Acta Endocrinologica*, **114**, 543–6.

Hayashi, Y., Tamai, J., Fukata, S., Hirota, Y., Katayama, S., Kuma, K., Kumagai, L.F. & Nagataki, S. (1985). A long term clinical, immunological, and histological follow-up study of patients with goitrous chronic lymphocytic thyroiditis. *Journal of Clinical Endocrinology and Metabolism*, **61**, 1172–8.

Hayslip, C.C., Baker, J.R., Wartofsky, L., Klein, T.A., Opsahl, M.S. & Burman, K.D. (1988). Natural killer cell activity and serum autoantibodies in women with postpartum thyroiditis. *Journal of Clinical Endocrinology and Metabolism*, **66**, 1089–93.

Hirayu, H., Seto, P., Magnusson, R.P., Filetti, S. & Rapoport, B. (1987). Molecular cloning and partial characterization of a new autoimmune thyroid disease-related antigen. *Journal of Clinical Endocrinology and Metabolism*, **64**, 578–84.

Hiromatsu, Y., Cardaso, L., Salvi, M. & Wall, J.R. (1990). Significance of cytotoxic eye muscle antibodies in patients with thyroid-associated ophthalmopathy. *Autoimmunity*, **5**, 205–13.

Hirose, W., Lahat, N., Platzer, M., Schmitt, D. & Davies, T.F. (1988). Activation of MHC-restricted rat T cells by syngeneic thyrocytes. *Journal of Immunology*, **141**, 1098–102.

Honda, K., Tamai, J., Morita, T., Kuma, K., Nishimura, Y., & Sasazuki, T. (1989). Hashimoto's thyroiditis and HLA in Japanese. *Journal of Clinical Endocrinology and Metabolism*, **69**, 1268–73.

How, J., Topliss, D.J., Lewis, M., Row, V.V. & Volpé, R. (1983). T lymphocyte sensitisation and suppressor T lymphocyte defect in patients long after treatment for Graves' disease. *Clinical Endocrinology*, **18**, 61.

Hutchings, P., Rayner, D.C., Champion, B.R., Marshall-Clarke, S., Macatonia, S., Roitt, I.M. & Cooke, A. (1987). High efficiency antigen presentation by thyroglobulin-primed murine splenic B cells. *European Journal of Immunology*, **17**, 393–8.

Hyjek, E. & Isaacson, P.G. (1988). Primary B cell lymphoma of the thyroid and its relationship to Hashimoto's thyroiditis. *Human Pathology*, **19**, 1315–26.

Iitaka, M., Iwatani, Y., Gerstein, H.C., Row, V.V. & Volpé, R. (1987). Immunomodulatory effect of the treatment of Graves' disease on antigen-specific monocyte procoagulant activity production. *Clinical Endocrinology*, **27**, 321–30.

Iitaka, M., Aguayo, J.F., Iwatani, Y., Row, V.V. & Volpé, R. (1988). Studies of the effect of suppressor T lymphocytes on the induction of antithyroid microsomal antibody-secreting cells in autoimmune thyroid disease. *Journal of Clinical Endocrinology and Metabolism*, **66**, 708–14.

Imahori, S. & Vladutiu, A.O. (1984). Evolution and host-dependent lesions in autoimmune thyroiditis: experimental study in inbred mice. *Clinical Immunology and Immunopathology*, **33**, 87–98.

Irvine, W.J. (1978). The immunology and genetics of autoimmune endocrine disease. In *Genetic Control of Autoimmune Disease*, ed. N.R. Rose, P.E. Bigazzi & N.L. Warner, pp. 77–97. Amsterdam: Elsevier/North-Holland.

Irvine, W.J., McGregor, A.G. & Stuart, A.E. (1962). The prognostic significance of thyroid antibodies in the management of thyrotoxicosis. *Lancet*, **ii**, 843–7.

Islam, M.N., Pepper, B.M., Briones-Urbina, R. & Farid, N.R. (1983). Biological activity of anti-thyrotropin anti-idiotypic antibodies. *European Journal of Immunology*, **13**, 1357–63.

Ito, M., Tanimoto, M., Kamura, H., Yoneda, M., Morishima, Y., Yamauchi, K., Itatsu, T., Takatsuki, K. & Saito, H. (1989). Association of HLA antigen and restriction fragment length polymorphism of T cell receptor β-chain gene with Graves' disease and Hashimoto's thyroiditis. *Journal of Clinical Endocrinology and Metabolism*, **69**, 100.

Iwatani, Y., Amino, N., Mori, H., Asari, S., Izumiguchi, Y., Kumahara, Y. & Miyai, K. (1983). T lymphocyte subsets in autoimmune thyroid diseases and subacute thyroiditis detected with monoclonal antibodies. *Journal of Clinical Endocrinology and Metabolism*, **56**, 251–4.

Iwatani, Y., Gerstein, H.C., Iitaka, M., Row, V.V. & Volpé, R. (1986). Thyrocyte HLA-DR expression and interferon-γ production in autoimmune thyroid disease. *Journal of Clinical Endocrinology and Metabolism*, **63**, 695–707.

Iwatani, Y., Amino, N., Kaneda, T., Ichihara, K., Tamaki, H., Tachi, J., Matsuzuka, F., Fukata, S., Kuma, K. & Miyai, K. (1989). Marked increase of CD5$^+$ B cells in hyperthyroid Graves' disease. *Clinical and Experimental Immunology*, **78**, 196–200.

Jacobson, D.H. & Gorman, C.A. (1984). Endocrine ophthalmopathy: current ideas concerning etiology, pathogenesis and treatment. *Endocrine Reviews*, **5**, 200–20.

Jansson, R., Karlsson, A. & Forsum, U. (1984a). Intrathyroidal HLA-DR expression and T lymphocyte phenotypes in Graves' thyrotoxicosis, Hashimoto's thyroiditis and nodular colloid goitre. *Clinical and Experimental Immunology*, **58**, 264–72.

Jansson, R., Bernander, S., Karlsson, A., Levin, K. & Nilsson, G. (1984b). Autoimmune thyroid dysfunction in the postpartum period. *Journal of Clinical Endocrinology and Metabolism*, **58**, 681–7.

Jansson, R., Tötterman, T.H., Sallstrom, J. & Dahlberg, P.A. (1984c). Intrathyroidal and circulating lymphocyte subsets in different stages of autoimmune postpartum thyroiditis. *Journal of Clinical Endocrinology and Metabolism*, **58**, 942–6.

Jansson, R., Säfwenberg, J. & Dahlberg, P.A. (1985). Influence of the HLA-DR4 antigen and iodine status on the development of autoimmune postpartum thyroiditis. *Journal of Clinical Endocrinology and Metabolism*, **60**, 168–73.

Jansson, R., Thompson, P.M., Clark, F. & McLachlan, S.M. (1986). Association between thyroid microsomal antibodies of subclass IgG-1 and hypothyroidism in autoimmune postpartum thyroiditis. *Clinical and Experimental Immunology*, **63**, 80–6.

Jansson, R., Dahlberg, P.A., Winsa, B., Meirik, O., Säfwenberg, J. & Karlsson, A. (1987). The postpartum period constitutes an important risk for the development of clinical Graves' disease in young women. *Acta Endocrinologica*, **116**, 321–5.

Jansson, R., Dahlberg, P.A. & Karlsson, F.A. (1988). Postpartum thyroiditis. *Ballière's Clinical Endocrinology and Metabolism*, **2**, 619–35.

Jin, S., Hornieck, F.J., Neylan, D., Zakarija, M. & McKenzie, J.M. (1986). Evidence that adenosine 3',5'-monophosphate mediates stimulation of thyroid growth in FRTL–5 cells. *Endocrinology*, **119**, 802–10.

Jolliffe, D.S., Gaylarde, P.M., Brock, A.P. & Sarkany, I. (1979). Pretibial myxoedema: stimulation of mucopolysaccharide production of fibroblasts by serum. *British Journal of Dermatology*, **101**, 557–60.

Kabel, P.J., Voorbij, H.A.M., Van Der Gaag, R.D., Wiersinga, W.M., De Haan, M. & Drexhage, H.A. (1987). Dendritic cells in autoimmune thyroid disease. *Acta Endocrinologica*, **281**, 42–8.

Kabel, P.J., Voorbij, J.A.M., De Haan, M., Van Der Gaag, R.D. & Drexhage, H.A. (1988). Intrathyroidal dendritic cells. *Journal of Clinical Endocrinology and Metabolism*, **66**, 199–207.

Kadlubowski, M., Irvine, W.J. & Rowland, A.C. (1986). The lack of specificity of ophthalmic immunoglobulins in Graves' disease. *Journal of Clinical Endocrinology and Metabolism*, **63**, 990–5.

Kadlubowski, M., Irvine, W.J. & Rowland, A.C. (1987). Anti-muscle antibodies in Graves' ophthalmopathy. *Journal of Clinical and Laboratory Immunology*, **24**, 105–11.

Kahaly, G., Schrezenmeir, J., Krause, U., Schweikert, B., Meuer, S., Muller, W., Dennebaum, R. & Beyer, J. (1986). Cyclosporin and prednisone v. prednisone in treatment of Graves' ophthalmopathy: a controlled, randomized and prospective study. *European Journal of Clinical Investigation*, **16**, 415–22.

Kämpe, O., Jansson, R. & Karlsson, F.A. (1990). Effects of L-thyroxine and iodide on the development of autoimmune postpartum thyroiditis. *Journal of Clinical Endocrinology and Metabolism*, **70**, 1014–18.

Kappelgaard, E., Nielsen, H., Bech, K., Bliddal, H., Feldt-Rasmussen, U. & Thomsen, M. (1983). Circulating immune complexes in Hashimoto's thyroiditis. *Allergy*, **38**, 433–9.

Karlsson, F.A., Tötterman, T.H. & Jansson, R. (1986). Subacute thyroiditis: activated HLA-DR and interferon-γ expressing T cytotoxic/suppressor cells in thyroid tissue and peripheral blood. *Clinical Endocrinology*, **25**, 487–93.

Karlsson, F.A., Dahlberg, P.A., Jansson, R., Westermark, K. & Enoksson, P. (1989). Importance of TSH receptor activation in the development of severe endocrine ophthalmopathy. *Acta Endocrinologica*, **121** (Suppl. 2), 132–41.

Kasajima, T., Yamakawa, M. & Imai, Y. (1987). Immunohistochemical study of intrathyroidal lymph follicles. *Clinical Immunology and Immunopathology*, **43**, 117–28.

Katz, D.K., Kite, J.H. & Albini, B. (1981). Immune complexes in tissues of Obese strain (OS) chickens. *Journal of Immunology*, **126**, 2296–301.

Katz, D.V., Albini, B. & Kite, J.H. (1986). Materno-embryonally transferred antibodies precipitate autoimmune thyroiditis in Obese strain (OS) chickens. *Journal of Immunology*, **137**, 542–5.

Katz, S.M. & Vickery, A.L. (1974). The fibrous variant of Hashimoto's thyroiditis. *Human Pathology*, **5**, 161–70.

Katzin, W.E., Fishleder, A.J. & Tubbs, R. (1989). Investigation of the clonality of lymphocytes in Hashimoto's thyroiditis using immunoglobulin and T-cell receptor gene probes. *Clinical Immunology and Immunopathology*, **51**, 264–74.

Kaufman, K.D., Filetti, S., Seto, P. & Rapoport, B. (1990). Recombinant human thyroid peroxidase generated in eukaryotic cells: a source of specific antigen for the immunological assay of antimicrosomal antibodies in the sera of patients with autoimmune thyroid disease. *Journal of Clinical Endocrinology and Metabolism*, **70**, 724–8.

Kaulfersch, W., Baker, J.R., Burman, K.D., Ahmann, A.J., D'Avis, J.C. & Waldmann, T.A. (1988). Immunoglobulin and T cell antigen receptor gene rearrangements indicate that the immune response in autoimmune thyroid disease is polyclonal. *Journal of Clinical Endocrinology and Metabolism*, **66**, 958–63.

Kendall-Taylor, P., Jones, D. & Atkinson, S. (1987). The specificity of autoantibodies in Graves' ophthalmopathy. *Acta Endocrinologica*, **115**, Suppl. 281, 330–3.

Kendall-Taylor, P., Stephenson, A., Stratton, A., Papiha, S.S., Perros, P. & Roberts, D.F. (1988). Differentiation of autoimmune ophthalmopathy from Graves' hyperthyroidism by analysis of genetic markers. *Clinical Endocrinology*, **28**, 601–10.

Kennedy, J.S. & Thomson, J.A. (1974). The changes in the thyroid gland after irradiation with ^{131}I or partial thyroidectomy for thyrotoxicosis. *Journal of Pathology*, **112**, 65–81.

Khalid, B.A.K., Hamilton, N.T. & Cauchi, M.N. (1976). Binding of thyroid microsomes by lymphocytes from patients with thyroid disease and normal subjects. *Clinical and Experimental Immunology*, **23**, 28–32.

Khoury, E.L., Hammond, L., Bottazzo, G.F. & Doniach, D. (1981). Presence of organ-specific 'microsomal' autoantigen on the surface of human thyroid cells in culture: its involvement in complement-mediated cytotoxicity. *Clinical and Experimental Immunology*, **45**, 316–28.

Khoury, E.L., Bottazzo, G.F., Pontes de Carvalho, L.C., Wick, G. & Roitt, I.M. (1982). Predisposition to organ-specific autoimmunity in Obese strain (OS) chickens: reactivity to thyroid, gastric, adrenal and pancreatic cytoplasmic antigens. *Clinical and Experimental Immunology*, **49**, 273–82.

Khoury, E.L., Bottazzo, G.F. & Roitt, I. (1984). The thyroid 'microsomal' antibody revisited. Its paradoxical binding *in vivo* to the apical surface of the follicular epithelium. *Journal of Experimental Medicine*, **159**, 577–89.

Kimura, S., Kotani, T., McBride, O.M., Unicki, K., Hirai, K., Nakeyama, T. & Ohtaki, S. (1987). Human thyroid peroxidase: complete cDNA and protein sequence, chromosome mapping and identification of two alternately spliced mRNAs. *Proceedings of the National Academy of Science, USA*, **84**, 5555–9.

Kinney, J.S., Hurwitz, E.S., Fishbein, D.B., Woolf, P.D., Pinsky, P.F., Lawrence, D.N., Anderson, G.P., Wilson, C.K., Loschen, D.J., Nordlund, H.M., Oldfather, J., Rodey, G.E., Stoesz, P.A. & Schonberger, L.B. (1988). Community outbreak of thyrotoxicosis: epidemiology, immunogenetic characteristics, and long-term outcome. *American Journal of Medicine*, **84**, 10–17.

Kitchin, F.D., Howel-Evans, W., Clarke, C.A., McConnell, R.B. & Sheppard, P.M. (1959). P.T.C. taste response and thyroid disease. *British Medical Journal*, **ii**, 1069–75.

Kiy, Y., Rezkallah-Iwasso, M.T., Peraçoli, M.T.S. & Mota, N.G.S. (1981). Immunological disturbances in toxic multinodular goitre and active Graves' disease. *Clinical Endocrinology*, **16**, 11–17.

Knight, J., Laing, P., Knight, A., Adams, D. & Ling, N. (1986). Thyroid-stimulating autoantibodies usually contain only λ-light chains: evidence for the 'forbidden clone' theory. *Journal of Clinical Endocrinology and Metabolism*, **62**, 342–7.

Kodama, K., Sikorska, H., Bandy-Dafoe, P., Bayly, R. & Wall, J.R. (1982). Demonstration of a circulating autoantibody against a soluble eye-muscle antigen in Graves' ophthalmopathy. *Lancet*, **ii**, 1353–6.

Kohno, Y., Hiyama, Y., Shimojo, N., Niimi, H., Nakajima, H. & Hosoya, T. (1986). Autoantibodies to thyroid peroxidase in patients with chronic thyroiditis: effect of antibody binding on enzyme activities. *Clinical and Experimental Immunology*, **65**, 634–41.

Kojima, A., Tanaka-Kojima, U., Sakakura, T. & Nishizuka, U. (1976a). Spontaneous development of autoimmune thyroiditis in neonatally thymectomized mice. *Laboratory Investigation*, **34**, 550–7.

Kojima, A., Tanaka-Kojima, Y., Sakakura, T. & Nishizuka, Y. (1976b). Prevention of post-thymectomy and autoimmune thyroiditis in mice. *Laboratory Investigation*, **34**, 601–5.

Kologlu, M., Fung, H., Darke, C., Richards, C.J., Hall, R. & McGregor, A.M. (1987). Postpartum thyroid dysfunction and HLA status. In *Thyroid Autoimmunity*, ed. A. Pinchera, S.H. Ingbar, J.M. McKenzie & G.F. Fenzi, pp. 441–3. New York: Plenum Press.

Kong, Y.M. (1986). The mouse model of autoimmune thyroid disease. In *Immunology of Endocrine Diseases*, ed. A.M. McGregor, pp 1–24. Lancaster: MTP Press.

Kong, Y.M., Giraldo, A.A., Waldmann, H., Cobbold, S.P. & Fuller, B.E. (1989). Resistance to experimental autoimmune thyroiditis: L3T4⁺ cells as mediators of both thyroglobulin-activated and TSH-induced suppression. *Clinical Immunology and Immunopathology*, **51**, 38–54.

Konishi, J., Herman, M.N. & Kriss, J.P. (1974). Binding of thyroglobulin and thyroglobulin–antithyroglobulin complex to extraocular muscle membrane. *Endocrinology*, **95**, 434–66.

Konishi, J., Iida, Y., Endo, K., Misaki, T., Nohara, Y., Matsuura, N., Mori, T. & Torizuka, K. (1983). Inhibition of thyrotropin-induced adenosine 3′,5′- monophosphate increase by immunoglobulins from patients with primary myxedema. *Journal of Clinical Endocrinology and Metabolism*, **57**, 544–9.

Kotani, T., Komuro, K., Yoshiki, T. & Aizawa, M. (1981). Spontaneous autoimmune thyroiditis in the rat accelerated by thymectomy and low doses of irradiation: mechanisms implicated in the pathogenesis. *Clinical and Experimental Immunology*, **45**, 329–37.

Kotani, T., Umeki, K., Matsunaga, S., Kato, E. & Ohtaki, S. (1986). Detection of autoantibodies to thyroid peroxidase in autoimmune thyroid diseases by micro-ELISA and immunoblotting. *Journal of Clinical Endocrinology and Metabolism*, **62**, 928–33.

Kotani, T., Umeki, K., Hirai, K. & Ohtaki, S. (1990). Experimental murine thyroiditis induced by porcine thyroid peroxidase and its transfer by the antigen-specific T cell line. *Clinical and Experimental Immunology*, **80**, 11–16.

Kozma, L., Stenszky, V., Kraszits, E., Balázs, C. & Farid, N.R. (1985). The association of IgG heavy-chain allotypes (Gm) with Graves' disease in Hungary. *Experimental and Clinical Immunogenetics*, **2**, 154–7.

Kraiem, Z., Lahat, N., Glaser, B., Baron, E., Sadeh, O. & Shienfeld, M. (1987a). Thyrotrophin receptor blocking antibodies: incidence, characterization and *in vivo* synthesis. *Clinical Endocrinology*, **27**, 409–21.

Kraiem, Z., Glaser, B., Yigla, M., Pauker, J., Sadeh, O. & Sheinfeld, M. (1987b). Toxic multinodular goiter: a variant of autoimmune hyperthyroidism. *Journal of Clinical Endocrinology and Metabolism*, **65**, 659–64.

Kriss, J.P. (1970). Radioisotopic thyroidolymphography in patients with Graves' disease. *Journal of Clinical Endocrinology and Metabolism*, **40**, 872–5.

Kriss, J.P., Pleshakov, V. & Chien, J.R. (1964). Isolation and identification of the long-acting thyroid stimulator and its relation to hyperthyroidism and circumscribed pretibial myxedema. *Journal of Clinical Endocrinology and Metabolism*, **24**, 1005–28.

Krömer, G., Sundick, R.S., Schauenstein, K., Hála, K. & Wick G. (1985). Analysis of lymphocytes infiltrating the thyroid gland of obese strain chickens. *Journal of Immunology*, **135**, 2452–7.

Kroemer, G. & Wick, G. (1989). The role of interleukin-1 in autoimmunity. *Immunology Today*, **10**, 246–51.

Lazarus, J.H., Burr, M.L., McGregor, A.M., Weetman, A.P., Ludgate, M., Woodhead, J.S. & Hall, R. (1984). The prevalence and progression of autoimmune thyroid disease in the elderly. *Acta Endocrinologica*, **106**, 341–7.

Lee, K.U., Pak, C.Y., Amano, K. & Yoon, J.W. (1988). Prevention of lymphocytic thyroiditis and insulitis in diabetes-prone BB rats by the depletion of macrophages. *Diabetologia*, **31**, 400–2.

Lervang, H.H., Pryds, O., Østergaard Kristensen, H.P., Jakobsen, B.K. & Svejgaard, A. (1984). Postpartum autoimmune thyroid disease associated with HLA-DR4? *Tissue Antigens*, **23**, 250–2.

Lervang, H.H., Pryds, O. & Østergaard Kristensen, H.P. (1987). Thyroid dysfunction after delivery: incidence and clinical course. *Acta Medica Scandinavica*, **222**, 369–74.

Lewis, M., Giraldo, A.A. & Kong, Y.M. (1987). Resistance to experimental autoimmune thyroiditis induced by physiologic manipulation of thyroglobulin level. *Clinical Immunology and Immunopathology*, **45**, 92–104.

Libert, F., Lefort, A., Gerard, C., Parmentier, M., Perret, J., Ludgate, M., Dumont, J.E. & Vassart, G. (1989). Cloning, sequencing and expression of the human thyrotropin (TSH) receptor: evidence for binding of antibodies. *Biochemical and Biophysical Research Communications*, **165**, 1250–5.

Lillehoj, H. & Rose, N.R. (1982). Humoral and cellular response to thyroglobulin in different inbred rat strains. *Clinical and Experimental Immunology*, **47**, 661–9.

Lloyd, R.V., Johnson, T.L., Blaivas, M., Sisson, J.C. & Wilson, B.S. (1985). Detection of HLA-DR antigens in paraffin-embedded thyroid epithelial cells with a monoclonal antibody. *Journal of Pathology*, **120**, 106–11.

Logtenberg, T., Kroon, A., Gmelig-Meyling, F.H.J. & Ballieux, R.E. (1986). Production of anti-thyroglobulin antibody by blood lymphocytes from patients with autoimmune thyroiditis, induced by the insolubilized autoantigen. *Journal of Immunology*, **136**, 1236–9.

Londei, M., Lamb, J.R., Bottazzo, G.F. & Feldmann, M. (1984). Epithelial cells expressing aberrant MHC call II determinants can present antigen to cloned human T cells. *Nature*, **312**, 639–41.

Londei, M., Bottazzo, G.F. & Feldmann, M. (1985). Human T cell clones from autoimmune thyroid glands: specific recognition of autologous thyroid cells. *Science*, **228**, 85–9.

Lonergan, C., Babiarz, D. & Burke, G. (1973). Isoelectric focusing of long-acting thyroid stimulator immunoglobulin G. *Endocrinology*, **36**, 439–44.

Ludgate, M., Dong, Q., Dreyfus, P.A., Zakut, H., Taylor, P., Vassart, G. & Soreq, H. (1989). Definition, at the molecular level, of a thyroglobulin-acetylcholinesterase shared epitope: study of its pathophysiological significance in patients with Graves' ophthalmopathy. *Autoimmunity*, **3**, 167–76.

Ludgate, M.E., McGregor, A.M., Weetman, A.P., Ratanchaiyavong, S., Hall, R., Lazarus, J.H. & Middleton, G.W. (1984). T cell subset analysis in Graves' disease: alterations associated with carbimazole therapy. *British Medical Journal*, **288**, 526–30.

Ludgate, M.E., Ratanachaiyavong, S., Weetman, A.P., Hall, R. & McGregor, A.M. (1985). Failure to demonstrate cell-mediated immune responses to thyroid antigens in Graves' disease using *in vitro* assays of lymphokine-mediated migration inhibition. *Journal of Clinical Endocrinology and Metabolism*, **60**, 98–102.

Lundell, G., Holm, L.E., Ljunggren, J.G. & Wasserman, J. (1981). Incidence of hypothyroidism after ^{131}I therapy for hyperthyroidism. Relation to pretherapy serum levels of T3, T4 and thyroid antibodies. *Acta Radiologica, Oncology*, **20**, 225–30.

Maagøe, H., Reintoft, I., Christensen, H.E., Simonsen, J. & Mogensen, E.F. (1977). Lymphocytic thyroiditis. *Acta Medica Scandinavica*, **202**, 469–73.

McConahey, W.M., Keating, F.R., Beahrs, O.H. & Woolner, L.B. (1962). On the increasing occurrence of Hashimoto's thyroiditis. *Journal of Clinical Endocrinology and Metabolism*, **22**, 542–44.

McGregor, A.M., McLachlan, S.M., Clark, F., Smith, B.R. & Hall, R. (1979a). Thyroglobulin and microsomal autoantibody production by cultures of Hashimoto peripheral blood lymphocytes. *Immunology*, **36**, 81–5.

McGregor, A.M., Petersen, M.M., Capiferri, R., Evered, D.C., Rees Smith, B. & Hall, R. (1979b). Effects of radioiodine on thyrotrophin binding inhibiting immunoglobulins in Graves' disease. *Clinical Endocrinology*, **11**, 437–44.

McGregor, A.M., McLachlan, S.M., Rees Smith, B. & Hall, R. (1979c). Effect of irradiation on thyroid autoantibody production. *Lancet*, **ii**, 442–4.

McGregor, A.M., Rees Smith, B., Hall, R., Petersen, M.M., Miller, M. & Dewar, P.J. (1980a). Prediction of relapse in hyperthyroid Graves' disease. *Lancet*, **i**, 1101–3.

McGregor, A.M., Petersen, M.M., McLachlan, S.M., Rooke, P., Rees Smith, B. & Hall, R. (1980b). Carbimazole and the autoimmune response in Graves' disease. *New England Journal of Medicine*, **303**, 302–7.

McGregor, A.M., Rees Smith, B., Hall, R., Collins, P.N., Bottazzo, G.F. & Petersen, M.M. (1982). Specificity of the immunosuppressive action of carbimazole in Graves' disease. *British Medical Journal*, **284**, 1750–1.

McKenna, R., Kearns, M., Sugrue, D., Drury, M.I. & McCarthy, C.F. (1982). HLA and hyperthyroidism in Ireland. *Tissue Antigens*, **19**, 97–9.

McKenzie, J.M. (1964). Neonatal Graves' disease. *Journal of Clinical Endocrinology and Metabolism*, **24**, 660–5.

MacKenzie, W.A., Schwartz, A.E., Friedman, E.W. & Davies, T.F. (1987). Intrathyroidal T cell clones from patients with autoimmune thyroid disease. *Journal of Clinical Endocrinology and Metabolism*, **64**, 818–23.

McLachlan, S.M., Rees Smith, B., Petersen, V.B., Davies, T.F. & Hall, R. (1977). Thyroid-stimulating antibody production *in vitro*. *Nature*, **270**, 447–9.

McLachlan, S.M., Wee, S.L., McGregor, A.M., Rees Smith, B. & Hall, R. (1980). *In vitro* studies on the control of thyroid autoantibody synthesis. *Journal of Laboratory and Clinical Immunology*, **3**, 15–21.

McLachlan, S.M., Bird, A.G., Weetman, A.P., Rees Smith, B. & Hall, R. (1981). Use of plaque assays to study human thyroglobulin autoantibody synthesis. *Scandinavian Journal of Immunology*, **14**, 233–42.

McLachlan, S.M., Fawcett, J., Atherton, M.C., Thompson, P., Baylis, P. & Rees Smith, B. (1983). Thyroid autoantibody synthesis by cultures of thyroid and peripheral blood lymphocytes. II.Effect of thyroglobulin on thyroglobulin antibody synthesis. *Clinical and Experimental Immunology*, **52**, 620–8.

McLachlan, S.M., Pegg, C.A.S., Atherton, M.C., Middleton, S., Young, E.T., Clark, F. & Rees Smith, B. (1985). The effect of carbimazole on thyroid autoantibody synthesis by thyroid lymphocytes. *Journal of Clinical Endocrinology and Metabolism*, **60**, 1237–42.

McLachlan, S.M., Pegg, C.A.S., Atherton, M.C., Middleton, S.L., Dickinson, A., Clark, F., Proctor, S.J., Proud, G. & Rees Smith, B. (1986a). Subpopulations of thyroid autoantibody secreting lymphocytes in Graves' and Hashimoto thyroid glands. *Clinical and Experimental Immunology*, **65**, 319–28.

McLachlan, S.M., Pegg, C.A.S., Atherton, M.C., Middleton, S.L., Young, E.T., Clark, F. & Rees Smith, B. (1986b). TSH receptor antibody synthesis by thyroid lymphocytes. *Clinical Endocrinology*, **24**, 223–9.

McLachlan, S.M., Taverne, J., Atherton, M.C., Cooke, A., Middleton, S., Pegg, C.A.S., Clark, F. & Rees Smith, B. (1990). Cytokines, thyroid autoantibody synthesis and thyroid cell survival in culture. *Clinical and Experimental Immunology*, **79**, 175–81.

Mahieu, P. & Winand, R. (1972). Demonstration of delayed hypersensitivity to retrobulbar and thyroid tissues in human exophthalmos. *Journal of Clinical Endocrinology and Metabolism*, **34**, 1090–2.

Malthiery, Y. & Lissitzky, S. (1987). Primary structure of human thyroglobulin deduced from the sequence of its 8448-base complementary DNA. *European Journal of Biochemistry*, **105**, 491–8.

Marcocci, C., Valente, W.A., Pinchera, A., Aloj, S.M., Kohn, L.D. & Grollman, E.F. (1983). Graves' IgG stimulation of iodide uptake in FRTL-5 rat thyroid cells: a clinical assay complementing FRTL-5 assays measuring adenylate cyclase and growth-stimulating antibodies in autoimmune thyroid disease. *Journal of Endocrinological Investigation*, **6**, 463–71.

Margolick, J.B., Hsu, S-M., Volkman, D.J., Burman, K.D. & Fauci, A.S. (1984). Immunohistochemical characterization of intrathyroid lymphocytes in Graves' disease. Interstitial and intraepithelial populations. *American Journal of Medicine*, **76**, 815–21.

Margolick, J.B., Weetman, A.P. & Burman, K.D. (1988). Immunohistochemical analysis of intrathyroidal lymphocytes in Graves' disease: evidence of activated T cells and production of interferon-gamma. *Clinical Immunology and Immunopathology*, **47**, 208–18.

Mariotti, S., Martino, E., Francesconi, M., Ceccarelli, C., Grasso, L., Lippi, F., Baschieri, L. & Pinchera, A. (1986). Serum thyroid autoantibodies as a risk factor for development of hypothyroidism after radioactive iodine therapy for a single thyroid 'hot' nodule. *Acta Endocrinologica*, **113**, 500–7.

Maron, R. & Cohen, I.R. (1979). Mutation at H-2K locus influences susceptibility to autoimmune thyroiditis. *Nature*, **279**, 715–16.

Maron, R., Zerubavel, R., Friedman, A. & Cohen, I.R. (1983). T lymphocyte line specific for thyroglobulin produces or vaccinates against autoimmune thyroiditis in mice. *Journal of Immunology*, **131**, 2316–21.

Marshall, N.J., & Ealey, P.A. (1986). Recent developments in the in vitro bioassay of TSH and thyroid-stimulating antibodies. In *Immunology of Endocrine Diseases*, ed. A.M. McGregor, pp. 25–49. Lancaster: MTP Press.

Martino, E., Aghini-Lombardi, F., Mariotti, S., Bartalena, L., Lenziardi, M., Ceccarelli, C., Bambini, G., Safran, M., Braverman, L.E. & Pinchera, A. (1987). Amiodarone iodine-induced hypothyroidism: risk factors and follow-up in 28 cases. *Clinical Endocrinology*, **26**, 227–37.

Mason, P.D., Weetman, A.P., Sissons, J.G.P. & Borysiewicz, L.K. (1988). Suppressive role of NK cells in pokeweed mitogen-induced immunoglobulin synthesis: effect of depletion/enrichment of Leu 11b$^+$ cells. *Immunology*, **65**, 113–18.

Matsuura, N., Yamada, Y., Nohara, Y., Konishi, J., Kasagi, K., Endo, K., Kojima, H. & Wataya, K. (1980). Familial neonatal transient hypothyroidism due to maternal TSH-binding inhibitor immunoglobulins. *New England Journal of Medicine*, **303**, 738–41.

Matsuura, N., Konishi, J., Fujieda, K., Kasagi, K., Iida, Y., Hagisawa, M., Fujimoto, S., Fukushi, M. & Takasugi, N. (1988). TSH-receptor antibodies in mothers with Graves' disease and outcome in their offspring. *Lancet*, **i**, 14–17.

Mauri, L., Meienberg, O., Roth, E. & Konig, M.P. (1984). Evaluation of endocrine ophthalmopathy with saccadic eye movements. *Journal of Neurology*, **231**, 182–7.

Mayr, W.R., Ludwig, H., Scherthaner, G. & Hofer, R. (1976). HLA-CW3 in thyrotoxicosis patients with and without endocrine ophthalmopathy. *Tissue Antigens*, **7**, 243–6.

Meek, J.C., Jones, A.E., Lewis, U.J. & Vanderhaan, W.P. (1964). Characterization of the long-acting thyroid stimulator of Graves' disease. *Proceedings of the National Academy of Sciences, USA*, **52**, 342–9.

Michie, W., Swanson Beck, J., Mahaffy, R.G., Honein, E.F. & Fowler, G.B. (1967). Quantitative radiological and histological studies of the thymus in thyroid disease. *Lancet*, **i**, 691–5.

Misaki, T., Konishi, J., Nakashima, T., Iiada, Y., Kasagi, K., Endo, K., Uchiyama, T., Kuma, K. & Torizuka, K. (1985). Immunohistological phenotyping of thyroid infiltrating lymphocytes in Graves' disease and Hashimoto's thyroiditis. *Clinical and Experimental Immunology*, **60**, 104–10.

Misrahi, M., Loosfelt, H., Atger, M., Sar, S., Guiochon-Mantel, A. & Milgrom, E. (1990). Cloning, sequencing and expression of human TSH receptor. *Biochemical and Biophysical Research Communications*, **166**, 394–403.

Miyazaki, A., Hanafusa, T., Itoh, N., Miyagawa, J., Kono, N., Tarui, S., Kiystaki, C. & Yostizaki, K. (1989). Demonstration of interleukin-1β on perifollicular endothelial cells in the thyroid glands of patients with Graves' disease. *Journal of Clinical Endocrinology and Metabolism*, **69**, 738–44.

Moens, H. & Farid, N.R. (1978). Hashimoto's thyroiditis is associated with HLA-DRw3. *New England Journal of Medicine*, **299**, 133–4.

Mori, H., Hamada, N. & DeGroot, L.J. (1985). Studies on thyroglobulin-specific suppressor T cell function in autoimmune thyroid disease. *Journal of Clinical Endocrinology and Metabolism*, **61**, 306–12.

Mortimer, R.H., Hill, G.E., Galligan, J.P., Bransden, A.I., Tyack, S.A. & Roeser, H.P. (1986). Hypothyroidism and Graves' disease after mantle irradiation: a follow up study. *Australian and New Zealand Journal of Medicine*, **16**, 347–51.

Mourant, A.E., Kopeć, A.C. & Domaniewska-Sobczak, K. (1978). *Blood Groups and Diseases. A Study of Associations of Diseases with Blood Groups and Other Polymorphisms*, pp. 38–41. Oxford: Oxford University Press.

Mukhtar, E.D., Smith, B.R., Pyle, G.A., Hall, R. & Vice, P. (1975). Relation of thyroid-stimulating immunoglobulins to thyroid function and effects of surgery, radioiodine and antithyroid drugs. *Lancet*, **i**, 713–15.

Mullin, B.R., Levinson, R.E., Friedman, A., Henson, D.E., Winand, R.J. & Kohn, L.D. (1977). Delayed hypersensitivity in Graves' disease and exophthalmos: identification of thyroglobulin in normal human orbital muscle. *Endocrinology*, **100**, 351–66.

Munro, D.S. (1984). Thyroid stimulating immunoglobulins. *Journal of the Royal College of Physicians of London*, **18**, 155–60.

Munro, R.E., Lamki, L., Row, V.V. & Volpé, R. (1973). Cell-mediated immunity in the exophthalmos of Graves' disease as demonstrated by the migration inhibition factor (MIF) test. *Journal of Clinical Endocrinology and Metabolism*, **37**, 286–92.

Murakami, M., Koizumi, Y., Aizawa, T., Yamada, T., Takahashi, Y., Watanabe, T. & Kamoi, K. (1988). Studies of thyroid function and immune parameters in patients with hyperthyroid Graves' disease in remission. *Journal of Clinical Endocrinology and Metabolism*, **66**, 103–8.

Nagayama, Y., Izumi, M., Ashizawa, K., Kiriyama, T., Yokoyama, N., Morita, S., Ohtakara, S., Fukuda, T., Eguchi, K., Morimoto, I., Okamoto, S., Ishikawa, N., Ito, K. & Nagataki, S. (1987). Inhibitory effect of interferon-γ on the response of human thyrocytes to thyrotropin

(TSH) stimulation: relationship between the response to TSH and the expression of DR antigen. *Journal of Clinical Endocrinology and Metabolism*, **64**, 949–53.

Nagayama, Y., Kaufman, K.D., Seto, P. & Rapoport, B. (1989). Molecular cloning, sequence and functional expression of the cDNA for the human thyrotropin receptor. *Biochemical and Biophysical Research Communications*, **165**, 1184–90.

Naito, N., Saito, K., Hosoya, T., Tarutani, O., Sakata, S., Nishikawa, T., Niimi, H. & Kohno, Y. (1990). Antithyroglobulin autoantibodies in sera from patients with chronic thyroiditis and from healthy subjects: differences in cross-reactivity with thyroid peroxidase. *Clinical and Experimental Immunology*, **80**, 4–9.

Nakao Y., Matsumoto, H., Miyazaki, T., Nishitani, H., Takatsuki, K., Kasukawa, R., Nakayama, S., Izumi, S., Fujita, T. & Tsuji K. (1980). IgG heavy chain allotypes (Gm) in autoimmune diseases. *Clinical and Experimental Immunology*, **42**, 20–6.

Nakao, Y., Matsumoto, H., Miyazaki, T. & Farid, N.R. (1982). IgG heavy chain allotypes (Gm) in atrophic and goitrous thyroiditis. *Journal of Immunogenetics*, **9**, 311–16.

Neu, N., Hála, K., Dietrich, H. & Wick, G. (1985). Spontaneous autoimmune thyroiditis in Obese strain chickens: a genetic analysis of target organ abnormalities. *Clinical Immunology and Immunopathology*, **37**, 397–405.

Nikolai, T.F., Turney, S.L. & Roberts, R.C. (1987). Postpartum lymphocytic thyroiditis. Prevalence, clinical course and long term follow-up. *Archives of Internal Medicine*, **147**, 221–4.

Nilsson, G. (1972). Lymphoid infiltration in toxic goitres studied with fine needle aspiration biopsy. *Acta Endocrinologica*, **71**, 480–90.

Noble, B., Yoshida, T., Rose, N.R. & Bigazzi, P.E. (1976). Thyroid antibodies in spontaneous autoimmune thyroiditis in the Buffalo rat. *Journal of Immunology*, **117**, 1447–55.

Noma, T., Yata, J., Shishiba, Y. & Inatsuki, B. (1982). *In vitro* detection of anti-thyroglobulin antibody forming cells from the lymphocytes of chronic thyroiditis patients and analysis of their regulation. *Clinical and Experimental Immunology*, **49**, 565–71.

Noppakun, N., Baucheun, K. & Chandraprasert, S. (1986). Unusual locations of localised myxoedema in Graves' disease: report of three cases. *Archives of Dermatology*, **122**, 85.

Nye, L., Pontes de Carvalho, L.P. & Roitt, I.M. (1980). Restrictions in the response to autologous thyroglobulin in the human. *Clinical and Experimental Immunology*, **41**, 252–63.

Nye, L., Pontes de Carvalho, L.P. & Roitt, I.M. (1981). An investigation of the clonality of human autoimmune thyroglobulin antibodies and their light chains. *Clinical and Experimental Immunology*, **46**, 161–70.

Ochi, Y., Nagamune, T., Nakajima, Y., Ishida, M., Kajita, Y., Hachiya, T. & Ogura, H. (1989). Anti-TSH antibodies in Graves' disease and their failure to interact with TSH receptor antibodies. *Acta Endocrinologica*, **120**, 773–7.

Okayasu, I., Kong, Y.M. & Rose, N.R. (1981). Effect of castration and sex hormones on experimental autoimmune thyroiditis. *Clinical Immunology and Immunopathology*, **20**, 240–5.

Okita, N., Kidd, A., Row, V.V. & Volpé, R. (1980). Sensitization of T-lymphocytes in Graves' and Hashimoto's diseases. *Journal of Clinical Endocrinology and Metabolism*, **51**, 316–20.

Okita, N., Topliss, D., Lewis, M., Row, V.V. & Volpé, R. (1981). T-lymphocyte sensitization in Graves' and Hashimoto's diseases confirmed by an indirect migration inhibition factor test. *Journal of Clinical Endocrinology and Metabolism*, **52**, 523–7.

Oksenberg, J.R., Sherritt, M., Begovitch, A.B., Erlich, H.A., Bernard, C.C., Cavalli-Sforza, L.L. & Steinman, L. (1989). T-cell receptor Vα and Cα alleles associated with multiple sclerosis and myasthenia gravis. *Proceedings of the National Academy of Sciences, USA*, **86**, 988–92.

Omar, M.A.K., Hammond, M.G., Desai, R.K., Motala, A.A., Aboo, N. & Seedat, M.A. (1990). HLA class I and II antigens in South African Blacks with Graves' disease. *Clinical Immunology and Immunopathology*, **54**, 98–102.

Othman, S., Phillips, D.I.W., Parkes, A.B., Richards, C.J., Harris, B., Fung, H., Darke, C., John, R., Hall, R. & Lazarus, J.H. (1990). A long-term follow-up of postpartum thyroiditis. *Clinical Endocrinology*, **32**, 559–64.

Pacini, F. & DeGroot, L.J. (1983). Studies of immunoglobulin synthesis in cultures of peripheral T and B lymphocytes: reduced T-suppressor cell activity in Graves' disease. *Clinical Endocrinology*, **18**, 219–32.

Papic, M., Stein-Streilen, J., Zakarija, M., McKenzie, J.M., Guffee, J. & Fletcher, M.A. (1987). Suppression of peripheral blood natural killer cell activity by excess thyroid hormone. *Journal of Clinical Investigation*, **79**, 404–8.

Parish, N.M., Rayner, D., Cooke, A. & Roitt, I.M. (1988). An investigation of the nature of induced suppression to experimental autoimmune thyroiditis. *Immunology*, **63**, 199–203.

Parkes, A.B., McLachlan, S.M., Bird, P. & Rees Smith, B. (1984). The distribution of microsome and thyroglobulin antibody activity among the IgG subclasses. *Clinical and Experimental Immunology*, **57**, 239–43.

Parmentier, M., Libert, F., Maenhaut, C., Lefort, A., Gerard, C., Perret, J., Van Sande, J., Dumont, J.E. & Vassart, G. (1989). Molecular cloning of the thyrotropin receptor. *Science*, **246**, 1620–23.

Pedersen, B.K., Perrild, H., Feldt-Rasmussen, U., Christensen, T., Klarlund, K. & Hansen, J.M. (1989). Suppressed natural killer cell activity in patients with euthyroid Graves' ophthalmopathy. *Autoimmunity*, **2**, 291–8.

Penhale, W.J., Farmer, A., McKenna, R.P. & Irvine, W.J. (1973). Spontaneous thyroiditis in thymectomized and irradiated Wistar rats. *Clinical and Experimental Immunology*, **15**, 225–36.

Penhale, W.J., Farmer, A., Urbaniak, S.J. & Irvine, W.J. (1975). Susceptibility of inbred rat strains to experimental thyroiditis: quantitation of thyroglobulin-binding cell and assessment of T cell function in susceptible and non-susceptible strains. *Clinical and Experimental Immunology*, **19**, 179–91.

Penhale, W.J., Irvine, W.J., Inglis, J.R. & Farmer, A. (1976). Thyroiditis and T-cell depleted rats: suppression of the autoallergic response by reconstitution with normal lymphoid cells. *Clinical and Experimental Immunology*, **25**, 6–26.

Penhale, W.J. & Ansar Ahmed, S. (1981). The effect of gonadectomy on the sex-related expression of autoimmune thyroiditis in thymectomized and irradiated rats. *American Journal of Reproductive Immunology*, **1**, 326–30.

Penhale, W.J. & Young, P.R. (1988). The influence of the normal microbial flora on the susceptibility of rats to experimental autoimmune thyroiditis. *Clinical and Experimental Immunology*, **72**, 288–92.

Pepper, B., Noel, E.P. & Farid, N.R. (1981). The putative anti-thyrotropin receptor antibodies of Graves' disease. I.Gm allotypes. *Journal of Immunogenetics*, **8**, 89–100.

Pfaltz, M. & Hediger, C.E. (1986). Abnormal basement membrane structures in autoimmune thyroid disease. *Laboratory Investigation*, **55**, 531–9.

Phillips, D., McLachlan, S., Stephenson, A., Roberts, D., Moffitt, S., McDonald, D., Ad'Hiah, A., Stratton, A., Young, E., Clark, F., Beever, K., Bradbury, J. & Rees Smith, B. (1990). Autosomal dominant transmission of autoantibodies to thyroglobulin and thyroid peroxidase. *Journal of Clinical Endocrinology and Metabolism*, **70**, 742–6.

Pinchera, A., Liberti, P., Martino, E., Fenzi, G.F., Grasso, L., Rovis, L., Baschieri, L. & Doria, G. (1969). Effects of antithyroid therapy on the long acting thyroid stimulator. *Journal of Clinical Endocrinology and Metabolism*, **29**, 231–8.

Pinchera, A., Fenzi, G.F., Bartalena, L., Chiovato, L., Marcocci, C. & Baschieri, L. (1980). Antigen-antibody systems involved in thyroid autoimmunity. In *Autoimmune Aspects of Endocrine Disease*, ed. A. Pinchera, D. Doniach, G.F. Fenzi & L. Baschieri, pp. 57–72. London: Academic Press.

Pontes de Carvalho, L. C., Wick, G. & Roitt, I.M. (1981). Requirement of T cells for the development of spontaneous autoimmune thyroiditis in obese strain (OS) chickens. *Journal of Immunology*, **126**, 750–3.

Pontes de Carvalho, L.P., Templeman, J., Wick, G. & Roitt, I.M. (1982). The role of self-antigen in the development of autoimmunity in obese strain chickens with spontaneous autoallergic thyroiditis. *Journal of Experimental Medicine*, **155**, 1255–66.

Pope, R.M., Ludgate, M.E. & McGregor, A.M. (1986). Observations on Graves' ophthalmopathy: pathology and pathogenesis. In *Immunology of Endocrine Diseases*, ed. A.M. McGregor, pp. 161–80. Lancaster: MTP Press.

Prummel, M.F., Mourits, M.P., Berghout, A., Krenning, E.P., Van der Gaag, R., Koornneef, L. & Wiersinga, W.M. (1989). Prednisone and cyclosporine in the treatment of severe Graves' ophthalmopathy. *New England Journal of Medicine*, **321**, 1353–9.

Prummel, M.F., Wiersinga, W.M., Mourits, M.P., Koornneef, L., Berghout, A. & Van der Gaag, R. (1990). Effect of abnormal thyroid function on the severity of Graves' ophthalmopathy. *Archives of Internal Medicine*, **150**, 1098–101.

Pryds, O., Lervang, H.H., Østergaard Kristensen, H.P., Jakobsen, B.K. & Svejgaard, A. (1987). HLA-DR factors associated with postpartum hypothyroidism: an early manifestation of Hashimoto's thyroiditis? *Tissue Antigens*, **30**, 34–7.

Pujol-Borrell, R., Hanafusa, T., Chiovato, L. & Bottazzo, G.F. (1983). Lectin induced expression of DR antigen on human cultured follicular thyroid cells. *Nature*, **304**, 71–3.

Raines, K.B., Baker, J.R., Lukes, Y.G., Wartofsky, L. & Burman, K.D. (1985). Antithyrotropin antibodies in the sera of Graves' disease patients. *Journal of Clinical Endocrinology and Metabolism*, **61**, 217–22.

Rajatanavin, R., Chailurkit, L., Tirarungsikul, K., Chalayondeja, W., Jittivanich, U. & Puapradit, W. (1990). Postpartum thyroid dysfunction in Bangkok: a geographical variation in the prevalence. *Acta Endocrinologica*, **122**, 283–7.

Ramsay, I.D. (1966). Muscle dysfunction in hyperthyroidism. *Lancet*, **ii**, 931–5.

Rapoport, B., Greenspan, F.S., Filetti, S. & Pepitone, M. (1984). Clinical experience with a human thyroid cell bioassay for thyroid-stimulating immunoglobulin. *Journal of Clinical Endocrinology and Metabolism*, **58**, 332–8.

Ratanachaiyavong, S. & McGregor, A.M. (1985). Immunosuppressive effects of antithyroid drugs. *Clinics in Endocrinology and Metabolism*, **14**, 449–66.

Rees Smith, B., McLachlan, S.M. & Furmaniak, J. (1988). Autoantibodies to the thyrotrophin receptor. *Endocrine Reviews*, **9**, 106–21.

Reinhardt, W., Paul, T.L., Allen, E.M., Alex, S., Yang, Y.N., Appel, M.C. & Braverman, L.E. (1988). Effect of L-thyroxine administration on the incidence of iodine induced and spontaneous lymphocytic thyroiditis in the BB/Wor rat. *Endocrinology*, **122**, 1179–81.

Reinwein, D., Benker, G., König, M.P., Pinchera, A., Schatz, H. & Schleusener, H. (1986). Hyperthyroidism in Europe: clinical and laboratory data of a prospective multicentre survey. *Journal of Endocrinological Investigation*, **9**(Suppl. 2), 1–35.

Rennie, D.P., McGregor, A.M., Keast, D., Weetman, A.P., Foord, S.M., Dieguez, C., Williams, E.D. & Hall, R. (1983). The influence of methimazole on thyroglobulin-induced autoimmune thyroiditis in the rat. *Endocrinology*, **112**, 326–30.

Roberts, I.M., Whittingham, S. & McKay, I.R. (1973). Tolerance to an autoantigen-thyroglobulin. Antigen-binding lymphocytes in thymus and blood in health and disease. *Lancet*, **ii**, 936–40.

Roitt, I.M., Doniach, D., Campbell, P.N. & Vaughan Hudson, R. (1956). Autoantibodies in Hashimoto's disease (lymphadenoid goitre). *Lancet*, **ii**, 820–1.

Romaldini, J.H., Bromberg, N., Werner, R.S., Tanaka, L.M., Rodrigues, H.F., Werner, M.C., Farah, C.S. & Reis, L.C.F. (1983). Comparison of effects of high and low dosage regimens of antithyroid drugs in the management of Graves' hyperthyroidism. *Journal of Clinical Endocrinology and Metabolism*, **57**, 563–70.

Romball, C.G. & Weigle, W.O. (1984). T cell competence to heterologous and homologous thyroglobulins during the induction of experimental autoimmune thyroiditis. *European Journal of Immunology*, **14**, 887–93.

Romball, C.G. & Weigle, W.O. (1987). Transfer of experimental autoimmune thyroiditis with T cell clones. *Journal of Immunology*, **138**, 1092–8.

Rose, N.R. & Witebsky, E. (1956). Studies in organ specificity. V Changes in the thyroid glands of rabbits following active immunization with rabbit thyroid extracts. *Journal of Immunology*, **76**, 417–27.

Rose, N.R., Bacon, L.D. & Sundick, R.S. (1976). Genetic determinations of thyroiditis in the obese strain chicken. *Transplantation Reviews*, **31**, 264.

Rose, N.R., Kong, Y.M., Okayasu, I., Giraldo, A.A., Beisel, K. & Sundick, R.S. (1981). T-cell regulation in autoimmune thyroiditis. *Immunological Reviews*, **55**, 299–314.

Rose, N.R., Outschoorn, I.M., Burek, C.L. & Kuppers, R.C. (1987). IgG subclass distribution of anti-Tg antibodies among thyroid disease patients and their relatives and in high and low responder mouse strains. In *Thyroid Autoimmunity*, ed. A. Pinchera, S.H. Ingbar, J.M. McKenzie & G.F. Fenzi, pp. 189–98. New York: Plenum Press.

Rotella, C.M., Zonefrati, R., Toccafondi, R., Valente, W.A. & Kohn, L.D. (1986). Ability of monoclonal antibodies to the thyrotropin receptor to increase collagen synthesis in human fibroblasts: an assay which appears to measure exophthalmogenic immunoglobulins in Graves' sera. *Journal of Clinical Endocrinology and Metabolism*, **62**, 357–67.

Rotella, C., Alvarez, F., Kohn, L.D. & Toccafondi, R. (1987). Graves' autoantibodies to extrathyroidal TSH receptor: their role in ophthalmopathy and pretibial myxoedema. *Acta Endocrinologica*, **281**, 344–7.

Roubaty, C., Bedin, C. & Charriere, J. (1990). Prevention of experimental autoimmune thyroiditis through the anti-idiotypic network. *Journal of Immunology*, **144**, 2167–72.

Rousset, B., Bernier-Valentin, K., Poncel, C., Orgiazzi, J., Madec, A-M., Mornier, J.C. & Mornex, R. (1983). Antitubulin antibodies in autoimmune thyroid disorders. *Clinical and Experimental Immunology*, **52**, 325–32.

Row, V.V. & Volpé, R. (1986). *In vitro* regulation of antithyroglobulin synthesis by lymphocytes of patients with Hashimoto's disease by an antigen-specific 'suppressor factor' derived from cultured normal human T-lymphocytes. *Journal of Clinical and Laboratory Immunology*, **21**, 159–63.

Sack, J., Baker, J.R., Weetman, A.P., Wartofsky, L. & Burman, K.D. (1986). Killer cell activity and antibody-dependent cell-mediated cytotoxicity are normal in Hashimoto's disease. *Journal of Clinical Endocrinology and Metabolism*, **62**, 1–6.

Sack, J., Zilberstein, D., Barile, M.F., Lukes, Y.G., Baker, J.R., Wartofsky, L. & Burman, K.D. (1989). Binding of thyrotropin to selected mycoplasma species: detection of serum antibodies against a specific mycoplasma membrane antigen in patients with autoimmune thyroid disease. *Journal of Endocrinological Investigation*, **12**, 77–86.

Sakaguchi, S., Fukuma, K., Kuribayashi, K. & Masuda, T. (1985). Organ-specific autoimmune diseases induced in mice by elimination of T cell subset. I Evidence for the active participation of T cells in natural self-tolerance; deficit of a T cell subset as a possible cause of autoimmune disease. *Journal of Experimental Medicine*, **161**, 72–87.

Sakaguchi, S. & Sakaguchi, N. (1989). Organ-specific disease induced in mice by elimination of T cell subsets. *Journal of Immunology*, **142**, 471–80.

Sakata, S., Nakamura, S. & Miura, K. (1985). Autoantibodies against thyroid hormones or iodothyronine. Implications in diagnosis, thyroid function, treatment, and pathogenesis. *Annals of Internal Medicine*, **103**, 579–89.

Salamero, J. & Charreire, J. (1983). Syngeneic sensitization of mouse lymphocytes on monolayers of thyroid epithelial cells. V The primary syngeneic sensitization is under I-A subregion control. *European Journal of Immunology*, **13**, 948–51.

Salamero, J., Michel-Bechet, M., Wietzerbin, J. & Charreire, J. (1985). Syngeneic sensitisation of mouse lymphocytes on monolayers of thyroid epithelial cells (TEC). VIII Gamma-interferon induced Ia expression on TEC cultures. *Tissue Antigens*, **25**, 266–77.

Salvi, M., Miller, A. & Wall, J.R. (1988). Human orbital tissue and thyroid membranes express a 64 kd protein which is recognised by autoantibodies in the serum of patients with thyroid associated ophthalmopathy. *FEBS Letters*, **232**, 135–9.

Salvi, M., Zhang, Z.G., Haegert, D., Woo, M., Liberman, A., Cadarso, L. & Wall, J.R. (1990). Patients with endocrine ophthalmopathy not associated with overt thyroid disease have multiple thyroid immunological abnormalities. *Journal of Clinical Endocrinology and Metabolism*, **70**, 89–94.

Sasazuki, T., Nishimura, Y., Muto, M. & Ohta, N. (1983). HLA-linked genes controlling immune response and disease susceptibility. *Immunological Reviews*, **70**, 51–73.

Sato, K., Satoh, T., Shizume, K., Ozawa, M., Han, D.C., Imamura, H., Tsushima, T., Dimura, H., Kanaji, Y., Ito, Y., Obara, T. & Fujimoto, Y. (1990). Inhibition of ^{125}I organification and thyroid hormone release by interleukin-1, tumor necrosis factor-α, and interferon-γ in human thyrocytes in suspension culture. *Journal of Clinical Endocrinology and Metabolism*, **70**, 1735–43.

Schermer, D.R., Roenigle, H.H., Schumacher, O.P. & McKenzie, J.M. (1970). Relationship of long-acting thyroid stimulator to pretibial myxoedema. *Archives of Dermatology*, **102**, 62–7.

Schleusener, H., Schernthaner, G., Mayr, W.R., Kotulla, P., Bogner, U., Finke, R., Meinhold, H., Koppenhagen, K. & Wenzel, K.W. (1983). HLA-DR3 and HLA-DR5 associated thyrotoxicosis – two different types of toxic diffuse goitre. *Journal of Clinical Endocrinology and Metabolism*, **56**, 781–5.

Schleusener, H., Schwander, J., Fischer, C., Holle, R., Holl, G., Badenhoop, K., Hensen, J., Finke, R., Bogner, U., Mayr, W.R., Schernthaner, G., Schatz, H., Pickardt, C.R. & Kotulla, P. (1989). Prospective multicentre study on the prediction of relapse after anti-thyroid drug treatment in patients with Graves' disease. *Acta Endocrinologica*, **120**, 689–701.

Sekino, T., Shishiba, Y., Inatsuki, B. & Yata, J. (1988). Heterogeneity of the immune status concerning anti-thyroglobulin antibody production among patients with Hashimoto's thyroiditis; an *in vitro* study. *Clinical and Experimental Immunology*, **71**, 486–92.

Sergott, R.C., Felberg, N.T., Savino, P.J., Blizzard, J.T., Schatz, N.J. & Sanford, C.A. (1983). Association of HLA antigen Bw35 with severe Graves' ophthalmopathy. *Investigative Ophthalmology and Visual Science*, **24**, 104–12.

Shen, D.C., Wu, S.Y., Chopra, I.J., Huang, H.W., Shian, L.R., Bian, T.Y., Jeng, C.Y. & Solomon, D.H. (1985). Long term treatment of Graves' hyperthyroidism with sodium ipodate. *Journal of Clinical Endocrinology and Metabolism*, **61**, 723–7.

Shenkman, L. & Bottone, E.J. (1976). Antibodies to *Yersinia enterocolitica* in thyroid disease. *Annals of Internal Medicine*, **85**, 735–9.

Shigemasa, C., Ueta, Y., Mitani, Y., Taniguchi, S., Urabe, K., Tanaka, T., Yoshida, A. & Mashiba, H. (1990). Chronic thyroiditis with painful tender thyroid enlargement and transient thyrotoxicosis. *Journal of Clinical Endocrinology and Metabolism*, **70**, 385–90.

Shine, B., Fells, P., Edwards, O.M. & Weetman, A.P. (1990). Association of Graves' ophthalmopathy and smoking. *Lancet*, **i**, 1261–3.

Shinozawa, T., Villadolid, M.C. & Ingbar, S.H. (1986). Detection and measurement of fat cell-binding immunoglobulins: a new method applicable to the diagnosis and study of Graves' disease. *Journal of Clinical Endocrinology and Metabolism*, **62**, 1–9.

Sikorska, H. & Wall, J.R. (1985). Failure to detect eye muscle membrane specific autoantibodies in Graves' ophthalmopathy. *British Medical Journal*, **291**, 604.

Silverman, D.A. & Rose, N.R. (1974). Neonatal thymectomy increases the incidence of spontaneous and methylcholanthrene enhanced thyroiditis in rats. *Science*, **184**, 162–4.

Silverman, D.A. & Rose, N.R. (1975). Spontaneous and methylcholanthrene-enhanced thyroiditis in Buf rats. I. The incidence and severity of disease, and the genetics of susceptibility. *Journal of Immunology*, **114**, 145–7.

Singer, P.A. & Gorsky, J.E. (1985). Familial postpartum transient hyperthyroidism. *Archives of Internal Medicine*, **145**, 240–2.

Sisson, J.C. & Vanderburg, J.A. (1972). Lymphocyte-retrobulbar fibroblast interaction: mechanisms by which stimulation occurs and inhibition of stimulation. *Investigative Ophthalmology*, **11**, 15–20.

Smith, B.R. & Hall, R. (1974). Thyroid-stimulating immunoglobulins in Graves' disease. *Lancet*, **ii**, 427–31.

Smith, H., Chen, I.-M., Kubo, R. & Tung, K.S. (1989). Neonatal thymectomy results in a repertoire enriched in T cells deleted in adult thymus. *Science*, **245**, 749–52.

Smith, T.J., Bahn, R.S. & Gorman, C.A. (1989). Connective tissue, glycosaminoglycans, and diseases of the thyroid. *Endocrine Reviews*, **10**, 366–91.

Sridama, V., Hara, Y., Fauchet, R. & DeGroot, L.J. (1987). HLA immunogenetic heterogeneity in Black American patients with Graves' disease. *Archives of Internal Medicine*, **147**, 229–31.

Steel, N.R., Weightman, D.R., Taylor, J.J. & Kendall-Taylor, P. (1984). Blocking activity to action of thyroid stimulating hormone in serum from patients with primary hypothyroidism. *British Medical Journal*, **288**, 1559–62.

Steel, N.R., Taylor, J.J., Young, E.T., Farndon, J.R., Holcombe, M. & Kendall-Taylor, P. (1987). The effect of subtotal thyroidectomy with propranolol preparation on antibody activity in Graves' disease. *Clinical Endocrinology*, **26**, 97–106.

Stenszky, V., Balázs, C., Kozma, L., Rochlitz, S., Bear, J.C. & Farid, N.R. (1983). Identification of subsets of patients with Graves' disease by cluster analysis. *Clinical Endocrinology*, **18**, 335–45.

Stenszky, V., Kozma, L., Balázs, C., Rochlitz, S., Bear, J.C. & Farid, N.R. (1985). The genetics of Graves' disease: HLA and disease susceptibility. *Journal of Clinical Endocrinology and Metabolism*, **61**, 735–40.

Stenszky, V., Balázs, C., Kraszits, E., Juhasz, F., Kozma, L., Balázs, G. & Farid, N.R. (1987). Association of goitrous autoimmune thyroiditis with HLA-DR3 in eastern Hungary. *Journal of Immunogenetics*, **14**, 143–8.

Stern, S.A. & Dau, P.C. (1987). Induction of *in vitro* autoimmune responses by mononuclear blood cells in Hashimoto's thyroiditis. *Clinical and Experimental Immunology*, **69**, 508–15.

Sternthal, E., Like, A., Sarantis, K. & Braverman, L. (1981). Lymphocytic thyroiditis and diabetes in the BB/W rat. *Diabetes*, **30**, 1058–61.

Sugihara, S., Izumi, Y., Yoshioka, T., Yagi, H., Tsujimura, T., Tarutani, O., Kohno, Y., Murakami, S., Hamaoka, T. & Fujiwara, H. (1988). Autoimmune thyroiditis induced in mice depleted of particular T cell subsets. *Journal of Immunology*, **141**, 105–13.

Sugihara, S., Maruo, S., Tsujimura, T., Tarutani, O., Kohno, Y., Hamaoka, T. & Fujiwara, H.

(1990). Autoimmune thyroiditis induced in mice depleted of particular T cell subsets. III. Analysis of regulatory cells suppressing the induction of thyroiditis. *International Immunology*, **2**, 344–51.

Sundick, R.S., Herdegen, D.M., Brown, T.R. & Bagchi, N. (1987). The incorporation of dietary iodine into thyroglobulin increases its immunogenicity. *Endocrinology*, **120**, 2078–84.

Swillens, S., Ludgate, M., Mercken, L., Dumont, J.E. & Vassart, G. (1986). Analysis of sequence and structure homologies between thyroglobulin and acetylcholinesterase: possible functional and clinical significance. *Biochemical and Biophysical Research Communications*, **137**, 142–8.

Tachi, J., Amino, N., Tamaki, H., Aozasa, M., Iwatani, Y. & Miyai, K. (1988). Long term follow-up and HLA associations in patients with postpartum thyroiditis. *Journal of Clinical Endocrinology and Metabolism*, **66**, 480–4.

Takata, I., Suzuki, Y., Saida, K. & Sato, T. (1980). Human thyroid stimulating activity and clinical state in antithyroid treatment of juvenile Graves' disease. *Acta Endocrinologica*, **94**, 46–52.

Tallstedt, L. & Norberg, R. (1988). Immunohistochemical staining of normal and Graves' extraocular muscle. *Investigative Ophthalmology*, **29**, 175–84.

Tamai, H., Uno, H., Hirota, Y., Matsubayashi, S., Kuma, K., Matsumoto, H., Kumagai, L.F., Sasazuki, T. & Nagataki, S. (1985). Immunogenetics of Hashimoto's and Graves' disease. *Journal of Clinical Endocrinology and Metabolism*, **60**, 62–7.

Tandon, N., Mehra, N.K., Taneja, V., Vaidya, M.C. & Kochupillai, N. (1990). HLA antigens in Asian Indian patients with Graves' disease. *Clinical Endocrinology*, **33**, 21–6.

Tandon, N., Zhang, L. & Weetman, A.P. (1991). HLA associations in Hashimoto's thyroiditis. *Clinical Endocrinology*, **34**, 383–6.

Tao, T.-W., Leu, S.-L. & Kriss, J.P. (1985). Peripheral blood lymphocytes from normal individuals can be induced to secrete immunoglobulin G antibodies against self-antigen thyroglobulin *in vitro*. *Journal of Clinical Endocrinology and Metabolism*, **60**, 279–82.

Tao, T.-W., Leu, S.-L. & Kriss, J.P. (1989). Biological activity of autoantibodies associated with Graves' dermopathy. *Journal of Clinical Endocrinology and Metabolism*, **69**, 90–9.

Teng, C.S.S. & Yeo, P.P.B. (1977). Ophthalmic Graves' disease: natural history and detailed thyroid function studies. *British Medical Journal*, **1**, 273–5.

Teng, W.P., Cohen, S.B., Posnett, D.N. & Weetman, A.P. (1990a). T cell receptor phenotypes in autoimmune thyroid disease. *Journal of Endocrinological Investigation*, **13**, 339–42.

Teng, W.P., Stark, R., Munro, A.J., McHardy-Young, S., Borysiewicz, L.K. & Weetman, A.P. (1990b). Peripheral blood T cell activation after radioiodine treatment for Graves' disease. *Acta Endocrinologica*, **122**, 233–40.

Thielemans, C., Vanhaelst, L., De Waele, M., Jonckheer, M. & Van Camp, B. (1981). Autoimmune thyroiditis: a condition related to a decrease in T-suppressor cells. *Clinical Endocrinology*, **15**, 259–63.

Thompson, C. & Farid, N.R. (1985). Post-partum thyroiditis and goitrous (Hashimoto's) thyroiditis are associated with HLA-DR4. *Immunology Letters*, **11**, 301–3.

Thomsen, M., Ryder, L.P., Bech, K., Bliddal, H., Feldt-Rasmussen, U., Mølholm, J., Kappelgaard, E., Nielsen, H. & Svejgaard, A. (1983). HLA-D in Hashimoto's thyroiditis. *Tissue Antigens*, **21**, 173–5.

Todd, I., Pujol-Borrell, R., Hammond, L.J., Bottazzo, G.F. & Feldmann, M. (1985). Interferon-γ induces HLA-DR expression by thyroid epithelium. *Clinical and Experimental Immunology*, **61**, 265–73.

Todd, I., Pujol-Borrell, R., Hammond, L.J., McNally, J.M., Feldmann, M. & Bottazzo, G.F. (1987). Enhancement of thyrocyte HLA Class II expression by thyroid stimulating hormone. *Clinical and Experimental Immunology*, **69**, 524–31.

Tomazic, V. & Rose, N.R. (1975). Autoimmune murine thyroiditis. VII. Induction of the thyroid lesions by passive transfer of immune serum. *Clinical Immunology and Immunopathology*, **4**, 511–18.

Topliss, D., How, J., Lewis, M., Row, V. & Volpé, R. (1983). Evidence for cell-mediated immunity and specific suppressor T lymphocyte dysfunction in Graves' disease and diabetes mellitus. *Journal of Clinical Endocrinology and Metabolism*, **57**, 700–5.

Topliss, D.J., Okita, N., Lewis, M., Row, V.V. & Volpé, R. (1981). Allosuppressor T lymphocytes abolish migration inhibition factor production in autoimmune thyroid disease: evidence from radiosensitivity experiments. *Clinical Endocrinology*, **15**, 335–41.

Tötterman, T.H., Andersson, L.C. & Hayry, P. (1979). Evidence for thyroid antigen-reactive T lymphocytes infiltrating the thyroid gland in Graves' disease. *Clinical Endocrinology*, **11**, 59–68.

Tötterman, T.H., Karlsson, F.A., Bengtsson, M. & Mendel-Hartvig, I. (1987). Induction of circulating activated suppressor-like T cells by methimazole therapy for Graves' disease. *New England Journal of Medicine*, **316**, 15–22.

Trokel, S.L. & Jakobiec, F.A. (1981). Correlation of CT scanning and pathologic features of ophthalmic Graves' disease. *Ophthalmology*, **88**, 553–64.

Trotter, W.R., Belyavin, G. & Wadhams, A. (1957). Precipitating and complement-fixing antibodies in Hashimoto's disease. *Proceedings of the Royal Society of Medicine*, **50**, 961–2.

Trudeu, J.L., Sundick, R.S., Levine, S. & Rose, N.R. (1983). The decreased growth rate of obese strain chicken thyroid cells provides *in vitro* evidence for a primary target organ abnormality in chickens susceptible to autoimmune thyroiditis. *Clinical Immunology and Immunopathology*, **29**, 294–305.

Tunbridge, W.M.G., Evered, D.C., Hall, R., Appleton, D., Brewis, M., Clark, F., Grimley-Evans, J., Young, E., Bird, T. & Smith, P.A. (1977). The spectrum of thyroid disease in the community; the Whickham survey. *Clinical Endocrinology*, **7**, 481–92.

Tunbridge, W.M.G., Brewis, M., French, J.M., Appleton, D., Bird, T., Clark, F., Evered, D.C., Evans, J.G., Hall, R., Smith, P., Stephenson, J. & Young, E. (1981). Natural history of autoimmune thyroiditis. *British Medical Journal*, **282**, 258–62.

Turner, M., Londei, M. & Feldmann, M. (1987). Human T cells from autoimmune and normal individuals can produce tumor necrosis factor. *European Journal of Immunology*, **17**, 1807–14.

Tweedle, D., Colling, A., Schardt, W., Green, E.M., Evered, D.C., Dickinson, P.H. & Johnston, I.D.A. (1977). Hypothyroidism following partial thyroidectomy for thyrotoxicosis and its relationship to thyroid remnant size. *British Journal of Surgery*, **64**, 445–8.

Ueki, Y.M., Eguchi, K., Otsubo, T., Kawabe, Y., Shimomura, C., Matsunaga, M., Tezuka, H., Nakao, H., Kawakami, A. & Izumi, M. (1988). Phenotypic analysis of concanavalin-A-induced suppressor cell dysfunction of thyroidal lymphocytes from patients with Graves' disease. *Journal of Clinical Endocrinology and Metabolism*, **67**, 1018–24.

Uno, H., Sasazuki, T., Tamai, H. & Matsumoto, H. (1981). Two major genes, linked to HLA and Gm, control susceptibility to Graves' disease. *Nature*, **292**, 768–70.

Valdiserri, R.O. & Borochovitz, D. (1980). Histologic changes in previously irradiated thyroid glands. *Archives of Pathology and Laboratory Medicine*, **104**, 150–2.

Valente, W.A., Vitti, P., Rotella, C.M., Vaughan, M.M., Aloj, S.M., Grollman, E.F., Ambesi-Impiombato, F.S. & Kohn, L.D. (1983). Antibodies that promote thyroid growth: a distinct population of thyroid-stimulating autoantibodies. *New England Journal of Medicine*, **309**, 1028.

Van der Gaag, R.D., Drexhage, H.A. & Dussault, J.H. (1985). Role of maternal immuno-globulins blocking TSH-induced thyroid growth in sporadic forms of congenital hypo-thyroidism. *Lancet*, **i**, 246–50.

Van Dyk, H.J.L. (1981). Orbital Graves' disease: a modification of the 'NO SPECS' classification. *Ophthalmology*, **88**, 479–83.

Van Liessum, P.A., De Mulder, P.H.M., Mattijssen, E.J.M., Corstens, F.H.M. & Wagener, D.J.T. (1989). Hypothyroidism and goitre during interleukin-2 therapy without LAK cells. *Lancet*, **i**, 224.

Van Welsum, M., Feltkamp, T.E.W., De Vries, M.J., Doctor, R., Van Zijl, J. & Hennemann, G. (1974). Hypothyroidism after thyroidectomy for Graves' disease: a search for an explanation. *British Medical Journal*, **iv**, 755–7.

Vargas, M.T., Briones-Urbina, R., Gladman, D., Papsin, F.R. & Walfish, P.G. (1988). Antithyroid microsomal autoantibodies and HLA-DR5 are associated with postpartum thyroid dysfunction: evidence supporting an autoimmune pathogenesis. *Journal of Clinical Endocrinology and Metabolism*, **67**, 327-33.

Vento, S., Bottazzo, G., Williams, R., Hegarty, J.E., Macchia, E. & Eddleston, A.L.W.F. (1984). Antigen-specific suppressor cell function in autoimmune chronic active hepatitis. *Lancet*, **ii**, 1200–5.

Vladutiu, A.O. (1982). Autoimmune thyroiditis: conversion of low-responder mice to high-responders by cyclophosphamide. *Clinical and Experimental Immunology*, **47**, 683–8.

Vladutiu, A.O. (1989). Experimental autoimmune thyroiditis in mice chronically treated from birth with anti-IgM antibodies. *Cellular Immunology*, **121**, 49–59.

Vladutiu, A. & Rose, N.R. (1971). Autoimmune murine thyroiditis: relation to histocompati-bility (H-2) complex. *Science*, **174**, 1137–9.

Volpé, R. (1981). Autoimmunity in thyroid disease. *Monographs in Endocrinology*, **20**, 19–111.

Volpé, R. (1985). Autoimmune thyroid disease. In *Autoimmunity and Endocrine Disease*, ed. R. Volpé. pp. 109–286. New York: Marcel Dekker.

Volpé, R. (1988). The immunoregulatory disturbance in autoimmune thyroid disease. *Autoimmunity*, **2**, 55–72.

Volpé, R., Karlsson, A., Jansson, R. & Dahlberg, P.A. (1986). Evidence that antithyroid drugs induce remissions in Graves' disease by modulating thyroid cellular activity. *Clinical Endocrinology*, **25**, 453–62.

Wall, J.R. (1986). Role of cellular mechanisms in the orbital autoimmunity of Graves' opthalmopathy. *Journal of Endocrinological Investigation*, **9** (Suppl. 3), 71.

Wall, J.R., Trewin, A., Fang, S.L., Ingbar, S.H. & Braverman, L.E. (1978). Studies of immunoreactivity to human lacrimal gland fractions in patients with ophthalmic Graves' disease. *Journal of Endocrinological Investigation*, **1**, 253–8.

Wall, J.R., Walters, B.A.J. & Grant, C. (1979). Leukocyte adherence inhibition in response to human orbital and lacrimal extracts in patients with Graves' ophthalmopathy. *Journal of Endocrinological Investigation*, **2**, 375–8.

Wall, J.R., Baur, R., Schleusener, H. & Bandy-Dafoe, P. (1983). Peripheral blood and intrathyroidal mononuclear cell populations in patients with autoimmune thyroid disorders enumerated using monoclonal antibodies. *Journal of Clinical Endocrinology and Metab-olism*, **56**, 164–9.

Wang, P.W., Hiromatsu, Y., Laryea, E., Wosu, L., How, J. & Wall, J.R. (1986). Immunologi-cally mediated cytotoxicity against human eye muscle cells in Graves' ophthalmopathy. *Journal of Clinical Endocrinology and Metabolism*, **63**, 316–22.

Warford, A., McLachlan, S.M., Malcolm, A.J., Young, E.T., Farndon, J.R. & Rees Smith, B. (1984). Characterisation of lymphoid cells in the thyroid of patients with Graves' disease. *Clinical and Experimental Immunology*, **57**, 626–32.

Weaver, D.K., Batsakis, J.G. & Nishiyama, R.H. (1969). Relationship of iodine to lymphocytic goitres. *Archives of Surgery*, **98**, 183–6.

Weetman, A.P (1986). Effect of the antithyroid drug methimazole on interleukin-1 and interleukin-2 levels in vitro. *Clinical Endocrinology*, **25**, 133.

Weetman, A.P. (1989). Autologous CD8-positive cells suppress T cell proliferation in response to thyroid antigens in Hashimoto's thyroiditis. *Clinical Immunology and Immunopathology*, **51**, 303–10.

Weetman, A.P., McGregor, A.M. & Hall, R. (1983a). Thyroglobulin uptake and presentation by macrophages in experimental autoimmune thyroiditis. *Immunology*, **50**, 315–18.

Weetman, A.P., McGregor, A.M. & Hall, R. (1983b). Methimazole inhibits thyroid autoantibody production by an action on accessory cells. *Clinical Immunology and Immunopathology*, **28**, 39–45.

Weetman, A.P. & McGregor, A.M. (1984). Autoimmune thyroid disease: developments in our understanding. *Endocrine Reviews*, **5**, 309–55.

Weetman, A.P., Hassman, R., McGregor, A.M. & Hall, R. (1984a). The tissue distribution of thyroglobulin-responsive B and T cells in experimental autoimmune thyroiditis (EAT). *Journal of Laboratory and Clinical Immunology*, **14**, 59–63.

Weetman, A.P., McGregor, A.M., Wheeler, M.H. & Hall, R. (1984b). Extrathyroidal autoantibody synthesis in Graves' disease. *Clinical and Experimental Immunology*, **56**, 330–6.

Weetman, A.P., McGregor, A.M. & Hall, R. (1984c). Evidence for an effect of antithyroid drugs on the natural history of Graves' disease. *Clinical Endocrinology*, **21**, 163–72.

Weetman, A.P., Holt, M.E., Campbell, A.K., Hall, R. & McGregor, A.M. (1984d). Methimazole inhibits generation by oxygen radical monocytes: a potential role in immunosuppression. *British Medical Journal*, **288**, 518.

Weetman, A.P., Volkman, D.J., Burman, K.D., Gerrard, T.J. & Fauci, A.S. (1985a). The *in vitro* regulation of human thyrocyte HLA-DR antigen expression. *Journal of Clinical Endocrinology and Metabolism*, **61**, 817–24.

Weetman, A.P., Volkman, D.J., Burman, K.D. & Fauci, A.S. (1985b). Activation, proliferation and differentiation of circulating B cells in autoimmune thyroid disease. *Journal of Immunology*, **135**, 3138–43.

Weetman, A.P., Volkman, D.J., Burman, K.D., Margolick, J.B., Petrick, P., Weintraub, B.D. & Fauci, A.S. (1986a). The production and characterisation of thyroid-derived T cell lines in Graves' disease and Hashimoto's thyroiditis. *Clinical Immunology and Immunopathology*, **39**, 131–50.

Weetman, A.P., Ratanachaiyavong, S., Middleton, G.W., Love, W., John, R., Owen, G.M., Darke, C., Lazarus, J.H., Hall, R. & McGregor, A.M. (1986b). Prediction of outcome in Graves' disease after carbimazole treatment. *Quarterly Journal of Medicine*, **59**, 409–19.

Weetman, A.P., So, A.K., Roe, C., Walport, M.J. & Foroni, L. (1987a). T cell receptor α chain V region polymorphism linked to primary autoimmune hypothyroidism but not Graves' disease. *Human Immunology*, **20**, 167–73.

Weetman, A.P., Green, C. & Borysiewicz, L.K. (1987b). Regulation of major histocompatibility complex class II antigen expression by the FRTL-5 rat thyroid cell line. *Journal of Endocrinology*, **115**, 481–7.

Weetman, A.P. & Brazier, D.M. (1988). Immunoglobulin allotypes in Graves' disease. *Tissue Antigens*, **32**, 71–3.

Weetman, A.P. & Rees, A.J. (1988). Synergistic effects of recombinant tumour necrosis factor (TNF) and gamma interferon on rat thyroid cell growth and Ia antigen expression. *Immunology*, **63**, 285–9.

Weetman, A.P., Bhandal, S.K., Burrin, J.M., Robinson, K. & McKenna, W. (1988a). Amiodarone and thyroid autoimmunity in the United Kingdom. *British Medical Journal*, **297**, 33.

Weetman, A.P., So, A.K., Warner, C.A., Foroni, L., Fells, P. & Shine, B. (1988b). Immunogenetics of Graves' ophthalmopathy. *Clinical Endocrinology*, **28**, 619–28.

Weetman, A.P., Cohen, S.B., Oleesky, D.A. & Morgan, B.P. (1989a). Terminal complement complexes and C1/C1 inhibitor complexes in autoimmune thyroid disease. *Clinical and Experimental Immunology*, **77**, 25–30.

Weetman, A.P., Cohen, S.B., Gatter, K.C., Fells, P. & Shine, B. (1989b). Immunohisto-chemical analysis of the retrobulbar tissues in Graves' ophthalmopathy. *Clinical and Experimental Immunology*, **75**, 222–7.

Weetman, A.P., Fells, P. & Shine, B. (1989c). T and B cell reactivity to extraocular and skeletal muscle in Graves' ophthalmopathy. *British Journal of Ophthalmology*, **73**, 323–7.

Weetman, A.P., Bright-Thomas, R. & Freeman, M. (1990a). Regulation of interleukin-6 release by human thyrocytes. *Journal of Endocrinology*, **127**, 357–61.

Weetman, A.P., Freeman, M.A. & Morgan, B.P. (1990b). Thyroid follicular cell function after non-lethal complement membrane attack. *Clinical and Experimental Immunology*, **82**, 69–74.

Weetman, A.P., Freeman, M., Borysiewicz, L.K. & Makgoba, M.W. (1990c). Functional analysis of intercellular adhesion molecule-1-expressing human thyroid cells. *European Journal of Immunology*, **20**, 271–5.

Weetman, A.P., Fung, H.Y.M., Richards, C.J. & McGregor, A.M. (1990d). IgG subclass distribution and relative functional affinity of thyroid microsomal antibodies in postpartum thyroiditis. *European Journal of Clinical Investigation*, **20**, 133–6.

Weetman, A.P., Zhang, L., Webb, S. & Shine B. (1990e). Analysis of HLA-DQB and HLA-DPB alleles in Graves' disease by oligonucleotide probing of enzymatically amplified DNA. *Clinical Endocrinology*, **33**, 65–71.

Weetman, A.P. Yateman, M.E., Ealey, P.A., Black, C.M., Reimer C.B., Williams, R.C., Shine, B. & Marshall, N.J. (1990f). An investigation of thyroid stimulating antibody activity between different IgG subclasses. *Journal of Clinical Investigation*, **86**, 723–7.

Weiser, W.Y., Temple, P.A., Witek-Giannotti, J.-A.S., Remold, H.G., Clark, S.C. & David, J.R. (1989). Molecular cloning of a cDNA encoding a human macrophage migration inhibitory factor. *Proceedings of the National Academy of Science, USA*, **86**, 7522–6.

Weiss, I. & Davies, T.F. (1981). Inhibition of immunoglobulin-secreting cells by antithyroid drugs. *Journal of Clinical Endocrinology and Metabolism*, **53**, 1223–8.

Weiss, M., Ingbar, S.H., Winblad, S. & Kaspar, D.L. (1983). Demonstration of a saturable binding site for thyrotropin in *Yersinia enterocolitica*. *Science*, **219**, 1331–3.

Weissel, M., Hofer, R., Zasmeta, H. & Mayr, W.R. (1980). HLA-DR and Hashimoto's thyroiditis. *Tissue Antigens*, **16**, 256–9.

Wenzel, B., Kotulla, P., Wenzel, K.W., Finke, R. & Schleusener, H. (1981). Mitogenic response of peripheral blood lymphocytes from patients with Graves' disease incubated with solubilized thyroid cell membranes containing TSH receptor and with thyroglobulin. *Immunobiology*, **160**, 302–10.

Wenzel, B.E., Heesemann, J., Wenzel, K.W. & Scriba, P.C. (1988). Antibodies to plasmid-encoded proteins of enteropathogenic Yersinia in patients with autoimmune thyroid disease. *Lancet*, **i**, 56.

Werner, S.C. & Platman, S.R. (1965). Remission of hyperthyroidism (Graves' disease) and altered pattern of serum-thyroxine binding induced by prednisone. *Lancet*, **ii**, 751–6.

Werner, S.C., Coleman, D.J. & Franzen, L.A. (1974). Ultrasonographic evidence of a consistent orbital involvement in Graves' disease. *New England Journal of Medicine*, **308**, 420–4.

Whitmore, D.B. & Irvine, W.J. (1977). Prevention of autoimmune thyroiditis in T cell-depleted rats by injections of crude thyroid extract. *Clinical and Experimental Immunology*, **29**, 474–9.

Wick, G., Kite, J.H. & Witebsky, E. (1970). Spontaneous thyroiditis in the Obese strain of chickens. III. The effect of thymectomy and thymo-bursectomy on the development of the disease. *Journal of Immunology*, **104**, 54–62.

Wick, G., Boyd, R., Hála, K., Thunold, S. & Kofler, H. (1982). Pathogenesis of spontaneous autoimmune thyroiditis in Obese strain (OS) chickens. *Clinical and Experimental Immunology*, **47**, 1–18.

Wick, G., Hála, K., Wolf, H., Boyd, R.L. & Schauenstein, K. (1984). Distribution and functional analysis of B-L/Ia positive cells in the chicken: expression of B-L/Ia antigens on thyroid epithelial cells in spontaneous autoimmune thyroiditis. *Molecular Immunology*, **12**, 1259–65.

Wick, G., Most, J., Schaenstein, K., Kromer, G., Dietrich, H., Ziemiecki, A., Fassler, R., Schwarz, S., Neu, N. & Hála, K. (1985). Spontaneous autoimmune thyroiditis – a bird's eye view. *Immunology Today*, **6**, 359–64.

Wiersinga, W.M., Smit, T., Van der Gaag, R. & Koornneef, L. (1988). Temporal relationship between onset of Graves' ophthalmopathy and onset of thyroidal Graves' disease. *Journal of Endocrinological Investigation*, **11**, 615–19.

Wilkin, T.J. & Casey, C. (1984). The distribution of immunoglobulin-containing cells in human autoimmune thyroiditis. *Acta Endocrinologica*, **106**, 490–8.

Williams, E.D. & Doniach, I. (1962). The post-mortem incidence of focal thyroiditis. *Journal of Pathology*, **83**, 255–64.

Williams, R.C., Marshall, N.J., Kilpatrick, K., Montano, J., Brickell, P.M., Shine, B., Ealey, P., Weetman, A.P. & Craig, R.K. (1988). Kappa/lambda immunoglobulin distribution of Graves' thyroid stimulating antibodies. Simultaneous analysis of Cλ gene polymorphisms. *Journal of Clinical Investigation*, **82**, 1306–12.

Wilson, R., McKillop, J.H., Chopra, M. & Thomson, J.A. (1988). The effect of antithyroid drugs on B and T cell activity *in vitro*. *Clinical Endocrinology*, **28**, 389–97.

Wilson, R., McKillop, J.H., Travers, M., Smith, J., Smith, E. & Thomson, J.A. (1990). The effects of antithyroid drugs on intracellular mediators. *Acta Endocrinologica*, **122**, 605–9.

Wood, L.C. & Ingbar, S.H. (1979). Hypothyroidism as a late sequela in patients with Graves' disease treated with antithyroid drugs. *Journal of Clinical Investigation*, **64**, 1429.

Wortsman, J., Dietrich, J., Traycoff, R.B. & Stone, S. (1981). Preradial myxedema in thyroid disease. *Archives of Dermatology*, **117**, 635–8.

Yoshida, H., Amino, N., Yagawa, K., Uemura, K., Satoh, M., Miyai, K. & Kumahara, Y. (1978). Association of serum antithyroid antibodies with lymphocytic infiltraton of the thyroid gland: Studies of seventy autopsied cases. *Journal of Clinical Endocrinology and Metabolism*, **46**, 859–62.

Young, R.J., Sherwood, M.B., Simpson, J.G., Nicol, A.G., Michie, W. & Swanson Beck, J. (1976). Histometry of lymphoid infiltrate in the thyroid of primary thyrotoxicosis patients. *Journal of Clinical Pathology*, **29**, 398–402.

Zakarija, M. (1983). Immunochemical characterisation of the thyroid-stimulating antibody (TSAb) of Graves' disease: evidence for restricted heterogeneity. *Journal of Clinical and Laboratory Immunology*, **10**, 77–85.

Zakarija, M. & McKenzie, J.M. (1978). Isoelectric focusing of thyroid-stimulating antibody of Graves' disease. *Endocrinology*, **103**, 1469–75.

Zakarija, M., McKenzie, J.M. & Banovac, K. (1980). Clinical significance of assay of thyroid-stimulating antibody in Graves' disease. *Annals of Internal Medicine*, **93**, 28–32.

Zakarija, M., McKenzie, J.M. & Hoffman, W.H. (1986). Prediction and therapy of intra-uterine and late-onset neonatal hyperthyroidism. *Journal of Clinical Endocrinology and Metabolism*, **62**, 368–71.

Zakarija, M., Jin, S. & McKenzie, J.M. (1988). Evidence supporting the identity in Graves' disease of thyroid-stimulating antibody and thyroid growth-promoting immunoglobulin G as assayed in FRTL$_5$ cells. *Journal of Clinical Investigation*, **81**, 879–84.

Zakarija, M., McKenzie, J.M. & Eidson, M.S. (1990). Transient neonatal hypothyroidism: characterization of maternal antibodies to the thyrotropin receptor. *Journal of Clinical Endocrinology and Metabolism*, **70**, 1239–46.

Zanetti, M., Barton, R.W. & Bigazzi, P.E. (1983). Anti-idiotypic immunity and autoimmunity. II. Idiotypic determinants of autoantibodies and lymphocytes in spontaneous and experimentally induced thyroiditis. *Cellular Immunology*, **75**, 292–9.

Zanetti, M. & Bigazzi, P.E. (1981). Anti-idiotypic immunity and autoimmunity. I. *In vitro* and *in vivo* effects of anti-idiotypic antibodies to spontaneously occurring autoantibodies to rat thyroglobulin. *European Journal of Immunology*, **11**, 187–95.

Zhang, Z.G., Medeiros-Neto, G., Iacona, A., Lima, N., Hiromatsu, Y., Salvi, M., Triller, H., Bernard, N. & Wall, J.R. (1989). Studies of cytotoxic antibodies against eye muscle antigens in patients with thyroid-associated ophthalmopathy. *Acta Endocrinologica*, **121** (Suppl. 2), 23–30.

Ziemiecki, A., Kroemer, G., Mueller, R., Hála, K. & Wick, G. (1988). ev 22, a new endogenous retrovirus found in chickens with spontaneous autoimmune thyroiditis. *Archives of Virology*, **100**, 267–71.

–4–
Type 1 diabetes mellitus

Two main forms of diabetes mellitus are recognised: type 1 (or insulin-dependent) and type 2 (or non-insulin dependent). The two have also been classified by their age of onset as juvenile or maturity onset, but there is some overlap in this characteristic, as indeed there is in the need for insulin. Only type 1 diabetes mellitus is the result of an autoimmune process and the simple term diabetes will be used throughout the Chapter to refer to this group. The disease has a high incidence (15.6 cases per 100 000 of the under 21 year old population in the UK annually: Bingley & Gale, 1989). It is unlike the other autoimmune endocrinopathies in that the patients are usually very young, hormone replacement cannot be given orally and chronic vascular complications result in major morbidity and mortality. These facts make the need for understanding and treating this disorder all the more pressing. However, a major problem has been the difficulty in examining events at the site of the lesion and attention has therefore focussed on two forms of diabetes which occur spontaneously in the mouse and rat. These models permit sequential analysis of the pancreatic infiltrate preceding the onset of diabetes and, of course, allow experimental modulation of the lymphocyte subpopulations *in vivo* as well as *in vitro*. Animals have also been used to explore the potential role of viruses in diabetes. The data which have accumulated are summarised in the next section.

Experimental autoimmune diabetes

The non-obese diabetic (NOD) mouse

Diabetes develops in about 75% of female and less than 25% of male NOD mice between weeks 12–30 of life, although there is some variation between colonies. These have all been derived by inbreeding from a cataract-forming substrain of outbred ICR mice (Makino *et al.*, 1980). There are close clinical and immunological similarities to the human disease (Table 4.1) and without insulin treatment the animals die within two months (reviewed by Lampeter *et al.*, 1989). The strong female preponderance is unlike human diabetes and

Table 4.1. *Clinical and immunological features of diabetes in the NOD mouse, BB rat and man*

	NOD mouse	BB rat	Man
Weight loss	Yes	Yes	Yes
Polydipsia/polyuria	Yes	Yes	Yes
Hyperglycaemia	Yes	Yes	Yes
Ketoacidosis	Possible	Common	Common
Insulin deficiency	Yes	Yes	Yes
Sex preponderance	F $\gg$ M	F = M	F = M
Lymphopenia	No	Usual	No
Insulitis	Yes	Yes	Yes
Ia$^+$ beta cells	Unclear	No	Yes
Islet cell antibodies	Yes	Yes	Yes
Insulin antibodies	Yes	Yes	Yes
Associated autoimmunity	Yes[a]	Yes[b]	Yes[c]

[a] Particularly thyroiditis and salivary gland lymphocytic infiltration.
[b] Particularly thyroiditis and antibodies against gastric parietal cells.
[c] Particularly thyroiditis and pernicious anaemia; see Chapter 8.

this appears to reflect environmental influences on the penetrance of susceptibility genes (see below).

Immunogenetics

At least three diabetogenic loci operate in NOD mice, based on backcross experiments with various non-susceptible strains (Wicker *et al.*, 1987; Prochazka *et al.*, 1987). Only one is MHC encoded. Although all three genes appear to behave in a recessive fashion, a small number of diabetic heterozygotes (bearing both the NOD and B10 strain haplotypes) have been described, suggesting that in fact there is a single dominant MHC-linked diabetic gene with low penetrance in heterozygotes (Wicker *et al.*, 1989). One of the two non-MHC genes acts early in disease to initiate insulitis (Hattori *et al.*, 1990). The T cell receptor genes of the NOD mice do not operate in an autosomal recessive fashion in the response against the beta cell and therefore are not candidates for this susceptibility locus (Winter *et al.*, 1990). The MHC-linked gene is not required for the development of insulitis but appears essential for progression of the initial lesion to beta cell destruction and diabetes, as does the second non-MHC locus. This late phase of operation for the MHC in regulating disease expression may explain how different beta cell insults produce diabetes under MHC-linked control.

The NOD strain expresses only I-A molecules: I-E is not expressed because of a deletion in the first exon. Selectively inducing the expression of I-E, by creating transgenic mice with intact I-E genes, prevents the development of insulitis (Nishimoto *et al.*, 1987). This apparently protective effect could be mediated by I-E-restricted induction of beta cell-specific T suppressor cells. However, recent experiments suggest that I-E influences the diabetogenic T cell repertoire: cloned $CD4^+$ and $CD8^+$ T cells from the islets of NOD mice were found to have $V\beta5$ gene segment-encoded T cell receptors, and many T cells bearing this family of receptors are deleted during development in I-E-expressing mice (Reich *et al.*, 1989). Furthermore, $V\beta5^+$ T cells from NOD islets were shown to transfer disease and their depletion prevented this. The I-Aα chain of NOD mice is the same as that on I-A^d molecules, but the β chain has a unique sequence. This includes the replacement of aspartate, which is negatively charged, at position 57 by neutral serine. This non-aspartate substitution is also encoded by the HLA-DQB genes associated with human diabetes, as discussed below (Todd, Bell & McDevitt, 1987).

Thus diabetes in the NOD mouse depends on both MHC and non-MHC genes. The homozygous combination of a unique I-A molecule and an absence of I-E expression confers full MHC-linked susceptibility, but non-MHC genes are also critical. Their contribution is most clearly demonstrated in the ILI and CTS sister strains of the NOD mouse, also derived from the ICR strain. These have the same I-Aβ chain and failure of I-E expression as NOD mice but do not develop diabetes (Koide & Yoshida, 1990).

Environmental factors

Despite their identical genetic background, diabetes does not develop in all NOD mice and the incidence of disease varies between colonies, indicating an environmental component to the aetiology. Lymphocytic choriomeningitis virus infection of NOD mice prevents diabetes through an effect on virally infected $CD4^+$ T cells, although general immune competence remains intact (Oldstone, 1988, 1990). Pathogen-free animals have a much higher incidence of disease and more nearly equal sex ratio than those reared conventionally, whereas non-specific immunostimulants like complete Freund's adjuvant reduce disease (Leiter, Serreze & Prochazka, 1990). Micro-organisms may therefore enhance immunoregulatory functions in precariously placed NOD mice. If an animal receives insufficient stimulation, disease results. Females possibly require a greater stimulus than males as an explanation for their predisposition to diabetes. This in turn is dependent on sex hormones, as shown by castration experiments (Leiter, Prochazka & Coleman, 1987).

The complexity of such phenomena is underlined by the observation that the onset of beta cell destruction correlates with the appearance of T cells specific for a 65 kd heat shock protein (hsp), found endogenously but cross-reacting with a 65 kd hsp from mycobacteria (Elias *et al.*, 1990). T cells specific for this hsp can transfer disease and 65 kd hsp antibodies can also be detected. Depending on dose and timing, administration of exogenous 65 kd hsp induced or prevented disease. Thus microbial hsp could have a spectrum of effects on disease. Moreover, diet may provide an additional influence, as mice maintained on a semipurified formula have a reduced incidence of disease (Coleman, Kuzara & Leiter, 1990). The diabetogenic agent in standard chow is lipoidal, as it can be extracted with chloroform and methanol.

T cell responses

Insulitis appears as early as four weeks after birth, initially as an mononuclear cell infiltrate around the islet, followed by intra-islet accumulation. The lesion finally resolves when the beta cells have disappeared. Changes may be asynchronous in different parts of the pancreas. There is no current agreement on the composition of the infiltrate, especially regarding the nature of Ia^+ mononuclear cells (Bedossa *et al.*, 1989; Signore *et al.*, 1989). B cells and T cells (predominantly $L3T4^+$ helper cells) are both present but monocytes and macrophages are probably the earliest and most important cell type to appear in insulitis (Signore *et al.*, 1989). The T cells are activated as judged by their expression of IL-2 receptors.

As already mentioned, specific NOD T cell clones can transfer diabetes and this is also the case with unfractionated splenocytes (Wicker, Miller & Mullen, 1986). The latter phenomenon has been exploited to produce an accelerated model of disease, but in such animals, co-transfer of $CD4^+$ spleen cells from those NOD mice which are not diabetic inhibits the development of diabetes, implying the existence of suppressor cells in this population (Boitard *et al.*, 1989). Further circumstantial evidence supporting T cell-mediated control of disease is provided by the results of thymectomy, which accelerates the onset of diabetes if performed within three weeks of birth, possibly as a result of suppressor cell loss (Dardenne *et al.*, 1989). These effects of thymectomy are age and sex dependent.

It is unclear whether NOD beta cells express Ia (or MHC class II) antigens *in vivo*. In one study, Ia expression was detected in all islets with insulitis and in half of those without (Hanafusa *et al.*, 1987), while more recent studies have concluded that all islet cells are Ia-negative, irrespective of the stage of disease (Signore *et al.*, 1989; Jacob *et al.*, 1990). This uncertainty casts doubt on a role for aberrant Ia expression as an initiating event in autoimmunity (Bottazzo *et al.*, 1989) at least for this model of diabetes. Moreover, transgenic mice expressing class II MHC molecules on their beta cells do not develop insulitis: paradoxically, such beta cells may induce peripheral tolerance, as discussed in Chapter 1 (Lo *et al.*, 1988). In other transgenic lines, T cells do not become tolerised to I-E antigens expressed by beta cells, but nonetheless autoimmune insulitis does not develop (Götz, Eibel & Köhler, 1990). Thus, aberrant MHC class II expression on beta cells alone is insufficient to provoke the development of autoimmune diabetes in mice. An alternative role for class II expression, if indeed it does occur in NOD islets, could be to permit beta cell recognition by $CD4^+$ cytotoxic T cells. NOD beta cells become Ia^+ *in vitro* after culture with γ-IFN, whereas those from (CBA × NOD) F_1 hybrids do not, due to a *trans*-acting regulatory factor on the CBA genome (Leiter *et al.*, 1989). Thus, NOD beta cells seem unusually susceptible to Ia expression. A novel Qa-like MHC antigen also appears on the beta cell surface under these conditions, which could participate in cytotoxic response, possibly mediated by $\gamma\delta$ receptor-bearing T cells.

B cell responses

Autoantibodies typical of human diabetes are found in NOD mice. About half of these animals have islet cell cytoplasmic or surface antibodies by 20 weeks, but these later disappear (Reddy, Bibby & Elliott, 1988) and antibodies against an islet cell-specific protein of 64 kd can be detected by immunoprecipitation in the majority of diabetic mice (Atkinson & Maclaren, 1988). Insulin antibodies are present long before disease and also occur in a quarter of young control mice, but in them do not persist (Michel, Boitard & Bach, 1989). A role for any of these antibodies in disease is unclear and *in vivo* B cell depletion has no effect on the successful transfer of diabetes, when performed on either the transferred effector cell population or the recipient animals (Bendelac *et al.*, 1988). Thus, B cell-mediated islet cell autoreactivity is probably a secondary event that is not essential to the inception of the disease. NOD mice also have cytotoxic antibodies against lymphocytes and increased serum levels of total IgG. The distribution of these phenomena in F_1 mice indicates a genetically determined predisposition to B cell polyclonal activation, which is independent of the cell-mediated processes leading to diabetes (Lehuen *et al.*, 1990).

Effector mechanisms

Although $L3T4^+$ T cells can transfer disease, this does not indicate they have a direct pathogenic role, as other effector cells could be recruited for this purpose in the recipient animal. Depletion experiments with mono-clonal antibodies against Lyt-2 have demonstrated the requirement for this

MHC class I-restricted cytotoxic/suppressor population to induce diabetes (Charlton, Bacelj & Mandel, 1988). A cytotoxic role is suggested by the fact that $CD8^+$ cells located within the islets of NOD mice with insulitis express the cytolytic protein, perforin, although these constitute only 5% of all $CD8^+$ cells present and have yet to be demonstrated destroying beta cells (Young et al., 1989). However, by in vitro stimulation with IL-2, Lyt-2^+ T cells can be derived from NOD islets which kill cultured islet cells in a tissue-specific and class-restricted fashion (Nagata et al., 1989), supporting the participation of cytotoxic T cells in disease pathogenesis.

Administration of silica inhibits macrophage function and NOD mice so treated fail to develop diabetes (Charlton et al., 1988). This could be because there is failure of antigen presentation, but silica may also prevent macrophage participation in the effector phase. For instance, a variety of cytokines from macrophages (and T cells) may modulate islet cell function. In particular, IL-1 and γ-IFN inhibit DNA synthesis and hormone release by transformed murine islet cells, although both alpha and beta cells are affected (Hamaguchi & Leiter, 1990). As discussed below, any proposal for a role of cytokines in diabetes must take into account the exquisite beta cell specificity of the disease process. Paradoxically, the systemic administration of IL-1 or TNF prevents diabetes in NOD mice (Jacob et al., 1990). This may be explicable if locally produced cytokines achieve concentrations within the islet which inhibit endocrine cell function, whereas high levels of circulating cytokines non-specifically stimulate the unhealthy immune system of these mice, an action resembling the previously described beneficial effects of certain micro-organisms or adjuvant.

The Bio Breeding (BB) rat

These animals originate from a colony of Wistar rats, supplied by Bio Breeding Laboratories in Canada, in which a spontaneous mutation presumably caused diabetes (Chappel & Chappel, 1983). Derived colonies are indicated by suffixes, e.g. the Worcester, Massachusetts colony is designated BB/W. Clinical disease appears in 40–70% of animals at two to four months of age and closely resembles diabetes in man (Table 4.1, above). These features have recently been reviewed in detail (Baird, 1989). A discordant feature of this model is frequent lymphopenia, which renders the animals susceptible to infection and lymphoproliferative disorders. Diabetes can develop in rats without lymphopenia (and vice versa), but the lymphopenia is an important predisposing factor in the aetiology of disease under normal circumstances (Yale, Grose & Marliss, 1985; Like, Guberski & Butler, 1986a). As in the NOD mouse, there is a prediabetic period characterised by the appearance of insulitis two weeks before the onset of disease (Logothetopoulos et al., 1984). Prior even to this, there is increased expression of MHC class I and II molecules on the vascular endothelium (Dean *et al.*, 1985; Baird, 1989).

Immunogenetics

BB rats bear the MHC RT1^u haplotype and one of the diabetogenic genes is linked to the (two) class II genes in these animals (Colle *et al.*, 1988). At least one such allele is essential for the development of diabetes, although the exact class II subregion responsible is unknown. As in the NOD mouse, there is a serine at position 57 of the RT1.B and RT1.D class II β chains in BB rats, but the same is true of non-diabetic BB animals and those of Lewis strain, which also does not develop diabetes (Chao *et al.*, 1989). Thus, these allelic forms of class II molecules, based on differences in the amino acid encoded for at position 57, are not directly responsible for disease suscepti-bility. Instead, class II-linked genes may be associated with diabetes because they control the level of expression of class II gene products. This is suggested by the appearance of increased RT1.D mRNA levels in splenic lymphocytes from BB animals, compared to those from histocompatible Wistar rats (Holowachuk, Greer & Martin, 1988). Non-MHC loci also contribute to disease susceptibility, including an important enhancing effect of the gene controlling lymphopenia. In non-lymphopenic animals, diabetes may appear as an alternative genetic syndrome if other genes substitute for the effect of lymphopenia. It is possible that the class II genes could operate after these unknown loci have induced insulitis, as in the NOD mouse, so that both non-MHC- and MHC-linked genes are necessary for full disease expression.

Environmental factors

The incomplete penetrance of disease in this strain echoes that in NOD mice and in monozygotic twins with diabetes, implying the additional effect of environmental factors on genetic predisposition. Spontaneous diabetes occurs in germ-free animals (Rossini *et al.*, 1979), but this does not exclude a role for infection mediated by endogenous viruses. By contrast, myco-plasma infection may reduce the incidence of diabetes, possibly by stimu-lating an unstable immune system (Baird, 1989). Sex hormones do not appear to influence disease, as there is no difference between males and females in the incidence of diabetes. Repeated substantial stress, provoked by restraint, rotation, crowding and resocialisation, leads to an earlier onset of diabetes, which may be mediated through neuroendocrine effects on the immune system (Carter *et al.*, 1987).

Again reflecting similar findings in the NOD mouse, a defined, semipuri-fied diet prevents insulitis and diabetes and improves the lymphopenia of BB rats (Scott *et al.*, 1985). A variety of factors may be involved in this effect. As well as toxins and antigens in the food, modulation of beta cell function by the diet composition could alter autoantigen expression by these cells. This has been explored further by giving neonatal BB rats glucose with glucagon or arginine to stimulate their immature beta cells, a manoeuvre which reduced the subsequent incidence of diabetes by two-thirds (Buschard *et al.*, 1990a). Early maturation of beta cells, for instance by exposure to hyperglycaemia during a diabetic pregnancy, may therefore protect against disease. The exact mechanism for this effect remains unclear.

T cell responses

The first cells to infiltrate the islets are macrophages, followed by predominantly $CD4^+$ T cells (Dean *et al.*, 1985; Walker *et al.*, 1988). Transfer of mitogen-activated splenocytes from animals with acute diabetes produces disease in young BB rats (Koevary *et al.*, 1983) and $CD4^+$ T cell lines have been isolated from the pancreas and spleen of diabetic rats which are specific for islet cell antigens (Prud'homme *et al.*, 1984). Further evidence for T cell-mediated disease is provided by the results of neonatal thymectomy, which prevents disease (Like *et al.*, 1982).

T cells are therefore critical for the development of disease. There also seems to be a thymic abnormality in these animals responsible for their lymphopenia (Plamondon *et al.*, 1990). Reduced numbers of intrathymic macrophages are found at birth in BB rats (Van Rees, Voorbij & Dijkstra, 1988) and diabetes can be prevented by transplantation of thymic antigen presenting cells from diabetes-resistant BB animals (Georgiou & Bellgrau, 1989). Abnormal thymic maturation results in loss of most of the $CD4^+$ and almost all the $CD8^+$ T cells (those which remain are NK cells). It may also lead to failure of intrathymic tolerance, preventing deletion of islet cell-specific T cells. Alternatively, the lymphopenia may result in inadequate levels of suppressor cells capable of down-regulating the autoimmune response. Transfusion of T cells from non-diabetic BB animals prevents disease, indicating the normal existence of lymphocytes in unaffected rats with the capacity to modulate the diabetogenic T cell repertoire of the diabetes-prone BB line (Rossini *et al.*, 1984).

In the rat, a proportion of $CD4^+$ and $CD8^+$ mature T cells expresses the RT6 differentiation molecule and it is this subset which is the most decimated in BB lymphopenia (Angelillo *et al.*, 1988). However, experimental depletion of $RT6^+$ cells alone is insufficient to induce diabetes in diabetes-resistant BB rats, although additional exogenous stimulation (with mitogens or sterile faecal suspension) will result in disease (Like, 1990). Another non-specific signal which modifies T cells is IL-2 and its administration to a low-responder line of BB rats increased disease incidence, although the opposite was true of high-responder animals (Zielasek *et al.*, 1990). It is possible that different levels of IL-2 inhibitors and thymic hormones in the two lines may explain these discordant results.

The potential role of Ia expression by pancreatic beta cells in stimulating T cells has been discussed already in regard to NOD mice. As in these animals, islet cells from diabetes-prone BB rats are far more susceptible to the induction of Ia expression by γ-IFN *in vitro* than islet cells from normal Wistar or diabetes-resistant BB animals (Walker *et al.*, 1986), but there is controversy over the existence of such class II expression by beta cells *in vivo*. Originally this was described as occurring late in disease, when in any case a major primary role in aetiology is unlikely (Dean *et al.*, 1985). However, a more detailed study by electron microscopy revealed that the Ia^+ cells staining immunohistochemically for insulin were in fact phagocytic leucocytes with intracellular insulin from destroyed and ingested beta cells (In't Veld & Pipeleers, 1988).

B cell responses

Antibodies recognising islet cell surface molecules, the islet cell 64 kd antigen and insulin are found in the prediabetic phase and in the majority of diabetic BB rats (Dyrberg *et al.*, 1982, 1984; Baekkeskov, Dyrberg & Lernmark, 1984; Laborie *et al.*, 1985; Dean *et al.*, 1987). There is little correlation between the antibodies, although islet cell surface antibodies are strongly associated with the development of diabetes. However, it is clear that diabetes may develop in some animals in the absence of any detectable antibodies, which could relate to assay insensitivity or the presence of other pathogenic autoantibodies. More likely, the humoral autoimmune response may only occur secondary to islet cell damage (see below). Antibodies against thyroglobulin and gastric parietal cells have been detected in some diabetic rats (Elder *et al.*, 1982; Chapter 8) and, like NOD mice, these animals also have lymphocyte antibodies, of uncertain significance but compatible with polyclonal activation (Dyrberg *et al.*, 1984).

Effector mechanisms

Islet cell surface antibodies fix complement and may be cytotoxic to beta but not alpha cells *in vitro* (Martin & Logothetopoulos, 1984; Laborie *et al.*, 1985). More recent analysis, relating such cytotoxicity to beta cell volume determined by biopsy, suggests that the appearance of these antibodies is a secondary reaction to ongoing loss of beta cells (Hehmke *et al.*, 1990). Whether humoral cytotoxicity participates in the rapid destruction of remaining beta cells after the onset of hyperglycaemia is not clear.

Administration of the Ox8 monoclonal antibody *in vivo*, which depletes $CD8^+$ cytotoxic T cells and NK cells, prevents the development of diabetes but not insulitis (Like *et al.*, 1986b). NK cell numbers and activity are increased in diabetes-prone animals compared to resistant BB lines (Woda & Biron, 1986). Another central effector cell is the macrophage. This is the initial and predominant cell type in the islet infiltrate and macrophage inactivation with silica prevents diabetes (Oschilewski, Kiesel & Kolb, 1985). Furthermore, islet cell killing by macrophages has been demonstrated *in vitro* and this activity is increased in the splenic macrophage population at the onset of diabetes, although there is much less correlation with the prior appearance of insulitis (Nagy *et al.*, 1989). These pathogenic effects may be mediated by cytokines, reactive oxygen metabolites or other active products released by macrophages. IL-1 has been investigated extensively in this regard, as discussed in the section on human disease, but the exquisite specificity of the autoimmune damage, which only affects the beta cells within the islet, is not readily explained by the known widespread effects of this and other cytokines.

While the injury is clearly beta cell-directed if it involves complement-fixing antibody, T cells or ADCC, it is unclear at present how this may be achieved for macrophage-mediated cytotoxicity. It is possible that beta cells are unusually prone to such non-specific damage, particularly if this operates in conjunction with sublethal injury produced in an antigen-specific fashion. It is interesting to note that systemic IL-1 at low doses actually prevents diabetes and thyroiditis in BB rats, whereas high-dose treatment accelerates the development of these disorders (Wilson *et al.*, 1990). These data do not support the idea that IL-1 is diabetogenic *per se,* suggesting instead that, systemically, it can modulate an ongoing immune response in a dose-dependent fashion. However, the local production of IL-1 and other cytokines could have powerful effects on beta cells which are not revealed by the indiscriminate form of delivery in these experiments.

Other forms of experimental autoimmune diabetes

Experimental diabetes has been described in many different settings but usually these models have derived from the exploration of potential environmental triggering factors, especially viruses. For example, Coxsackie B virus will induce diabetes in genetically predisposed mice, especially the C57BL/KS *db/db* mutant, although this differs from the human disease as there is an associated pancreatitis affecting the exocrine but not endocrine portion of the gland (Webb *et al.*, 1976). In the uninfected *db/db* mouse, hyperglycaemia and insulin insensitivity are notable features but even these may involve autoimmune mechanisms, as T cells and antibodies directed against islets appear before the onset of diabetes (Debray-Sachs *et al.*, 1983). This form of diabetes seems to depend on production of type C retrovirus by beta cells, accompanied by the presence of macrophages in close association with virus-expressing cells and by a perivascular and ductular infiltrate of lymphocytes (Leiter, 1985). Turning to the Coxsackie virus effect in this model, it has been shown that such infection generally decreases beta cell protein synthesis but enhances production of the 64 kd islet autoantigen two- to three-fold (Gerling, Nejman & Chatterjee, 1988). Therefore in certain situations, this picornavirus could enhance expression of a key autoantigen by injured beta cells, which may then engender an autoimmune response sufficient to administer the coup de grace. In such a scenario, the provocative virus may have already departed by the time such a culprit is sought.

Encephalomyocarditis virus induces strain-dependent diabetes in mice which can be the result of either direct damage to the beta cell or, in the BALB/cBy mouse, subclinical beta cell injury followed by autoimmune T cell-mediated destruction and hyperglycaemia (Jordan & Cohen, 1987). Diabetes in man may be triggered by congenital rubella virus infection, discussed below. This virus, when passaged in beta cells, can produce a similar diabetic syndrome in neonatal golden Syrian hamsters (Rayfield, Kelly & Yoon, 1986). Within a week of infection, the animals develop sustained hyperglycaemia and hypoinsulinaemia. These clinical manifestations are associated with the appearance of insulitis and islet cell cytoplasmic antibodies in about a third of animals, as well as viral localisation within the beta cell. Another example of experimental diabetes with an autoimmune component occurs with murine reovirus type 1 infection (Onodera et al., 1981, 1982). Insulitis has been documented in these animals and the disease can be prevented by immunosuppression. Infected mice also develop multiple tissue-reactive autoantibodies but their exact specificity and pathogenic relevance are unclear.

A sufficient dose of streptozotocin (an antineoplastic antibiotic) generally causes acute degeneration of beta cells, whereas repeated smaller doses in certain strains of mice produces a delayed but progressive increase in blood glucose, associated with insulitis and beta cell destruction. This syndrome may depend on the induction of endogenous retroviruses within the beta cell (Appel et al., 1978). Treatment with monoclonal antibodies directed against either the $L3T4^+$ or $Lyt-2^+$ T cell subset prevents the development of diabetes in this model, and indeed both T lymphocyte populations are present in the islet infiltrate, together with a large number of macrophages (Kantwerk et al., 1987).

The evidence from these models shows that autoimmune responses against the beta cell can be induced by a variety of viruses and a chemical toxin, streptozotocin, which in turn produce similar forms of diabetes, (although the histology in some cases is unlike that seen in typical disease in man). An important role for endogenous retroviruses is also suggested by these models. The specificity of such agents for the beta cell may explain why only these cells within the islets are damaged in diabetes.

Summary

Considerable insight has been gained from animals with spontaneous and induced disease into the complexity of the processes which may injure the beta cells in diabetes. Both spontaneous models closely resemble human diabetes despite important differences such as the profound lymphopenia in BB rats and the female preponderance in diabetic NOD mice. Data have accumulated in both strains in a parallel fashion and the results are remarkably similar. The importance of MHC and non-MHC genes in determining susceptibility is clearly evident, although the concept of an all-pervasive importance of amino acid substitutions at position 57 in MHC class II beta chains has had to be modified by recent data in these animals. A variety of environmental factors modify disease expression to give incomplete penetrance of disease and variation in incidence between colonies. Especially noteworthy are the suppressive rather than stimulatory effects of some infectious agents and a significant role for dietary constituents. Both $CD4^+$ and $CD8^+$ T cells play a part in disease initiation and evolution, whereas a role for islet cell and insulin autoantibodies in pathogenesis is much less clear. Considerable emphasis has been placed on a role for Ia expression by beta cells as an initiating event in diabetes and other auto-immune disorders, but experiments with transgenic mice suggest that this may actually tolerise T cells in some circumstances and fail to provoke autoreactivity in others. Moreover, in neither the NOD nor BB animal models is there unequivocal evidence of beta cells expressing Ia, despite histological features which otherwise seem similar to the human disease, and there are no data to show that beta cells can present antigen. Macrophages appear early and constitute a major proportion of the islet infiltrate. Because their functional impairment with silica prevents experimental diabetes, it seems likely that these are important autoantigen presenting cells. They may also have an effector role.

Human diabetes

As in animals, diabetes in man is caused by a combination of genetic and environmental factors. This interaction is illustrated by the wide range of incidence in divergent areas and ethnic groups (Diabetes Epidemiology Research International Group, 1988). The age-adjusted annual incidence in children aged under 15 years ranges from 1.7 per 100 000 in Japan to 29.5 per 100 000 in Finland. While some of this disparity seems due to genetic differences, the distribution of known HLA-D region markers are similar in European patients in whom there may be considerable inequality of risk depending on their country of origin. British cohort birth studies suggest that diabetes is now manifest at an earlier age in susceptible subjects and tends to occur in socially advantaged families (Kurtz, Peckham & Ades, 1988). Together with information from migrant studies and temporal changes in incidence in other countries (Diabetes Epidemiology Research International Group, 1988), this indicates an important contribution from environmental factors.

It is also possible that such ethnic, social and temporal heterogeneity may reflect the occurrence of several discrete diabetic syndromes which appear clinically to be a single entity. Certain patients have histopathological features in keeping with this idea, as discussed below. In addition, patients have been divided into two groups, 1a, in which the autoimmune disease follows viral infections and 1b, in which there is a primary autoimmune aetiology (Bottazzo et al., 1978). However, the distinction between these two types is unclear and subsequent immunogenetic analysis has not supported any obvious heterogeneity. Diabetic patients generally have a much higher than expected prevalence of autoantibodies, besides those directed against the islet (reviewed by Drell & Notkins, 1987), and may develop polyendocrine autoimmune disease (Chapter 8). Although this may well be related to a genetically determined increase in susceptibility, it is also conceivable that environmental triggers (e.g. a virus) or the disease process itself may contribute to enhanced autoreactivity.

Access to the diabetic pancreas is obviously exceedingly difficult in man and determining the pathology of the disorder has relied on post-mortem analysis. Lymphocytic infiltration of the islets of Langerhans has been observed in 78% of 60 patients dying with disease of less than one year's duration and was only present in those islets with surviving beta cells (Foulis et al., 1986). The distribution of lesions may be patchy and sampling error could therefore account for some of the remaining patients without insulitis. Alternatively, the lesions could have already disappeared at the time of death, while in four young patients the histopathology suggested a different disease to classical type 1 diabetes, as beta cell numbers were normal and there was no insulitis. In the majority of diabetic patients, however, the earliest occurrence of lymphocytes is at the periphery of islets with a normal complement of beta cells. Thereafter, a diffuse inflammatory infiltrate within the islet and a marked drop in beta cell numbers are found. Later still, islets contain no beta cells, although the proportion of cells containing glucagon, somatostatin and pancreatic polypeptide is probably normal, and the insulitis disappears. This complete process may take up to six years from diagnosis. There may also be a focal or diffuse lymphocytic infiltrate in the exocrine pancreas, affecting 10–20% of patients.

Immunogenetics

Genetic susceptibility to diabetes is an important but not inexorable component of the disorder. Monozygotic twins are only 36% concordant for diabetes and less than 10% of the non-identical twins and sibs of an affected patient develop the disease (Leslie & Pyke, 1986). Even with identical MHC haplotypes, the sibling risk for diabetes is 12.9%, falling to 4.5% if one haplotype is shared and 1.8% if neither haplotype is common, although this is still more than four-fold higher than the risk in a random population (Thomson *et al.*, 1988). Thus several genes, including some lying outside the MHC, contribute to genetic susceptibility. Many studies have examined the immunogenetics of diabetes, reviewed extensively elsewhere (Wassmuth & Lernmark, 1989). The emphasis in the present section will be on more recent developments in this area.

The first reported MHC associations were with HLA-B15 and HLA-B8 in Caucasians (Singal & Blajchman, 1973; Cudworth & Woodrow, 1975). However, it soon became apparent that a stronger association exists with DR3 and DR4, DR3 being in linkage disequilibrium with B8 and DR4 with B15 (Platz *et al.*, 1981). Numerous studies have confirmed this. About 95% of Caucasian diabetics are HLA-DR3 and/or -DR4, compared to 45–55% of controls (Tiwari & Terasaki, 1985). Furthermore, there is synergy between DR3 and DR4, the relative risk for DR3/4 heterozygotes being higher than for DR3 or DR4 homozygotes or individuals who have one of these alleles in combination with other types (Rotter *et al.*, 1983; Wolf, Spencer & Cudworth, 1983). Extensive family studies of affected siblings have confirmed this effect of DR3/4 heterozygosity (Thomson *et al.*, 1988). In non-heterozygotes, there may be independent dominant- and recessive-like modes of inheritance for DR4 and DR3 respectively, although further data are required to confirm this, as there may be a more complex pattern of DR4 inheritance in particular.

Together, these findings suggest that in Caucasians two separate susceptibility genes exist, which are MHC-encoded and in linkage disequilibrium with DR3 and DR4. After allowing for the susceptibility produced by DR3 and DR4, there is also a weak, positive association of HLA-DR1 with diabetes. An additional feature revealed by HLA typing is the apparently protective effect of certain MHC haplotypes (Tiwari & Terasaki, 1985). In particular, HLA-DR2 is rare in diabetic patients and a weaker negative association has been noted with DR5. Until recently it was difficult to distinguish between the possible protective action of these alleles and their simple diminution relative to the excess of DR3 and DR4 in the diabetic population. As discussed below, the absence of only certain haplotypes associated with these DR alleles suggests a protective effect rather than a result due to non-specific overtransmission of other alleles.

The HLA-DR associations in non-Caucasians are somewhat similar but not identical. Because different haplotypes may be associated with particular alleles in certain ethnic groups, these studies have provided useful data for trans-racial mapping of susceptibility loci. In Japan the strongest association is with DR4/9 heterozygotes, giving a relative risk of 5.7, which is about twice that for one allele without the other (Kida *et al.*, 1989). DR3 and DR9 are associated with diabetes in Chinese patients (relative risks 8.1 and 2.0) and again, individuals (aged less than 20 years) heterozygous for both alleles have an enhanced susceptibility, the relative risk being 17 (Hawkins *et al.*, 1987). In Blacks (predominantly Jamaican) resident in the UK, there are associations with DR3, 4, 7 and 9, but that with DR3 is weak (relative risk 1.8). The association is strongest for DR4 (relative risk 20), while DR2 is negatively associated (Fletcher *et al.*, 1988).

However, the DR subregion does not itself contain the key disease susceptibility locus. Only certain DR3 or DR4 haplotypes are associated with diabetes in Caucasians (Raum *et al.*, 1984; Tuomilehto-Wolf *et al.*, 1989), suggesting that the whole haplotype may be important in determining susceptibility and that other genes in linkage disequilibrium with DR3 or DR4 could confer even greater susceptibility. This latter possibility was initially explored and confirmed by RFLP analysis. A DQB *Bam* HI restriction fragment of 3.7 kb, associated with DR4, was present in a third of controls yet almost absent in diabetics (Owerbach *et al.*, 1983; Michelsen *et al.*, 1985) and subsequent studies using a DQB probe with various restriction enzymes found other RFLP patterns that were significantly associated with the DR4-related susceptibility to diabetes (Cohen-Hagenauer *et al.*, 1985; Bohme *et al.*, 1986; Festenstein *et al.*, 1986; Nepom *et al.*, 1986). In particular, two main DQB1 loci, DQw7 and DQw8 (previously termed DQw3.1 and DQw3.2) are in linkage disequilibrium with DR4 but only DQw8 has a positive association with diabetes, that with DQw7 being negative. It also became clear from RFLP analysis that the negative association of DR2 with diabetes was due to the absence of a particular haplotype, as a normal, DR2-associated *Bam* H1 fragment hybridising with a DQB probe was almost undetectable in diabetics (Cohen *et al.*, 1984). Further studies have established that most DR2-positive diabetics belong to a particular haplotype, now termed the DRw16 subgroup of DR2 (originally identified by the cellular specificity DwAZH), while the DRw15 subgroup is negatively associated with diabetes (Cohen-Hagenauer *et al.*, 1985; Bohme *et al.*, 1986). These DR and DQ associations are summarised in Table 4.2. It is important to note that an already complex issue has been made more so by the introduction of new nomenclature for some of the alleles. The key changes with regard to diabetes are also shown in Table 4.2.

The next major step in determining the nature of these positive and negative DQB1 gene associations came from direct sequence analysis (Todd

Table 4.2. *Main HLA-DR and -DQ haplotypes and their association with diabetes in Caucasians (Todd et al., 1987)*

HLA-DR[a]	HLA-DQ[b]	Association	Position 57 on DQβ chain[c]
1	w1.1 (w5)[d]	Positive	Valine
2 (w15)	w1.2 (w6)	Negative	Aspartic acid
2 (w16)	w1.AZH (w5)	Positive	Serine
3 (w17)	w2	Positive	Alanine
4	w3.1 (w7)	Negative/neutral	Aspartic acid
4	w3.2 (w8)	Positive	Alanine
5	w3.1 (w7)	Negative/neutral	Aspartic acid
w6 (w13)	w1.18 (w6)	Negative	Aspartic acid
w6 (w13)	w1.19 (w6)	Positive	Valine
7	w2	Neutral	Alanine

[a] Only the major HLA-DR alleles are shown.
[b] HLA-DQB1 gene in linkage disequilibrium with DR allele producing the haplotype.
[c] Amino acid encoded by each DQB1 gene at position 57 on the β chain first domain.
[d] Designations in parenthesis are recently applied names; the other terms were used up to about 1989 (WHO-HLA Nomenclature Committee, 1988).

et al., 1987). The first domains of the DRB1, DQA1 and DQB1 genes in diabetics were identical to healthy controls, ruling out mutant class II alleles as a reason for MHC-linked susceptibility. By focussing on the two main DR4-linked DQB1 genes (there are no DQA1 gene differences), it became apparent that four discordant amino acids are encoded by the DQw7 and DQw8 alleles. Only one of these, at position 57, correlated with disease susceptibility or resistance when other DQB1 genes were analysed. All of the DQB1 alleles positively associated with diabetes (DR4-DQw8, DR3-DQw2, DR1-DQw5 and DR2-DQw5) encode alanine, valine or serine (conservative substitutions) at this position, whereas all those with a neutral or negative association (DR4-DQw7, DR2-DQw6, DRw13–DQw6) encode a negatively charged aspartate (Asp) residue at this position (Table 4.2).

This dichotomy was confirmed by DQB1 typing, using PCR enzymatic amplification of the DQB1 first domain and oligonucleotide probes specific for the sequences encoding the position 57 amino acid. The results from this study suggested that this position on the DQβ chain played a critical role in determining susceptibility. In particular, individuals heterozygous for Asp at this position had a relatively low risk of diabetes, whereas Asp-57 homozygosity provided almost complete protection. On the other hand, homozygosity for two Asp-57-negative DQB1 alleles appeared necessary, but not sufficient, for disease susceptibility. This amino acid residue is probably situated on the alpha helix and in the antigen-binding groove of the assembled DQ molecule. At this site it may be critical to the interaction between the α and β chains, affecting both the structure and function of the dimer.

Since this landmark study, a number of observations have indicated that additional factors are involved in the HLA associations with diabetes, as indeed originally proposed by Todd *et al.* (1987). Several lines of evidence argue for this. For instance, DR7 is neutral in its association with diabetes in Caucasians, yet shares the same DQw2 haplotype with DR3, which is positively associated. On the other hand, DR1 has only a weak positive association despite being non-Asp-57. Sequence comparison of DQB1 homologues in the BB rat or NOD mouse with non-diabetic strains originally suggested similar protective or susceptibility associations based on the presence or absence of Asp-57 (Todd *et al.*, 1987), but further analysis has revealed exceptions, as detailed above.

The applicability of the Asp-57 rule to different racial groups has also been investigated, as direct involvement of the DQB1 locus in susceptibility should operate in all situations if it is these, rather than linked genes, which determine susceptibility. However, the unique diabetogenic DR7 haplotype in Blacks (Fletcher *et al.*, 1988) shares the same DQB1 sequence as the DR7 haplotype in Caucasians which has no association with diabetes (Todd *et al.*, 1989). Furthermore, Asp-57 does not protect against diabetes in Japanese and Chinese patients and non-Asp-57 containing alleles of DQB1 (particularly DQw8) are no more frequent in Japanese patients compared to controls (Yamagata *et al.*, 1989; Erlich *et al.*, 1990; Todd *et al.*, 1990). While it is possible that the high frequency of Asp-57 DQB1 alleles in Japanese and Chinese populations could account for the low prevalence of diabetes in these populations (Bao *et al.*, 1989), these results clearly rule out the provision of complete protection by Asp-57 and suggest the influence of other loci besides DQB1 on disease susceptibility.

Investigation has therefore extended to the contribution made by DQA1 as well as DQB1 genes to DQ-related susceptibility. For instance, one possible explanation for the increased susceptibility of DR3/4 heterozygotes is that hybrid DQ molecular dimers could form, comprised of α and β chains encoded in *trans* (i.e. on the two separate haplotypes: see Chapter 2). Such hybrid DQ molecules have been found in diabetes, but whether these recognise novel determinants, or even have a role in disease, is unknown (Nepom *et al.*, 1987). Involvement of the DQA1 locus does provide an explanation for a paradox previously mentioned, namely that the DR7 haplotype confers no positive risk in Caucasians, despite sharing the same DQB1 locus as DR3. In contrast, a unique DR7 haplotype is associated with diabetes in Jamaican Black patients (Table 4.3). The only difference between the two races in their DR7 haplotypes is at the DQA1 locus, the A2

Table 4.3. *Association of diabetes with various haplotypes in Caucasian and Black populations (Todd et al.*, 1989)

Race	Haplotype			Association
	DQA1[a]	DQB1[a]	DRB1[a]	
Caucasian	A2	DQw2	DR7	Neutral
Black	A3	DQw2	DR7	Positive[b]
Caucasian	A3	DQw9	DR9	Neutral
Black	A3	DQw2	DR9	Positive[c]
Caucasian/Black	A4	DQw2	DR3	Positive
Black	A4	DQw4	DR3	Neutral[d]

[a] Expressed genes on the haplotypes: see Fig. 2.2
[b] Association correlates with the DQA1 A3 allele on this haplotype
[c] Association correlates with the Asp-57-negative β chain encoded by the DQB1 DQw2 allele
[d] DQB1 DQw4 encodes an Asp-57. This is in linkage disequilibrium with DRw18 (DR3) on some Black haplotypes. DQw2 encodes an alanine residue at position 57 and is in linkage with DRw17 (DR3) on all Caucasian and some Black haplotypes. Other differences on the two haplotypes could also play a role.

allele being present on the Caucasian haplotype and A3 on the Black (Todd *et al.*, 1989). The A3 allele is also present on the DR9, DQw2 haplotype, again associated with diabetes in Black subjects, whereas this particular DR9 haplotype is very rare in the Caucasian population, explaining why DR9 has a neutral effect in this group. On the other hand, A3 is found on Caucasian DR4 haplotypes, where it could exert an effect in combination with the appropriate DQB1 allele, DQw8. In the Japanese population, the effect of the A3 allele is even more striking, conferring a relative risk of 19.7, which is greater than any other MHC class II allele (Todd *et al.*, 1990). In essence, it is now apparent that DQA1 and DQB1 alleles combine to confer susceptibility and, because of race-specific haplotypes, their associations with diabetes will differ between ethnic groups.

Further attention has also been paid to the protective effect of Asp-57 haplotypes in Caucasians. A family study of 172 members of 27 diabetic families showed that such haplotypes were significantly increased among non-diabetic subjects, whereas only one of 26 diabetics was heterozygous Asp/non-Asp (Morel *et al.*, 1988). This suggests a dominant protective effect of Asp-57, confirmed in a population study of 266 unrelated diabetics, although in contrast to previous reports, only DQw6 (previously called DQw1.2) rather than other Asp-57 alleles appeared to be relevant in this respect (Baisch *et al.*, 1990). While the DR4, DQw8 haplotype conferred susceptibility in a dominant fashion as before (Todd *et al.*, 1987; Thomson *et al.*, 1988), the results also showed that the protective effect of DQw6 predominated over the predisposition created by DQw8, as the relative risk for diabetes in heterozygous DQw6/DQw8 subjects was 0.37 (i.e. below 1.0).

The mechanism for the protective effect of Asp-57 alleles has not been established. Arguments have been advanced for these acting as immune suppression genes controlling the generation and function of beta cell-specific T suppressor cells, but the evidence for this so far is circumstantial (Oliveira & Peters, 1990). A more likely effect, compatible with the data from NOD mice, is that diabetogenic T cells may be deleted by Asp-57 alleles, although direct analysis of the T cell repertoire will be needed to confirm this. As discussed in Chapter 1, such negative selection is unlikely to be flawless, which would account for the incomplete protection observed.

This scrutiny of DQ genes was the result of observations on DR-linked haplotypes and studies recently have focussed back on the contribution made by non-DQ loci in these diabetogenic haplotypes. An added role for DR genes has been suggested by subtyping of DR4 alleles. Statistical analysis of various diabetic haplotypes thus identified indicated that maximal risk was produced by the appropriate combination of alleles at both the DQB1 and DRB1 loci (Sheehy *et al.*, 1989). This is comparable with the NOD mouse in which susceptibility is conferred by a null allele at I-E (equivalent to DR) and a particular susceptibility allele at I-A (DQ analogue). Two separate effects were proposed to explain the DR3 association with diabetes. As well as being associated with a non-Asp-57 DQB1 allele, DR3 has a non-specific enhancing effect on the immune system. This has already been discussed in Chapter 2 and may apply to many other autoimmune diseases, including most of those affecting the endocrine system.

A further possibility is that DR3 may be in linkage disequilibrium with yet other MHC genes conferring susceptibility. Both the HLA-B8, -DR3 haplotype and B18, DR3 haplotype have been associated with diabetes. In DR3/4 heterozygous French patients, Dw25 (associated with the B18, DR3 haplotype) confers an increased risk over Dw24 (associated with B8, DR3: Martell *et al.*, 1990). Another study, which highlighted associations with genes lying telomeric to the D region, examined C4 complement allotypes encoded in the class III region (Fig. 2.1). A significant association of diabetes with the C4A3 and C4B3 markers was found in DR3/4 heterozygotes when compared with DR3/4 controls (Thomsen *et al.*, 1988). The reasons for this are unknown. However, TNF is encoded between the HLA-B and C4 loci and genetically determined variability in TNF production might be important in diabetes pathogenesis and thus explain these extended haplotypes. A RFLP of the TNF gene has recently been described which differed in distribution between diabetics and healthy subjects in a family study (Badenhoop *et al.*, 1989), supporting this possibility. Finally, a new susceptibility haplotype (A2, Cw1, Bw56, w6, DR4) has been described as the third most common in Finnish diabetics and was the most frequent haplotype transmitted from diabetic parent to affected proband (Tuomilehto-Wolf et al., 1989). This may explain the high incidence of diabetes in Finns and such results also emphasise the importance of considering the whole haplotype in this disorder.

There is no consensus on the role of DP loci, which lie centromeric to the D region, and show little or no linkage disequilibrium with DR or DQ genes. An abnormal distribution of DP alleles was found in one study by RFLP analysis that was independent of any DR3 or DR4 effect (Easteal et al., 1990). However, these patients were unusually old at age of onset (median 23 years) and thus may differ from the typical patient, explaining why a DP association has not been noted previously (Thomsen et al., 1988). Perhaps it is also worth mentioning at this point that temporal changes, as well as patient heterogeneity, may play a role in producing discordant results. In Finland, the association of diabetes with DR3 has decreased strikingly over the last three decades, particularly when this was not part of the B8, DR3 haplotype (Kontiainen et al., 1988). This change in genetically determined susceptibility may be linked to the increasing incidence of diabetes or alterations in environmental factors.

In both the NOD mouse and the BB rat, non-MHC genes are important determinants of susceptibility. The results already quoted at the beginning of this section, showing a relatively low risk of diabetes in siblings with shared MHC haplotypes, suggest that non-MHC genes are also important in man. As with thyroid autoimmunity, interest has so far focussed on immunoglobulin allotypes and RFLP analysis of the T cell receptor. There is some evidence that certain Gm allotypes may be associated with diabetes, possibly by interaction with HLA-encoded antigens (Dizier et al., 1986; Tait et al., 1986; Field, 1986). Heterozygosity for a T cell receptor $C\beta$ genotype detected by RFLP has been linked with diabetes in Caucasians, especially in concordant twins (Millward et al., 1987). However the allelic frequencies were similar in the patient and control groups. In a subsequent Japanese study, the allelic frequencies were different in diabetics and controls and an interaction with HLA-DR4 was apparent in diabetes (Ito et al., 1988). In contrast, a group of Finnish patients showed no association of disease with this $C\beta$ RFLP (Reijonen et al., 1990).

In summary, the MHC associations with diabetes are complex, reflecting disease heterogeneity, but exciting developments recently have unravelled some of the mysteries. The main reason for the observed DR associations is that DQ genes in linkage disequilibrium have a major role in determining susceptibility. DQB1 genes encoding Asp-57 exert an important protective effect which may be particularly restricted to certain alleles (e.g. DQw6). The high frequency of Asp-57 in the Japanese may explain their lower prevalence of diabetes. Nonetheless, possession of Asp-57 is not a complete guarantee against developing the disease. Other amino acids encoded by DQB1 at position 57 confer varying degrees of susceptibility, DQw8 being notably diabetogenic in Caucasians. As evident in other races, DQA1 genes make an important contribution to susceptibility. Other genes besides those in the DQ region are also involved. HLA-DR3 may be associated with diabetes because it non-specifically modifies the immune response or because certain DR3 haplotypes contain other loci which influence susceptibility, such as genes encoding and regulating TNF. Finally, non-MHC loci seem very likely to play a role in determining diabetogenic potential and there are preliminary data which suggest that immunoglobulin and T cell receptor genes may be involved, although this may depend on ethnic background. Further understanding of the immunogenetics of diabetes may allow individual screening to predict the likelihood of disease developing. This will be vital if therapy is to be given early enough to have a chance of curing disease (see below). Such developments are likely to emerge as future studies reveal the functional basis for the associations noted.

Environmental factors

Observations in experimental autoimmune diabetes clearly define an important role for the interaction of a number of environmental factors in determining whether or not disease develops. Epidemiological studies mentioned in the introduction to this section point to such a possibility in human diabetes, as does the low concordance in monozygotic twins. Some of this non-genetically determined variability in the incidence of diabetes could be due to stochastic events occurring during rearrangements of T cell receptor or immunoglobulin genes (Chapter 2). For instance, only one twin may produce an appropriate T cell receptor capable of beta cell recognition. However, this mechanism alone seems unlikely to account for the marked heterogeneity noted in family and population studies. Moreover, there is accumulating positive evidence for the involvement of environmental factors in the aetiology of diabetes.

Most attention has focussed on viruses and early studies are reviewed elsewhere, including evidence for seasonal variations, 'outbreaks' of diabetes and familial clustering (Notkins, 1977). Several mechanisms could lead viruses to induce diabetes, including (i) alteration of beta cell structure or function after direct infection, (ii) molecular mimicry, in which sequence homology between a viral epitope and a beta cell determinant results in an antiviral immune response also directed against beta cells and (iii) breakdown of tolerance as a result of (i) and (ii). The potential for viral infections to cause diabetes is demonstrated in transgenic mice whose beta cells express influenza virus haemagglutinin: about 20% of these animals develop hyperglycaemia, insulitis and islet cell antibodies (Roman *et al.*, 1990). A major problem in implicating viruses aetiologically in human disease is that a long prediabetic period exists, during which it is assumed active beta cell destruction occurs (Gorsuch *et al.*, 1981). Only when the remaining beta cell mass reaches a critical level (around 10% of normal) does clinically apparent diabetes supervene. Viral studies at this time may indicate the presence of an infection which, as a non-specific stress, precipitates ultimate decompensation – the straw that breaks the camel's back – but such analysis gives no information regarding earlier initiating events. For instance, in the UK, high titre antibodies to Coxsackie B4 were present more frequently in diabetics within three months of diagnosis than controls (Gamble *et al.*, 1969). This was supported by a combined study in England, Austria and Australia which also demonstrated that these were acute infections (Banatvala *et al.*, 1985). An excess of antibodies against mumps, rubella or cytomegalovirus was not detected.

Mumps virus has been implicated in other studies (Hyöty, Huupponen & Leinikki, 1985). An inverse correlation between islet cell and insulin autoantibodies and age was found in Finnish diabetic children, in whom there was also an inverse correlation between the presence of these autoantibodies and serological evidence of Coxsackie B4 or mumps virus infection (Karjalainen *et al.*, 1988). This observation raises another possible type of heterogeneity in diabetics by suggesting that a particular set of autoimmune responses may be critical in younger children, whereas viruses (presumably triggering other autoimmune mechanisms) may be more important with increasing age. Explicit evidence for virally-induced diabetes was provided by the isolation of Coxsackie B4 from the pancreas of a 10 year old child presenting with fatal diabetic ketoacidosis (Yoon *et al.*, 1979). Autopsy revealed insulitis plus beta cell necrosis and serological studies ante-mortem indicated a rise in virus neutralising antibodies from undetectable levels at the onset of illness. Furthermore, the isolated virus produced insulitis and hyperglycaemia on subsequent inoculation in SJL mice. This case is of extreme interest, but there were atypical clinical features in the presentation, particularly the coexistence of encephalitis which may have contributed to death.

All these studies have examined viruses in relation to the onset of disease; perhaps, as already discussed, a more critical aetiological role for viruses operates at the inception of the autoimmune process. A well-defined example of this occurs in the congenital rubella syndrome. Patients have a 40% prevalence of diabetes and many of the characteristic immunological features of classical diabetes, including the presence of circulating islet cell surface antibodies and susceptibility associated with HLA-DR3 and DR4, but not HLA-DR2 (Ginsberg-Fellner *et al.*, 1984). Congenital cytomegalovirus infection may also be associated with diabetes and a strong association has been described between the presence of islet cell antibodies in newly diagnosed diabetes and the detection of cytomegalovirus genome by *in situ* hybridisation in their peripheral blood lymphocytes (Pak *et al.*, 1988). However, the specificity and sensitivity of the hybridisation assay used have been questioned (Morris, Kimpton & Corbitt, 1988) and in any case further work would be required to substantiate a primary role for this virus in causing diabetes. In contrast to the animal models of diabetes, no human studies have examined the possibility that infection by viruses and other micro-organisms may be negatively associated with diabetes.

Dietary factors have also been implicated and these may explain differences between socio-economic groups in diabetes prevalence, as well as the increasing incidence in some countries. A prospective case-control study of recently diagnosed diabetic children revealed significant differences from controls in their dietary intake of protein, carbohydrates and nitrosamine compounds (Dahlquist *et al.*, 1990). Surveys such as this may be prone to errors in recall, but no obvious trend in this regard was observed and a clear effect of diet is apparent in experimental diabetes. Children born to diabetic mothers have only one-third the risk of developing diabetes compared to those whose fathers are diabetic, and there is no evidence to support selective loss of susceptible fetuses in diabetic mothers as an explanation for this phenomenon (Warram, Krolewski & Kahn, 1988). Although genetic mechanisms cannot be ruled out completely (Tuomilehto-Wolf *et al.*, 1989), this finding does suggest an environmental influence. Ia^+ and $4F2^+$ T cells are found in the cord blood of neonates born to diabetic mothers, markers of abnormal activation of the immune system in these fetuses (Di Mario *et al.*, 1987). A plausible but unproven possibility is suggested by the previously cited experiment in BB rats, namely that maternal hyperglycaemia stimulates fetal beta cells. These become less prone to subsequent autoimmune attack because increased beta cell autoantigen expression *in utero* increases tolerance induction. In this regard, it is notable that high glucose concentrations stimulate expression of the 64 kd autoantigen by islets *in vitro* (Kämpe *et al.*, 1989).

T cell responses

As already indicated in the introduction, insulitis is a characteristic feature of most patients with diabetes and T cells invade the islets in experimental diabetes. One factor which may perpetuate the infiltration is IL-6 production by beta cells (Campbell *et al.*, 1989a). As in the thyroid, this is enhanced by cytokines such as γ-INF and TNF, and local IL-6 secretion *in vivo* may then costimulate autoreactive T and B cells within the islets. In one patient who died within 24 hours of diagnosis, the islet infiltrate consisted of both $CD4^+$ and $CD8^+$ T cells, together with NK and B cells but apparently no macrophages (Bottazzo *et al.*, 1985). By contrast, insulitis was not seen in seven remarkable patients with newly diagnosed diabetes who consented to laparoscopic pancreatic biopsy (Hanafusa *et al.*, 1990), vividly illustrating the major problem that a long prediabetic period imposes on interpreting immunological responses tested after diagnosis. At this stage, some auto-immune phenomena may be secondary to beta cell destruction and others may be the result of the metabolic disturbances, while it is obvious that the response within the islet will have evolved considerably from the initial lesion.

Activated T cells are increased in the peripheral blood of newly diagnosed diabetics, identified by their expression of Ia or IL-2 receptor; in one study, the majority of these appeared to be $CD4^+$ (Jackson *et al.*, 1982; Hayward & Herberger, 1984; De Berardinis *et al.*, 1988a). There is no consensus on a decrease in CD4:CD8 ratio or abnormalities in the distribution of $CD45RA^+$ and $CD29^+$ subsets (Mandrup-Poulsen, 1988; De Berardinis *et al.*, 1988a; Faustman *et al.*, 1989). In a group of six prediabetic subjects, identified by screening the first degree relatives of patients, five had a decrease in CD4 : CD8 ratio in the year or two before diagnosis (Al-Sakkaf *et al.*, 1989). Activated T cells were observed in only two of these patients. Such changes in the phenotypes of circulating T cells may reflect the ongoing autoimmune process, but this is incomplete and totally non-specific.

Functional studies on T cells have been rather limited. Non-specific suppressor cell activity, assessed by blastogenic responses to concanavalin A and theophylline, was decreased in diabetic patients apparently in pro-portion to the impairment of their metabolic control (Crosti *et al.*, 1986). T cell sensitisation to a mixture of pancreatic antigens has been shown in about half of the diabetics tested by assays of MIF production (Nerup *et al.*, 1971). A decrease in islet cell antigen-specific suppressor activity has also been suggested, using the same MIF assay method as in autoimmune thyroiditis (Topliss *et al.*, 1983). Again, only about half the patients gave a positive MIF response to pancreatic antigen prior to the addition of putative suppressor cells. The nature of these responder and suppressor cells and the antigen recognised has not been identified. A variety of cytotoxic $CD4^+$ T cell clones have been obtained from the circulation of a newly diagnosed diabetic patient, one of which appeared to lyse histocompatible Ia^+ islet cells specifically, although the antigen, or even cell type, recognised was not defined (De Berardinis *et al.*, 1988b). Other $CD4^+$ clones have been derived which proliferate in response to insulin secretory granule proteins (Roep *et al.*, 1990). It is possible that such T cells could interact with the proteins expressed on the beta cell surface, but a formal pathological role has yet to be defined. Further analysis of autoreactive T cell clones and the autoanti-gens recognised by them will contribute greatly to the understanding of diabetic pathophysiology.

Considerable interest has been generated by the idea, discussed in Chapter 3, that Ia expression by endocrine cells may initiate autoimmunity (Bottazzo et al., 1989). MHC class II expression has been detected by immunohistochemistry on insulin-containing islet cells in diabetics (Bottazzo et al., 1985; Foulis & Farquharson, 1986; Hanafusa et al., 1990). This was observed in the presence or absence of insulitis, but was never found on other islet cell types. These Ia^+ cells also showed increased expression of class I molecules and in many patients heightened class I and II antigen staining was seen on the endothelium of blood vessels around the islet. The Ia^+ islet cells have been assumed to be beta cells, since there was no morphological evidence of necrosis or macrophage infiltration. However, this has not been subjected to the same ultrastructural scrutiny as in the BB rat, where a similar appearance was actually due to phagocytosis of beta cells by macrophages (In't Veld & Pipeleers, 1988). It is also doubtful that beta cells in NOD mice express Ia. Even if diabetic beta cells are Ia^+ in man, the observations made to date cannot define whether this expression precedes or follows the autoimmune response.

In vitro, class II expression can be induced on about 50% of normally Ia^- beta cells by the combination of γ-IFN and TNF or lymphotoxin; γ-IFN alone enhances class I expression but has no effect on Ia (Campbell et al., 1986; Pujol-Borrell et al., 1987). However, alpha and delta islet cells, containing glucagon and somatostatin respectively, also become Ia^+ with γ-IFN plus TNF, whereas Ia^+ cells containing these hormones have not been observed in diabetic islets. This at least questions the notion that γ-IFN and TNF induce beta cell Ia expression in vivo, unless there is differential sensitivity within the islet to these cytokines or their delivery is somehow directed to the beta cells. Autoantigen presentation by Ia^+ beta cells to T cells has not been demonstrated and transgenic mice expressing Ia on their beta cells do not develop autoimmune insulitis, although diabetes does occur in these animals, even if the entire class II molecule is not expressed (Lo et al., 1988; Götz et al., 1990). Diabetes also occurs, again without insulitis, in mice with transgenes causing beta cell overexpression of class I molecules (Allison et al., 1988).

The cause of diabetes in these animals is unknown but the results suggest that increased production of MHC molecules by beta cells damages the function of these cells. Thus, rather than triggering an autoimmune response, beta cell hyperexpression of class I and II MHC molecules, in response to so far undefined viruses, toxins or endogenous cytokines, could be a (non-immune) mechanism for beta cell failure (Harrison et al., 1989). In such a scheme, insulitis may not be required subsequently to produce diabetes (in keeping with histological evidence in some patients), or it could mediate a separate or additional pathway of beta cell destruction. This hypothesis leaves unexplained the predilection of beta cells for destruction, unless the initiating factors have tropism for these cells. It is also based on the assumption that the lifelong hyperexpression of MHC molecules in transgenic mice is quantitatively and qualitatively the same as in human diabetes, which intuitively seems unlikely. Furthermore, insulitis and beta cell-specific autoimmune responses are found in most diabetics and, if some of the transgenic mouse models of diabetes apply to man, the initial appearance of Ia molecules on beta cells would be expected to induce tolerance rather than autoimmunity. This is an area of intense interest which has produced some unexpected and exciting findings, but more data are required to build up a complete picture of the role for MHC molecule expression by beta cells in diabetes. At present, it is possible to hypothesise a number of consequences, ranging from tolerance induction to the initiation of autoimmunity; it is also conceivable that the phenomena observed *in vivo* are secondary events with little relevance to the pathogenesis of diabetes.

B cell responses

As indicated, little is known about the beta cell antigens recognised by autoreactive T cells in diabetes, but there is more information on the autoantigens which provoke antibody responses. The key autoantibodies are those against islet cell cytoplasm (ICAb), islet cell surface antigens (ICSAb), a 64 kd islet protein (64 kd Ab) and insulin. Antibodies to the insulin receptor are rare (<2% of patients) in type 1 diabetes (Rochet *et al.*, 1990), although these can cause the unusual diabetic syndrome of Type B insulin resistance when present in sufficient concentration, as discussed in Chapter 8.

ICAb are generally of low titre and detected by indirect immunofluorescence on sections of normal human pancreas (Bottazzo, Florin-Christensen & Doniach, 1974). This method causes problems in comparing studies from different laboratories, as the concordance between centres in ICAb detection ranges from 52% to over 90%, depending on the antibody concentration, due in part to variations in the pancreatic substrate (Bottazzo & Gleichmann, 1986). Inclusion of standard sera in assays now permits a certain degree of quantitation and precision, results being expressed in Juvenile Diabetes Foundation (JDF) units (Bonifacio *et al.*, 1990). The pathogenic relevance of these antibodies is questionable, since the antigen is not located on the cell surface and is present in all islet cell types, rather than exclusively in beta cells. A separate group of ICAb has been reported which bind complement (Bottazzo *et al.*, 1980), but this now simply appears to reflect the activity of conventional ICAb present in such sera at high concentrations (Bruining *et al.*, 1984).

Despite these caveats, ICAb are clearly related in some way to the autoimmune process in diabetes, as their detection in first degree diabetics'

relatives often, but not inevitably, correlates with the subsequent development of diabetes or impaired insulin responses to glucose (Srikanta et al.,
1985; Dean et al., 1986; Bonifacio et al., 1990). About a third of relatives
with detectable ICAb develop diabetes over a 10 year period, compared to
less than 1% of those without ICAb, and those with the highest ICAb titres
are at the greatest risk. The coexistence of insulin antibodies further
increases susceptibility (Dean et al., 1986; Betterle et al., 1987). At diagnosis, about 80% of diabetics have ICAb, although this later falls to 30%
after three to five years: those patients with the highest ICAb tend to lose
residual beta cell function the fastest (Peig et al., 1989).

ICSAb have been detected by immunofluorescence using human or rat
insulinoma or islet cells. In most newly diagnosed patients, these antibodies
bind exclusively to beta cells, but other cell types may also be stained by sera
from older diabetics and some healthy controls (Van De Winkel et al.,
1982). ICSAb are present in about two-thirds of newly diagnosed diabetics
and can occur in the presence or absence of ICAb (Lernmark et al., 1981).
Like ICAb, ISCAb tend to disappear in the years after diagnosis. One-third
of diabetics have antibodies which, in the presence of complement, are
cytotoxic to a rat insulinoma cell line, RINm 5F, as well as a somatostatin-
containing cell line, RINm 14B (Eisenbarth, Morris & Scearce, 1981).
Antibodies against RINm 5F cells can also be detected by flow cytometry in
the same proportion of newly diagnosed diabetics and tend to be associated
with the simultaneous occurrence of insulin antibodies (Lander et al., 1989).
However, the fact that these ICSAb also bind to a delta cell line makes their
pathogenic significance unclear.

Antibodies which immunoprecipitate a 64 kd protein from human islets
were first described in eight of 10 newly diagnosed diabetic children
(Baekkeskov et al., 1982). These 64 kd Ab were detectable in 11 of 14
diabetics 4–91 months before the onset of clinical diabetes, such patients
being followed because they were twins or first degree relatives of a diabetic
(Baekkeskov et al., 1987). Of 61 controls, including patients with thyroid
autoimmunity and SLE, the only positive subject had a diabetic sibling. This
predictive power of 64 kd Ab has recently been confirmed in a study showing
that such antibodies appear before ICAb or insulin antibodies in pre-
diabetes and are more frequently detectable than them (Atkinson et al.,
1990). The 64 kd antigen is primarily located in beta cells and may be
expressed on the cell surface (Christie et al., 1990). It appeared to be related
to an endogenous 65 kd hsp, based on (i) the recognition of the 64 kd antigen
by monoclonal antibodies against this hsp and (ii) the increase in 64 kd
antigen expression after cytokine treatment, suggesting that it is itself a
stress protein (Jones, Hunter & Duff, 1990). Although matched by similar
findings in the NOD mouse (Elias et al., 1990), subsequent work has shown
that the human 65 kd hsp is not islet cell specific and is physically separate

from the 64 kd protein, while sera from diabetic patients do not immuno-precipitate islet cell-derived 72, 75 and 90 kd hsp (Atkinson, Maclaren & Scharp 1990; Kämpe *et al.*, 1990). Moreover, recent studies indicate that the 64 kd antigen is the γ-aminobutyric acid-synthesising enzyme, glutamic acid decarboxylase, definitively separating this protein from a hsp (Baekkeskov *et al.*, 1990). Of interest, antibodies to this enzyme, located in γ-aminobutyric acid-secreting neurones, are found in the rare neurological condition, the stiff man syndrome, and patients with this disorder have a high prevalence of diabetes. It remains to be established whether cellular immune mechanisms may be involved in a response to the 65 kd (or any other) hsp in diabetes.

Insulin antibodies and their relationship to diabetes have been extensively reviewed elsewhere (Wilkin, 1990). Both radiobinding assays and ELISA have been used to detect insulin antibodies; there are some sera which react in one assay but not the other. In the first report of insulin antibodies in diabetes, about a third of newly diagnosed patients were found to be positive (Palmer *et al.*, 1983). Crucially, these antibodies were detectable before insulin therapy had begun and so could not have been due to an immune response against injected heterologous insulin. A similar prevalence of insulin antibodies has been discovered in other surveys and unaffected twins of long-standing diabetics may also have high but fluctuating levels (Wilkin *et al.*, 1985). These non-diabetic twins had little risk of developing disease, so it is clear that insulin antibodies are not very sensitive or specific markers. However, the presence of insulin antibodies predicts future diabetes in over 50% of first degree relatives and this risk is greater if ICAb are also positive (Ziegler *et al.*, 1989). Once positive for insulin antibodies, subjects usually remain so, irrespective of outcome. It is relatively easy in the detection assays to examine sera for the presence of anti-idiotypes, but these have not been detected (Kyner *et al.*, 1989). A high frequency of B cells committed to producing IgG insulin antibodies has been found in the circulation of newly diagnosed diabetics; such antibodies are monoreactive and have high affinity (Casali *et al.*, 1990).

Insulin autoantibodies are occasionally detected in other autoimmune disorders, particularly thyroiditis and connective tissue diseases. Drugs such as methimazole, penicillamine and hydrallazine have also been associated with their occurrence (Wilkin, 1989). Besides their association with diabetes, insulin antibodies can very rarely be responsible for spontaneous hypoglycaemia (usually reactive, occasionally fasting) in the so-called insulin autoimmune syndrome. This condition is reviewed extensively by Taylor *et al.* (1989). Originally described in Japan, the syndrome has been identified in Caucasians and affects both sexes at a wide variety of ages (Goldman *et al.*, 1979). In one recently studied patient, the antibodies were shown to be of monoclonal origin and the autoantigenic epitope of the insulin B-chain was identified (Uchigata *et al.*, 1989). Besides the hypoglycaemia, which draws attention to the syndrome, impaired glucose tolerance may also be seen. The mechanism for the hypoglycaemia seems to be slow release of insulin from a large pool bound to the antibody, which is not under feedback control: glucose intolerance results from rapid binding of released insulin after a glucose challenge. Although rare (123 cases reported up to 1987), this syndrome is important to identify as some patients, misdiagnosed as having an insulinoma, have undergone pancreatectomy.

Effector mechanisms

Whatever causes beta cell destruction in diabetes must be specific for these particular islet cells and must operate over a prolonged period to affect individual islets asynchronously. The evidence that T cells and antibodies may be involved has already been mentioned and, for obvious reasons, is nowhere near as extensive as in experimental diabetes. Both humoral and T cell-mediated cytotoxicity to islet cells *in vitro* have been demonstrated and therefore some role for these mechanisms seems credible. It remains unclear whether they operate in the initiation phase of disease or simply perpetuate the process. Leaving aside questions of beta cell specificity, the presence of islet-reactive antibodies in individuals who are unlikely to develop diabetes and their absence in a sizeable proportion of diabetic patients both suggest that humoral mechanisms are unlikely to be prime movers. All islet cells express ICAM-1 *in vitro* in response to γ-IFN or TNF and this could increase the potential for their recognition and killing by cytotoxic T and NK cells (Campbell *et al.*, 1989b).

The results in NOD mice and BB rats described previously suggest a major role for macrophages (and NK cells) in experimental diabetes, at least partly mediated by cytokines. The specificity of such effector cells and cytokines would depend on heightened sensitivity of the beta cells, compared with alpha and delta cells, unless ADCC were involved. In man, most attention has focussed on the islet cell injury produced *in vitro* by cytokines, particularly IL-1 (Mandrup-Poulsen, 1988). IL-1β, but not IL-1α, reduces beta cell insulin content and release, whereas lymphotoxin and γ-IFN have no effect (Bendtzen *et al.*, 1986). TNF has only a weak inhibitory action. The inhibition of insulin release by IL-1 requires relatively high concentrations of this cytokine (2–6 ng/ml) and lower concentrations actually stimulate insulin release (Spinas *et al.*, 1986). These dual activities have been confirmed in assays of glucose-stimulated insulin secretion by islets *in vitro* (Comens *et al.*, 1987). Actual destruction of rat islet cell monolayers has been observed after culture with a combination of TNF and γ-IFN (Pukel, Baquerizo & Rabinovitch, 1988). Furthermore, ultrastructural degenerative changes induced by IL-1 alone have been described, specifically affecting

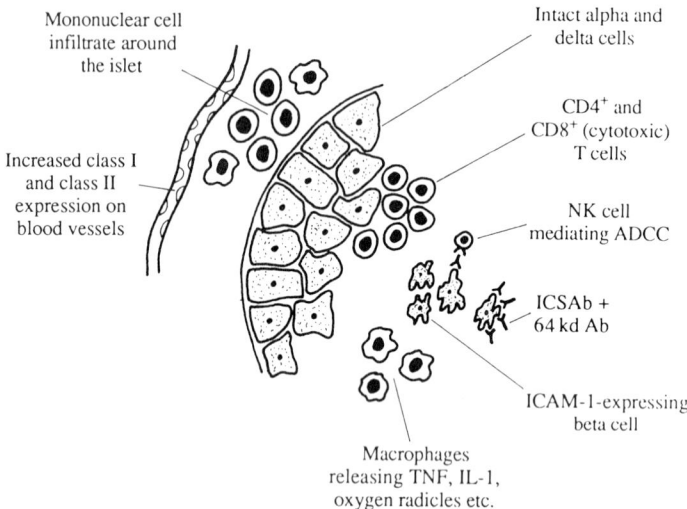

Fig. 4.1   Possible effector mechanisms working in concert in diabetes.
See text for details.

the beta cells within isolated rat and human islets (Mandrup-Poulsen, 1988).
Indirect evidence suggests that IL-1 could be selectively toxic by inducing
reactive oxygen metabolite formation, to which beta cells are very sensitive
(Sumoski, Baquerizo & Rabinovitch, 1989).

In contrast to these observations, IL-1 and TNF were each found to inhibit
human alpha and beta cell function and, when added together, were
cytotoxic for both cell types (Rabinovitch et al., 1990). γ-IFN synergised
with these two cytokines but had no effect alone. This lack of islet cell
specificity mirrors that shown by cytokine-induced ICAM-1 and Ia expression in vitro. Exogenous IL-6 stimulates insulin synthesis and secretion
but paradoxically produces ultrastructural beta cell changes which resemble
those induced by IL-1 (Buschard et al., 1990b). How this relates to beta cell-
derived IL-6 (Campbell et al., 1989a), which could presumably act in an
autocrine fashion, is not clear. Finally, γ-IFN may play some unique role, as
transgenic mice with γ-IFN-producing beta cells develop diabetes and
insulitis (Sarvetnick et al., 1988). However, the exact mechanism for these
changes and their relevance to human diabetes, in which local γ-IFN will
only be derived from lymphocytes, remain unknown.

In summary, cytokines have a variety of effects on beta cells, increasing
ICAM-1 and MHC molecule expression, modulating hormone synthesis
and release and, in some cases, producing cytotoxicity. These actions are
probably not specific for the beta cell and it remains to be shown that any of
these effects are diabetogenic in vivo. However, beta cell specificity need
not be a prerequisite for cytokine-mediated cytotoxicity if these cells prove

to be unusually susceptible to such effects, or if the cytokines are directed to the beta cells by the binding of specific lymphocytes. Macrophage products may also operate as part of an effector cascade (Fig. 4.1). In such a scheme, beta cell destruction would only occur if several effector mechanisms were operating at once within the islet, perhaps together with a necessary trigger such as virally infected beta cells. This would explain the long prediabetic period, the asynchronous involvement of islets and the existence of some markers of beta cell-specific autoimmunity in individuals who never progress to full-blown disease. The findings in experimental diabetes are in keeping with the additive involvement of multiple effector mechanisms and different mixtures of these could result in the histopathological and clinical heterogeneity which is apparent.

Treatment

Until recently, insulin replacement has been the only form of therapy for diabetes but this does not prevent the development of major complications, including retinopathy and nephropathy, nor is the administration of insulin itself trouble-free. Pancreas transplantation may be one answer (Sutherland, 1990). However, the realisation that autoimmune mechanisms cause diabetes has led to trials using a variety of immunologically directed therapy in experimental and human diabetes. In NOD mice the poly-ADP-ribose synthetase inhibitor, nicotinamide, reduces the incidence of insulitis and diabetes (Yamada *et al.*, 1982). Cyclosporin A also ameliorates the severity of insulitis in NOD mice and in the BB rat prevents diabetes (Lampeter *et al.*, 1989; Laupacis *et al.*, 1983). Subtherapeutic doses of cyclosporin A are effective in curing BB rats with diabetes, if given with a monoclonal antibody against the IL-2 receptor (Hahn *et al.*, 1987). This approach is of interest as cyclosporin A is quite a toxic compound and strategies which can reduce the dose given are desirable. The IL-2 receptor antibody appears to block activated T cells, including those with autoreactivity. A new immuno-suppressive agent, FK 506, also prevents diabetes and insulitis in BB rats (Murase *et al.*, 1990). However, as with cyclosporin A, some of the animals develop disease once treatment is stopped, so that total cure is not accomplished.

A variety of immunological treatments have also been tried in human diabetes but, with the exception of cyclosporin A, these have proved disappointing (Table 4.4). Age, sex, HLA phenotype and the presence of autoantibodies are not predictors of a response to cyclosporin A, but mild disease of short duration prior to treatment is associated with a better outcome. There is no consensus regarding any effect of this treatment on ICAb. It is striking that the most recent trial of cyclosporin A for four months (Chase *et al.*, 1990) showed no clinical effect, explicable by the

Table 4.4. *Immunotherapy for diabetes*

Trial	Treatment	Number of patients treated	Controlled trial	Outcome
Cobb et al., 1980	Levamisole	3	N[a]	No effect
Elliott et al., 1981	Prednisone	9	Y	4 remissions in treated group (0 in controls)
Ludvigsson et al., 1983	Plasma exchange	10	Y	Extended partial remission in 4[b]
Leslie et al., 1985	Prednisone, azathioprine, anti-lymphocyte globulin + plasma exchange	5	N	No clear effect
Heinze et al., 1985	Pooled gamma globulin	6	N	Extended partial remission in 4
Vague et al., 1987	Nicotinamide	7	Y	3 remissions (0 in controls)
Mendola et al., 1989	Nicotinamide	10	Y	No significant effect
Herskowitz et al., 1989	Nicotinamide	3	N	No clear effect
Chatenoud et al., 1989	Anti-CD3 monoclonal antibody	7	N	Amelioration – no further details
Harrison et al., 1985	Azathioprine	13	N	6 remissions[c]; all relapsed within 3 years

Study	Treatment	n	Y/N[a]	Effect
Cook et al., 1989	Azathioprine	24	Y	No significant effect
Stiller et al., 1984	Cyclosporin A (mean 7–8 months)	41	N	18 remissions
Assan et al., 1985	Cyclosporin A (3–4 months)[d]	12	N	4 remissions, 4 partial remissions
Bougneres et al., 1988	Cyclosporin A (>6 months)	40	N	24 remissions (at 6 months)
Feutran et al., 1986	Cyclosporin A (>6 months)	63	Y	No significant difference from controls at 6 months; significantly more remissions at 9 months[e] (24% vs 6% in controls)
Canadian–European Randomized Control Trial Group, 1988	Cyclosporin A (12 months)[d]	93	Y	Significantly more remissions (33% vs 21% in controls)
Chase et al., 1990	Cyclosporin A (4 months)	22	Y	No significant effect

[a]N = no, Y = yes.
[b]Partial remission = sustained C-peptide production/low insulin requirement.
[c]Remission = no requirement for insulin.
[d]Treatment stopped by 3 months if no remission, otherwise continued.
[e]Treatment continued in those in remission at 6 months.

higher than expected remission rate in control subjects, as well as the short duration of treatment. Of course, all such untreated patients eventually will require insulin, but these results in the controls are in keeping with the natural history of a slow decline in beta cell function (Tarn *et al.*, 1987). Perhaps with earlier diagnosis of diabetes, partial or complete remission for a period of time ('diabetic honeymoon') has become more frequent and this has implications in interpreting the uncontrolled trials listed in Table 4.4. Comparison between trials is also hampered by the lack of agreed standards for determining outcome, particularly clinical remission (Kolb *et al.*, 1989). Moreover, cyclosporin A only appears to delay the onset of disease: when it is stopped, patients become diabetic (Assan *et al.*, 1988).

So few beta cells remain by the time of diagnosis that cyclosporin A, or indeed any other agent, is unlikely to produce reliable benefit and this accords with the better outcome in the least severely affected patients, who presumably have more beta cells to start with. A major step forward would be the availability of sensitive and specific markers to predict which individuals will go on to develop diabetes. In first degree relatives of diabetics, the combination of high titre ICAb, insulin antibodies and an impaired first phase insulin response to glucose strongly predict the subsequent onset of disease within three years (Ziegler *et al.*, 1990). Immunological intervention in these prediabetic subjects would probably increase the chances of successfully aborting the disease. Immunosuppressive treatment remains a tantalising possibility in diabetes but currently seems unjustifiable except as part of a research protocol. Further developments will depend on the emergence of reliable predictors of diabetes and new or additional forms of treatment, as cyclosporin A has a high risk to benefit ratio.

Summary

The aetiology and pathogenesis of diabetes are beginning to be understood as a result of several recent advances, critically supplemented by the insights gained from experimental models of diabetes. Epidemiological and histological data suggest that type 1 diabetes is heterogenous, probably comprising several entities with separate precipitating factors which result in the typical, but not universal, picture of insulitis and beta cell destruction. Major developments in understanding the immunogenetics at a molecular level reveal a very complex interaction of loci both within the MHC and outside it. Genes in the DQ subregion play a major role in determining susceptibility or conferring protection. However, there is a hierarchy, depending on haplotype, for these effects, which may relate to other loci that are in linkage disequilibrium, like those regulating TNF. Much less is known of the influence of non-MHC genes, although by analogy with experimental diabetes, these may be critical to the emergence of disease. This is underlined by relatively low concordance in HLA-identical siblings, compared to monozygotic twins, but in turn, the occurence of diabetes in only 40% of subjects with an affected identical twin indicates the importance of environmental factors. Viruses have some role, most clearly shown in the congenital rubella syndrome; much further work is required to identify how other viral infections may contribute to the initiation of disease. T cell cloning is beginning to elucidate the nature of beta cell-specific T cell autoimmune responses. Several beta cell autoantigens have been identified, although none has been fully characterised and, apart from insulin, these are not completely beta cell-specific. Autoantibodies to the 64 kd antigen seem the most promising marker for diabetes: their pathogenic importance is uncertain.

The beta cell may contribute to its own destruction by hyperexpression of MHC class I and II molecules and by the synthesis of ICAM-I and IL-6, all in response to cytokines. Autoantigen presentation by class II-expressing beta cells has not been demonstrated and this hypothetical function is not supported by experiments with transgenic mice. Cytokines like IL-1 and TNF may be important in beta cell destruction, intra-islet specificity possibly being achieved because beta cells are already damaged or are particularly susceptible to this type of injury. Immunosuppressive treatment has on the whole been disappointing. The most promising agent, cyclosporin A, produces a modest increase in insulin-free remissions but these are only temporary and there are major side effects of prolonged therapy. One possible strategy to improve outcome would be commencement of immunomodulatory treatment before presentation, when around 90% of the beta cells are already destroyed. This depends on the availability of reliable prediabetic markers and recent progress suggests that such screening may soon be feasible.

References

Allison, J., Campbell, I.J., Morahan, G., Mandel, T.E., Harrison, L.C. & Miller, J.F.A.P. (1988). Diabetes in transgenic mice resulting from over-expression of class I histocompatibility molecules in pancreatic β cells. *Nature*, **333**, 529–33.

Al-Sakkaf, L., Pozzilli, P., Tarn, A.C., Schwarz, G., Gale, E.A.M. & Bottazzo, G.F. (1989). Persistent reduction of CD4/CD8 lymphocyte ratio and cell activation before the onset of type I (insulin-dependent) diabetes. *Diabetologia*, **32**, 322–5.

Angellilo, M., Greiner, D.L., Mordes, J.P., Handler, E.S., Nakamura, N., McKeever, U. & Rossini, A. (1988). Absence of RT6.1[+] T cells in diabetes-prone BioBreeding/Worcester rats is due to genetic and cell developmental defects. *Journal of Immunology*, **141**, 4146–51.

Appel, M.C., Rossini, A.A., Williams, R.M. & Like, A.A. (1978). Viral studies in streptozotocin-induced pancreatic insulitis. *Diabetologia*, **15**, 327–36.

Assan, R., Debray-Sachs, M., Laborie, C., Chatenoud, L., Feutren, G., Quiniou-Debrie, M.C., Thomas, G. & Bach, J.F. (1985). Metabolic and immunological effects of cyclosporin in recently diagnosed type I diabetes mellitus. *Lancet*, **i**, 67–71.

Assan, R., Feutren, G. & Sirmai, J. (1988). Cyclosporine trials in diabetes: updated results of the French experience. *Transplantation Proceedings*, **20**, 178–83.

Atkinson, M.A. & Maclaren, N.R. (1988). Autoantibodies in non-obese diabetic mice immunoprecipitate 64,000-M_r islet antigen. *Diabetes*, **37**, 1587–90.

Atkinson, M.A., Maclaren, N.R., Scharp, D.W., Lacy, P.E. & Riley, W.J. (1990). 64,000 M_r autoantibodies as predictors of insulin-dependent diabetes. *Lancet*, **335**, 1357–60.

Atkinson, M.A., Maclaren, N.R. & Scharp, D.W. (1990). No role for 65 kd heat-shock protein in diabetes. *Lancet*, **336**, 1250–1.

Badenhoop, K., Schwarz, G., Trowsdale, J., Lewis, V., Usadel, K.H., Gale, E.A.M. & Bottazzo, G.F. (1989). TNF-α gene polymorphisms in Type 1 (insulin-dependent) diabetes mellitus. *Diabetologia*, **32**, 445–8.

Baekkeskov, S., Nielsen, J.H., Marner, B., Bilde, T., Ludvigsson, J. & Lernmark, Å. (1982). Autoantibodies in newly diagnosed diabetic children immunoprecipitate human pancreatic islet cell proteins. *Nature*, **298**, 167–9.

Baekkeskov, S., Dyrberg, T. & Lernmark, Å. (1984). Autoantibodies to a 64 kilodalton islet cell protein precede the onset of spontaneous diabetes in the BB rat. *Science*, **224**, 1348–50.

Baekkeskov, S., Landin, M., Kristensen, J.K., Srikanta, S., Bruining, G.J., Mandrup-Poulsen, T., De Beaufort, C., Soeldner, J.S., Eisenbarth, G.S., Lindgren, F., Sundquist, G. & Lernmark, Å. (1987). Autoantibodies to a 64,000 M_r human islet cell antigen precede the clinical onset of insulin-dependent diabetes. *Journal of Clinical Investigation*, **79**, 926–34.

Baekkeskov, S., Jan-Aanstoot, H., Christgau, S., Reetz, A., Solimena, M., Cascalho, M., Foli, F., Richter-Olsen, H. & Camilli, P.-D. (1990). Identification of the 64 K autoantigen in insulin-dependent diabetes as the GABA-synthesizing enzyme glutamic acid decarboxylase. *Nature*, **347**, 151–6.

Baird, J.D. (1989). Relevance of the BB rat as a model for human insulin-dependent (Type I) diabetes mellitus. In *Recent Advances in Endocrinology and Metabolism*, Volume 3, ed. C.R.W. Edwards & D.W. Lincoln. pp. 253–80. Edinburgh: Churchill Livingstone.

Baisch, J.M., Weeks, T., Giles, R., Hoover, M., Stastny, P. & Capra, J.D. (1990). Analysis of HLA-DQ genotypes and susceptibility in insulin-dependent diabetes mellitus. *New England Journal of Medicine*, **322**, 1836–41.

Banatvala, J.E., Bryant, J., Schernthaner, G., Borkenstein, M., Schober, E., Brown, D., De Silva, L.M., Menser, M.A. & Silink, M. (1985). Coxsackie B, mumps, rubella, and cytomegalovirus specific IgM responses in patients with juvenile-onset insulin-dependent diabetes mellitus in Britain, Austria, and Australia. *Lancet*, **ii**, 1409–12.

Bao, M.-Z., Wang, J.-X., Dorman, J.S. & Trucco, M. (1989). HLA-DQβ non-Asp-57 allele and the incidence of diabetes in China and the USA. *Lancet*, **ii**, 497–8.

Bedossa, P., Bendelac, A., Bach, J.F. & Carnaud, C. (1989). Syngeneic T cell transfer of diabetes into NOD newborn mice: in situ studies of the autoimmune steps leading to insulin-dependent diabetes. *European Journal of Immunology*, **19**, 1947–51.

Bendelac, A., Boitard, C., Bedossa, P., Bazin, H., Bach, J.F. & Carnaud, C. (1988). Adoptive T cell transfer of autoimmune non-obese diabetic mouse diabetes does not require recruitment of host B lymphocytes. *Journal of Immunology*, **141**, 2625–8.

Bendtzen, K., Mandrup-Poulsen, M., Nerup, J., Nielsen, J.H., Dinarello, C.A. & Svenson, M. (1986). Cytotoxicity of human pI 7 interleukin–1 for pancreatic islets of Langerhans. *Science*, **232**, 1545–7.

Betterle, C., Presotto, F., Pedini, B., Moro, L., Slack, R.S., Zanette, F. & Zanchetta, R. (1987). Islet cell and insulin autoantibodies in organ-specific autoimmune patients. Their behaviour and predictive value for the development of Type 1 (insulin-dependent) diabetes mellitus. A follow-up study. *Diabetologia*, **30**, 292–7.

Bingley, P.J. & Gale, E.A.M. (1989). Incidence of insulin-dependent diabetes in England: a study in the Oxford region, 1985–6. *British Medical Journal*, **298**, 558–60.

Bohme, J., Carlson, B., Wallin, J., Moller, E., Persson, B., Peterson, P.A. & Rask, L. (1986). Only one DQ-β restriction fragment pattern of each DR specificity is associated with insulin-dependent diabetes. *Journal of Immunology*, **137**, 941–7.

Boitard, C., Yasunami, R., Dardenne, M. & Bach, J.F. (1989). T cell-mediated inhibition of the transfer of autoimmune diabetes in NOD mice. *Journal of Experimental Medicine*, **169**, 1669–80.

Bonifacio, E., Bingley, P.J., Shattock, M., Dean, B.M., Dunger, D., Gale, E.A.M. & Bottazzo, G.F. (1990). Quantification of islet-cell antibodies and prediction of insulin-dependent diabetes. *Lancet*, **335**, 147–9.

Bottazzo, G.F., Florin-Christensen, A. & Doniach, D. (1974). Islet-cell antibodies in diabetes mellitus with autoimmune polyendocrine deficiencies. *Lancet*, **ii**, 1279–83.

Bottazzo, G.F., Cudworth, A.G., Moul, D.J., Doniach, D. & Festenstein, H. (1978). Evidence for a primary autoimmune type of diabetes mellitus. *British Medical Journal*, **2**, 1253–5.

Bottazzo, G.F., Dean, B.M., Gorsuch, A.N., Cudworth, A.G. & Doniach, D. (1980). Complement-fixing islet-cell antibodies in type 1 diabetes: possible monitors of active beta-cell damage. *Lancet*, **i**, 668–72.

Bottazzo, G.F., Dean, B.M., NcNally, J.M., MacKay, E.H., Swift, P.G.F. & Gamble, D.R. (1985). *In situ* characterization of autoimmune phenomena and expression of HLA molecules in the pancreas in diabetic insulitis. *New England Journal of Medicine*, **313**, 353–60.

Bottazzo, G.F. & Gleichmann, H. (1986). Immunology and diabetes workshops: report of the first international workshop on the standardisation of cytoplasmic islet cell antibodies. *Diabetologia*, **29**, 125–6.

Bottazzo, G.F., Bosi, E., Bonifacio, E., Mirakian, R., Todd, I. & Pujol-Borrell, R. (1989). Pathogenesis of type I (insulin-dependent) diabetes: possible mechanisms of autoimmune damage. *British Medical Bulletin*, **45**, 37–57.

Bougneres, P.F., Carel, J.C., Castano, L., Boitard, C., Gardin, J.P., Landais, J., Hors, J., Mihatsch, M.J., Paillard, M., Chaussain, J.L. & Bach, J.F. (1988). Factors associated with early remission of type 1 diabetes in children treated with cyclosporine. *New England Journal of Medicine*, **318**, 663–70.

Bruining, G.J., Molenaar, J., Tuk, C.W., Lindeman, J., Bruining, H.A. & Marner, B. (1984). Clinical time-course and characteristics of islet cell cytoplasmic antibodies in childhood diabetes. *Diabetologia*, **26**, 24–9.

Buschard, K., Aaen, K., Horn, T., Van Damme, J. & Bentdzen, K. (1990a). Interleukin 6: a functional and structural *in vitro* modulator of beta cells from islets of Langerhans. *Autoimmunity*, **5**, 185–94.

Buschard, K., Jorgensen, M., Aaen, K., Bock, T. & Josefsen, K. (1990b). Prevention of diabetes mellitus in BB rats by neonatal stimulation of β cells. *Lancet*, **335**, 134–5.

Campbell, I.L., Bizilj, K., Colman, P.G., Tuch, B.E. & Harrison, L.C. (1986). Interferon-γ induces the expression of HLA-A,B,C, but not HLA-DR on human pancreatic β-cells. *Journal of Clinical Endocrinology and Metabolism*, **62**, 1101–9.

Campbell, I.L., Cutri, A., Wilson, A. & Harrison, L.C. (1989a). Evidence for IL-6 production by and effects on the pancreatic β-cell. *Journal of Immunology*, **143**, 1188–91.

Campbell, I.L., Cutri, A., Wilkinson, D., Boyd, A.W. & Harrison, L.C. (1989b). Intercellular adhesion molecule-1 is induced on isolated endocrine islet cells by cytokines but not by reovirus infection. *Proceedings of the National Academy of Science, USA*, **86**, 4282–6.

Canadian–European Randomized Control Trial Group (1988). Cyclosporin-induced remission of IDDM after early intervention. Association of 1 yr of cyclosporin treatment with enhanced insulin secretion. *Diabetes*, **37**, 1574–82.

Carter, W.R., Herrman, J., Stokes, K. & Cox, D.J. (1987). Promotion of diabetes onset by stress in the BB rat. *Diabetologia*, **30**, 674–5.

Casali, P., Nakamura, M., Ginsberg-Fellner, F. & Notkins, A.B. (1990). Frequency of B cells committed to the production of antibodies to insulin in newly diagnosed patients with insulin-dependent diabetes mellitus and generation of high affinity human monoclonal IgG to insulin. *Journal of Immunology*, **144**, 3741–7.

Chao, N.J., Timmerman, L., McDevitt, H.O. & Jacob, C.O. (1989). Molecular characterization of MHC class II antigens (β domain) in the BB diabetes-prone and -resistant rat. *Immunogenetics*, **29**, 231–4.

Chappel, C.I. & Chappel, W.R. (1983). The discovery and development of the BB rat colony: an animal model of spontaneous diabetes mellitus. *Metabolism*, **32** (Supplement 1), 8–10.

Charlton, B., Bacelj, A. & Mandel, T.E. (1988). Administration of silica particles or anti-Lyt2 antibody prevents β-cell destruction in NOD mice given cyclophosphamide. *Diabetes*, **37**, 930–5.

Chase, H.P., Butler-Simon, N., Garg, S.K., Hayward, A., Klingensmith, G.J., Hamman, R.F. & O'Brien, D. (1990). Cyclosporine A for the treatment of new-onset insulin-dependent diabetes mellitus. *Pediatrics*, **85**, 241–5.

Chatenoud, L., Ferran, C. & Bach, J.F. (1989). *In-vivo* anti-CD3 treatment of autoimmune patients. *Lancet*, **ii**, 164.

Christie, M.R., Pipeleers, D.G., Lernmark, Å. & Baekkeskov, S. (1990). Cellular and subcellular localization of an M_r 64,000 protein autoantigen in insulin-dependent diabetes. *Journal of Biological Chemistry*, **265**, 376–81.

Cobb, W.E., Molitch, M. & Reichlin, S. (1980). Levamisole in insulin-dependent diabetes mellitus. *New England Journal of Medicine*, **303**, 1065–7.

Cohen, D., Cohen, O., Marcadet, A., Massart, C., Lathrop, M., Deschamps, I., Hors, J., Schuller, E. & Dausset, J. (1984). Class II HLA-DC β-chain DNA restriction fragments differentiate among HLA-DR2 individuals in insulin-dependent diabetes and multiple sclerosis. *Proceedings of the National Academy of Science, USA*, **81**, 1774–8.

Cohen-Hagenauer, O., Robbins, E., Massart, C., Busson, M., Deschamps, I., Hors, J., Lalouel, J.M., Dausset, J. & Cohen, D.A. (1985). A systematic study of HLA class II-β DNA restriction fragments in insulin-dependent diabetes mellitus. *Proceedings of the National Academy of Science, USA*, **82**, 3335–9.

Coleman, D.L., Kuzara, J.E. & Leiter, E.H. (1990). Effect of diet on incidence of diabetes in non-obese diabetic mice. *Diabetes*, **39**, 432–6.

Colle, E., Ono, S.J., Fuks, A., Guttmann, R.D. & Seemayer, T.A. (1988). Association of susceptibility to spontaneous diabetes in rats with genes of the major histocompatibility complex. *Diabetes*, **37**, 1438–43.

Comens, P.G., Wolf, B.A., Unanue, E.R., Lacy, P.E. & McDaniel, M.L. (1987). Interleukin 1 is potent modulator of insulin secretion from isolated rat islets of Langerhans. *Diabetes*, **36**, 963–70.

Cook, J.J., Hudson, I., Harrison, L.C., Dean, B., Colman, P.G., Werther, G.A., Warne, G.L. & Court, J.M. (1989). Double-blind controlled trial of azathioprine in children with newly diagnosed type I diabetes. *Diabetes*, **38**, 779–83.

Crosti, F., Secchi, A., Ferrerro, E., Falqui, L., Inverardi, L., Pontiroli, A.E., Cibbodo, G.F., Pavoni, D., Protti, R., Rugarli, C. & Pozza, G. (1986). Impairment of the lymphocyte suppressive system in recent-onset insulin-dependent diabetes mellitus. Correlation with metabolic control. *Diabetes*, **35**, 1053–7.

Cudworth, A.G. & Woodrow, J.C. (1975). Evidence for HL-A-linked genes in 'juvenile' diabetes mellitus. *British Medical Journal*, **3**, 133–5.

Dahlquist, G.G., Blom, L.G., Persson, L.-K., Sandstrom, A.I.M. & Wall, S.G.I. (1990). Dietary factors and the risk of developing insulin dependent diabetes in childhood. *British Medical Journal*, **300**, 1302–6.

Dardenne, M., Lepault, F., Bendelac, A. & Bach, J.F. (1989). Acceleration of the onset of diabetes in NOD mice by thymectomy at weaning. *European Journal of Immunology*, **19**, 889–95.

Dean, B.M., Walker, R., Bone, A.J., Baird, J.D. & Cooke, A. (1985). Pre-diabetes in the spontaneously diabetic BB/E rat: lymphocyte subpopulations in the pancreatic infiltrate and expression of rat MHC class II molecules in endocrine cells. *Diabetologia*, **28**, 464–6.

Dean, B.M., Becker, F., McNally, J.M., Tarn, A.C., Schwartz, G., Gale, E.A.M. & Bottazzo, G.F. (1986). Insulin autoantibodies in the pre-diabetic period: correlation with islet cell antibodies and development of diabetes. *Diabetologia*, **29**, 339–42.

Dean, B.M., Bone, A.J., Varey, A.M., Walker, R., Baird, J.D. & Cooke, A. (1987). Insulin autoantibodies, islet cell surface antibodies and the development of spontaneous diabetes in the BB Edinburgh rat. *Clinical and Experimental Immunology*, **69**, 308–13.

De Berardinis, P., Londei, M., Kahan, M., Balsano, F., Kotiainen, S., Gale, E.A.M., Bottazzo, G.F. & Feldmann, M. (1988a). The majority of the activated T cells in the blood of insulin-dependent diabetes mellitus (IDDM) patients are CD4$^+$. *Clinical and Experimental Immunology*, **73**, 255–9.

De Berardinis, P., Londei, M., James, R.F.L., Lake, S.P., Wise, P.H. & Feldmann, M. (1988b). Do CD4-positive cytotoxic T cells damage islet β cells in type 1 diabetes? *Lancet*, **ii**, 823–4.

Debray-Sachs, M., Sai, P., Boitard, C., Assan, R. & Hamburger, J. (1983). Antipancreatic immunity in genetically susceptible mice. *Clinical and Experimental Immunology*, **51**, 1–7.

Diabetes Epidemiology Research International Group (1988). Geographic patterns of child-hood insulin-dependent diabetes mellitus. *Diabetes*, **37**, 1113–19.

Di Mario, U., Dotta, F., Gargiulo, P., Sutherland, J., Andreani, D., Guy, K., Pachi, A. & Fallucca, F. (1987). Immunology in diabetic pregnancy: activated T cells in diabetic mothers and neonates. *Diabetologia*, **30**, 66–71.

Dizier, M.H., Deschamps, I., Hors, J., Blanc, M., Rivat, L. & Clerget-Darpoux, F. (1986). Interactive effect of HLA and Gm tested in a study of 135 juvenile insulin-dependent diabetic families. *Tissue Antigens*, **27**, 269–78.

Drell, D.W & Notkins, A.L. (1987). Multiple immunological abnormalities in patients with Type 1 (insulin-dependent) diabetes mellitus. *Diabetologia*, **30**, 132–43.

Dyrberg, T., Nakhooda, A.F., Baekkeskov, S., Lernmark, Å., Poussier, P. & Marliss, E.B. (1982). Islet cell surface antibodies and lymphocyte antibodies in the spontaneously diabetic BB Wistar rat. *Diabetes*, **31**, 278–81.

Dyrberg, T., Poussier, P., Nakhooda, F., Marliss, E.B. & Lernmark, Å. (1984). Islet cell surface and lymphocyte antibodies often precede the spontaneous diabetes in the BB rat. *Diabetologia*, **26**, 159–65.

Easteal, S., Kohonen-Corish, M.R.J., Zimmet, P. & Serjeantson, S.W. (1990). HLA-DP variation as additional risk factor in IDDM. *Diabetes*, **39**, 855–7.

Eisenbarth, G.S., Morris, M.A. & Scearce, R.M. (1981). Cytotoxic antibodies to cloned rat islet cells in serum of patients with diabetes mellitus. *Journal of Clinical Investigation*, **67**, 403–8.

Elder, M., Maclaren, N., Riley, W. & McConnell, T. (1982). Gastric parietal cell and other autoantibodies in the BB rat. *Diabetes*, **31**, 313–18.

Elias, D., Markovits, D., Reshef, T., Van Der Zee, R. & Cohen, I.R. (1990). Induction and therapy of autoimmune diabetes in the non-obese diabetic (NOD/Lt) mouse by a 65 kDa heat shock protein. *Proceedings of the National Academy of Science, USA*, **87**, 1576–80.

Elliott, R.B., Crossley, J.R., Berryman, C.C. & James, A.G. (1981). Partial preservation of pancreatic beta-cell function in children with diabetes. *Lancet*, **ii**, 1–4.

Erlich, H.A., Bugawan, T.L., Scharf, S., Nepom, G.T., Tait, B. & Griffith, R.L. (1990). HLA-DQB sequence polymorphism and genetic susceptibility to IDDM. *Diabetes*, **39**, 96–103.

Faustman, D., Eisenbarth, G., Daley, J. & Breitmeyer, J. (1989). Abnormal T-lymphocyte subsets in type I diabetes. *Diabetes*, **38**, 1462–8.

Festenstein, H., Awad, J., Hitman, G.A., Cutbush, S., Groves, A.V., Cassell, P., Ollier, W. & Sachs, J.A. (1986). New HLA DNA polymorphisms associated with autoimmune diseases. *Nature*, **322**, 64–7.

Feutran, G., Papoz, L., Assan, R., Vialettes, B., Karsenty, G., Vexiau, P., Du Rostu, H., Rodier, M., Sirmai, J., Lallemand, A. & Bach, J.F. (1986). Cyclosporin increases the rate and length of remissions in insulin-dependent diabetes of recent onset. Results of a multicentre double-blind trial. *Lancet*, **ii**, 119–24.

Field, L.L. (1986). No interaction between HLA and Gm in type 1 diabetes? *Journal of Immunogenetics*, **13**, 373–5.

Fletcher, J., Mijovic, C., Odugbesan, O., Jenkins, D., Bradwell, A.R. & Barnett, A.H. (1988). Trans-racial studies implicate HLA-DQ as a component of genetic susceptibility to Type 1 (insulin-dependent) diabetes. *Diabetologia*, **31**, 864–70.

Foulis, A.K. & Farquharson, M.A. (1986). Aberrant expression of HLA-DR antigens by insulin-containing cells in recent-onset type 1 diabetes mellitus. *Diabetes*, **35**, 1215–24.

Foulis, A.K., Liddle, C.N., Farquharson, M.A., Richmond, J.A. & Weir, R.S. (1986). The histopathology of the pancreas in type I (insulin-dependent) diabetes mellitus: a 25-year review of deaths in patients under 20 years of age in the United Kingdom. *Diabetologia*, **29**, 267–74.

Gamble, D.R., Kinsley, M.L., Fitzgerald, M.G., Bolton, R. & Taylor, K.W. (1969). Viral antibodies in diabetes mellitus. *British Medical Journal*, **iii**, 627–30.

Georgiou, H.M. & Bellgrau, D. (1989). Thymus transplantation and disease prevention in the diabetes-prone Bio-Breeding rat. *Journal of Immunology*, **142**, 3400–5.

Gerling, I., Nejman, C. & Chatterjee, N.K. (1988). Effect of coxsackie B4 infection in mice on expression of 64,000-M_r autoantigen and glucose sensitivity of islets before development of hyperglycaemia. *Diabetes*, **37**, 1419–25.

Ginsberg-Fellner, F., Witt, M.E., Yagihashi, S., Doberson, M.J., Taub, F., Fedun, B., McEvoy, R.C., Roman, S.H., Davies, T.F., Cooper, L.Z., Rubinstein, P. & Notkins, A.L. (1984). Congenital rubella syndrome as a model for Type 1 (insulin-dependent) diabetes mellitus: increased prevalence of islet cell surface antibodies. *Diabetologia*, **27**, 87–9.

Goldman, J., Baldwin, D., Rubenstein, A.H., Klink, D.D., Blackard, W.G., Fisher, L.K., Roe, T.F. & Schnure, J.J. (1979). Characterization of circulating insulin and proinsulin-binding antibodies in autoimmune hypoglycaemia. *Journal of Clinical Investigation*, **63**, 1050–9.

Gorsuch, A.N., Lister, J., Dean, B.M., Spencer, K.M., McNally, J.M. & Bottazzo, G.F. (1981). Evidence for a long prediabetic period in type I (insulin-dependent) diabetes mellitus. *Lancet*, **i**, 1363–5.

Götz, J., Eibel, H. & Köhler, G. (1990). Non-tolerance and differential susceptibility to diabetes in transgenic mice expressing major histocompatibility class II genes on pancreatic β cells. *European Journal of Immunology*, **20**, 1677–83.

Hahn, H.J., Lucke, S., Klöting, I., Volk, H.D., Baehr, R.V. & Diamanstein, T. (1987). Curing BB rats of freshly manifested diabetes by short-term treatment with a combination of a monoclonal anti-interleukin 2 receptor antibody and a subtherapeutic dose of cyclosporin A. *European Journal of Immunology*, **17**, 1075–8.

Hamaguchi, K. & Leiter, E.H. (1990). Comparison of cytokine effects on mouse pancreatic α-cell and β-cell lines. Viability, secretory function, and MHC antigen expression. *Diabetes*, **39**, 415–25.

Hanafusa, T., Fujino-Kurihara, H., Miyazaki, A., Yamada, K., Nakajima, H., Miyagawa, J., Kono, N. & Tarui, S. (1987). Expression of class II major histocompatibility complex antigens on pancreatic β cells in the NOD mouse. *Diabetologia*, **30**, 104–8.

Hanafusa, T., Miyazaki, A., Miyagawa, J., Tamura, S., Inada, M., Yamada, K., Shinji, Y., Katsura, H., Yamagata, K., Itoh, N., Asakawa, H., Nakagawa, C., Otsuka, A., Kawata, S., Kono, N. & Tarui, S. (1990). Examination of islets in the pancreas biopsy specimens from newly diagnosed Type 1 (insulin dependent) diabetic patients. *Diabetologia*, **33**, 105–11.

Harrison, L.C., Colman, P.G., Dean, B., Baxter, R. & Martin, F.I.R. (1985). Increase in remission rate in newly diagnosed type I diabetic subjects treated with azathioprine. *Diabetes*, **34**, 1306–8.

Harrison, L.C., Campbell, I.L., Allison, J. & Miller, J.F.A.P. (1989). MHC molecules and β-cell destruction. Immune and nonimmune mechanisms. *Diabetes*, **38**, 815–18.

Hattori, M., Fukuda, M., Ichikawa, T., Baumgartl, H.J., Katoh, H. & Makino, S. (1990). A single recessive non-MHC diabetogenic gene determines the development of insulitis in the presence of an MHC-linked diabetogenic gene in NOD mice. *Journal of Autoimmunity*, **3**, 1–10.

Hawkins, B.R., Lam, K.S.L., Ma, J.T.C., Low, L.C.K., Cheung, P.T., Serjeantson, S.W. & Yeung, R.T.T. (1987). Strong association of HLA-DR3/DRw9 heterozygosity with early-onset insulin-dependent diabetes mellitus in Chinese. *Diabetes*, **36**, 1297–300.

Hayward, A.R. & Herberger, M. (1984). Culture and phenotype of activated T-cells from patients with type I diabetes mellitus. *Diabetes*, **33**, 319–23.

Hehmke, B., Lucke, S., Schröder, D., Klöting, I. & Kohnert, K.-D. (1990). Complement-dependent antibody-mediated cytotoxicity in the spontaneously diabetic BB/OK rat: association with β cell volume density. *European Journal of Immunology*, **20**, 1091–6.

Heinze, E., Thon, A., Vetter, U., Gaedicke, G. & Zuppinger, K. (1985). Gamma-globulin therapy in 6 newly diagnosed diabetic children. *Acta Paediatrica Scandinavica*, **74**, 605–6.

Herskowitz, R.D., Jackson, R.A., Soeldner, J.S. & Eisenbarth, G.S. (1989). Pilot trial to prevent type I diabetes: progression to overt IDDM despite oral nicotinamide. *Journal of Autoimmunity*, **2**, 733–7.

Holowachuk, E.W., Greer, M.K. & Martin, D.R. (1988). Elevated mRNA levels of major histocompatibility complex class II genes in lymphocytes of autoimmune BB rats. *Diabetes*, **37**, 1637–40.

Hyöty, H., Huupponen, T. & Leinikki, P. (1985). Humoral immunity against viral antigens in insulin-dependent diabetes mellitus (IDDM): altered IgA class immune response against mumps virus. *Clinical and Experimental Immunology*, **60**, 139–44.

In't Veld, P.A. & Pipeleers, D.G. (1988). *In situ* analysis of pancreatic islets in rats developing diabetes. Appearance of nonendocrine cells with surface MHC class II antigens and cytoplasmic insulin immunoreactivity. *Journal of Clinical Investigation*, **82**, 1123–8.

Ito, M., Tanimoto, M., Kamura, H., Yoneda, M., Morishima, Y., Takatsuki, K., Itatsu, T. & Saito, H. (1988). Association of HLA-DR phenotypes and T-lymphocyte-receptor β-chain-region RFLP with IDDM in Japanese. *Diabetes*, **37**, 1633–6.

Jackson, R.A., Morris, M.A., Haynes, B.F. & Eisenbarth, G.S. (1982). Increased circulating Ia antigen bearing T cells in type I diabetes mellitus. *New England Journal of Medicine*, **306**, 785–8.

Jacob, C.O., Aiso, S., Michie, S.A., McDevitt, H.O. & Acha-Orbea, H. (1990). Prevention of diabetes in nonobese diabetic mice by tumor necrosis factor (TNF): similarities between TNF-α and interleukin-1. *Proceedings of the National Academy of Science, USA*, **87**, 968–72.

Jones, D.B., Hunter, N.R. & Duff, G.W. (1990). Heat-shock protein 65 as a β cell antigen of insulin-dependent diabetes. *Lancet*, **336**, 583–5.

Jordan, G.W. & Cohen, S.H. (1987). Encephalomyocarditis virus-induced diabetes mellitus in mice: model of viral pathogenesis. *Reviews of Infectious Diseases*, **9**, 917–24.

Kämpe, O., Andersson, A., Björk, E., Hallberg, A. & Karlsson, F.A. (1989). High-glucose stimulation of 64,000-M$_r$ islet cell autoantigen expression. *Diabetes*, **38**, 1326–8.

Kämpe, O., Velloso, L., Andersson, A. & Karlsson, A. (1990). No role for 65 KD heat-shock protein in diabetes. *Lancet*, **336**, 1250.

Kantwerk, G., Cobbold, S., Waldmann, H. & Kolb, H. (1987). L3T4 and Lyt-2 T cells are both involved in the generation of low-dose streptozotocin-induced diabetes in mice. *Clinical and Experimental Immunology*, **70**, 585–92.

Karjalainen, J., Knip, M., Hyöty, H., Leinikki, P., Ilonen, J., Käär, M.L. & Åkerblom, H.K. (1988). Relationship between serum insulin autoantibodies, islet cell antibodies and Coxsackie-B4 and mumps virus-specific antibodies at the clinical manifestation of Type 1 (insulin-dependent) diabetes. *Diabetologia*, **31**, 146–52.

Kida, K., Mimura, G., Kobayashi, T., Nakamura, K., Sonoda, S., Inouye, H. & Tsuji, K. (1989). Immunogenetic heterogeneity in type I (insulin-dependent) diabetes among Japanese – HLA antigens and organ-specific autoantibodies. *Diabetologia*, **32**, 34–9.

Koevary, S., Rossini, A., Stoller, W., Chick, W. & Williams, R.M. (1983). Passive transfer of diabetes in the BB/W rat. *Science*, **220**, 727–8.

Koide, Y. & Yoshida, T.O. (1990). The unique nucleotide sequence of the Aβ gene in the NOD mouse is shared with its non-diabetic sister strains, the ILI and the CTS mouse. *International Immunology*, **2**, 189–92.

Kolb, H., Bach, J.F., Eisenbarth, G.S., Harrison, L.C., Maclaren, N.K., Pozzilli, P., Skyler, J.S. & Stiller, C.R. (1989). Criteria for immune trials in type I diabetes. *Lancet*, **ii**, 686.

Kontiainen, S., Scheinin, T., Schlenzka, A., Mäenpää, J., Groop, L. & Koskimies, S. (1988). Differences in HLA types in children with insulin-dependent diabetes diagnosed in 1960s, 1970s, and 1980s. *Lancet*, **ii**, 219.

Kurtz, Z., Peckham, C.S. & Ades, A.E. (1988). Changing prevalence of juvenile-onset diabetes mellitus. *Lancet*, **ii**, 88–90.

Kyner, J.L., Peine, C.A., Alward, K.A. & Abdou, N.I. (1989). Immunoregulation of anti-islet cell antibody in insulin-dependent diabetes: failure to detect anti-idiotypic antibody following seroconversion. *Clinical Immunology and Immunopathology*, **53**, 321–8.

Laborie, C., Sai, P., Feutren, G., Debray-Sachs, M., Quiniou-Debrie, M.C., Poussier, P., Marliss, E.B. & Assan, R. (1985). Time course of islet cell antibodies in diabetic and non-diabetic BB rats. *Diabetes*, **34**, 904–10.

Lampeter, E:F., Signore, A., Gale, E.A.M. & Pozzilli, P. (1989). Lessons from the NOD mouse for the pathogenesis and immunotherapy of human Type 1 (insulin-dependent) diabetes mellitus. *Diabetologia*, **32**, 703–8.

Lander, T., Nerl, C., Held, M., Standl, E. & Mehnert, H. (1989). Flow-cytometric detection of human anti-islet insulinoma antibodies in relation to anti-human islet cell and anti-insulin antibodies. Recognition of distinct antigens by antibodies in early type I diabetes. *Diabetes*, **38**, 1557–66.

Laupacis, A., Gardell, C., Dupré, J., Stiller, C.R., Keown, P., Wallace, A.C. & Thibert, P. (1983). Cyclosporin prevents diabetes in BB Wistar rats. *Lancet*, **i**, 10–12.

Lehuen, A., Bendelac, A., Bach, J.F. & Carnaud, C. (1990). The non-obese diabetic mouse model. Independent expression of humoral and cell-mediated autoimmune features. *Journal of Immunology*, **144**, 2147–51.

Leiter, E.H. (1985). Type C retrovirus production by pancreatic beta cells. Association with accelerated pathogenesis in C3H-db/db (diabetes) mice. *American Journal of Pathology*, **119**, 22–32.

Leiter, E.H., Prochazka, M. & Coleman, D.L. (1987). Animal models of human disease. The non-obese diabetic mouse. *American Journal of Pathology*, **128**, 380–3.

Leiter, E.H., Christianson, G.J., Serreze, D.V., Ting, A.T. & Worthen, S.M. (1989). MHC antigen induction by interferon-γ on cultured mouse pancreatic β cells and macrophages. Genetic analysis of strain differences and discovery of an 'occult' class I-like antigen in NOD/Lt mice. *Journal of Experimental Medicine*, **170**, 1243–62.

Leiter, E.H., Serreze, D.V. & Prochazka, M. (1990). The genetics and epidemiology of diabetes in NOD mice. *Immunology Today*, **11**, 147–9.

Lernmark, Å., Hägglöf, B., Freedman, Z., Irvine, J., Ludvigsson, J. & Holmgren, G. (1981). A prospective analysis of antibodies reacting with pancreatic islet cells in insulin-dependent diabetic children. *Diabetologia*, **20**, 471–4.

Leslie, R.D.G., Pyke, D.A. & Denman, A.D. (1985). Immunosuppressive therapy in diabetes. *Lancet*, **i**, 516.

Leslie, R.D.G. & Pyke, D.A. (1986). The genetics of diabetes. In *The Diabetes Annual*, Volume 3, ed. K.G.M.M. Alberti & L.P. Krall, pp. 39–54. Amsterdam: Elsevier.

Like, A. (1990). Depletion of RT6.1+ T lymphocytes alone is insufficient to induce diabetes in diabetes-resistant BB/Wor rats. *American Journal of Pathology*, **136**, 565–74.

Like, A.A., Kislauskis, E., Williams, R.M. & Rossini, A.A. (1982). Neonatal thymectomy prevents spontaneous diabetes mellitus in the BB/W rat. *Science*, **216**, 644–6.

Like, A.A., Guberski, D.L. & Butler, L. (1986a). Diabetic BioBreeding/Worcester (BB/Wor) rats need not be lymphopenic. *Journal of Immunology*, **136**, 3254–8.

Like, A.A., Biron, C.A., Weringer, E.J., Byman, K., Sroczynski, E. & Guberski, D.L. (1986b). Prevention of diabetes in BioBreeding/Worcester rats with monoclonal antibodies that recognize T lymphocytes or natural killer cells. *Journal of Experimental Medicine*, **164**, 1145–59.

Lo, E., Burkly, L.C., Widera, G., Cowing, C., Flavell, R.A., Palmiter, R.D. & Brinster, R.L. (1988). Diabetes and tolerance in transgenic mice expressing class II molecule in pancreatic beta cells. *Cell*, **53**, 159–68.

Logothetopoulos, J., Valiquette, N., Madura, E. & Cvet, D. (1984). The onset and progression of pancreatic insulitis in the overt, spontaneously diabetic, young adult BB rat studied by pancreatic biopsy. *Diabetes*, **33**, 33–6.

Ludvigsson, J., Heding, L., Lieden, G., Marner, B. & Lernmark, Å. (1983). Plasmapheresis in the initial treatment of insulin-dependent diabetes mellitus in children. *British Medical Journal*, **286**, 176–8.

Makino, S., Kunimoto, K., Muraoka, Y., Mizushima, Y., Katagiri, K. & Tochino, Y. (1980). Breeding of a non-obese diabetic strain of mice. *Experimental Animals (Tokyo)*, **29**, 1–13.

Mandrup-Poulsen, T. (1988). On the pathogenesis of insulin-dependent diabetes mellitus. *Danish Medical Bulletin*, **35**, 438–60.

Martell, M., Marcadet, A., Moine, A., Boitard, C., Deschamps, I., Dausset, J., Bach, J.F. & Cohen, D. (1990). Heterogeneity of HLA genetic factors in IDDM susceptibility. *Immunogenetics*, **31**, 233–40.

Martin, D.R. & Logothetopoulos, J. (1984). Complement-fixing islet cell antibodies in the spontaneously diabetic BB rat. *Diabetes*, **33**, 93–6.

Mendola, G., Casanitjana, R. & Gomis, R. (1989). Effect of nicotinamide therapy on β cell function in newly diagnosed Type I (insulin-dependent) diabetic patients. *Diabetologia*, **32**, 160–2.

Michel, C., Boitard, C. & Bach, J.F. (1989). Insulin autoantibodies in non-obese diabetic (NOD) mice. *Clinical and Experimental Immunology*, **75**, 457–60.

Michelsen, B., Kastern, W., Lernmark, Å. & Owerbach, D. (1985). Identification of an HLA-DQ β-chain related genomic sequence associated with insulin-dependent diabetes. *Biomedicine et Biochimica Acta*, **44**, 33–6.

Millward, B.A., Welsh, K.I., Leslie, R.D.G., Pyke, D.A. & Demaine, A.G. (1987). T cell receptor beta chain polymorphisms are associated with insulin-dependent diabetes. *Clinical and Experimental Immunology*, **70**, 152–7.

Morel, P.A., Dorman, J.S., Todd, J.A., McDevitt, H.O. & Trucco, M. (1988). Aspartic acid at position 57 of the DQ β chain protects against type I diabetes: a family study. *Proceedings of the National Academy of Science, USA*, **85**, 8111–15.

Morris, D.J., Kimpton, C. & Corbitt, G. (1988). Persistent virus infection and type 1 diabetes. *Lancet*, **ii**, 450.

Murase, N., Lieberman, I., Nalesnik, M., Mintz, D., Todo, S., Drash, A.L. & Starzl, T.E. (1990). Prevention of spontaneous diabetes in BB rats with FK 506. *Lancet*, **336**, 373–4.

Nagata, M., Yokono, K., Hayakawa, M., Kawase, Y., Hatamori, N., Ogawa, W., Yonezawa, K., Shii, K. & Baba, S. (1989). Destruction of pancreatic islet cells by cytotoxic T lymphocytes in non-obese diabetic mice. *Journal of Immunology*, **143**, 1155–62.

Nagy, M.V., Chan, E.K., Teruya, M., Forrest, L.E., Likhite, V. & Charles, M.A. (1989). Macrophage-mediated islet cell cytotoxicity in BB rats. *Diabetes*, **38**, 1329–31.

Nepom, B.S., Palmer, J., Kim, S.J., Hansen, J.A., Holbeck, S.L. & Nepom, G.T. (1986). Specific genomic markers for the HLA-DQ subregion discriminate between DR4+ insulin-dependent diabetes mellitus and DR4+ seropositive juvenile rheumatoid arthritis. *Journal of Experimental Medicine*, **164**, 345–50.

Nepom, B.S., Schwarz, D., Palmer, J.P. & Nepom, G.T. (1987). Transcomplementation of HLA genes in IDDM. HLA-DQα- and β-chains produce hybrid molecules in DR3/4 heterozygotes. *Diabetes*, **36**, 114–17.

Nerup, J., Andersen, O.O., Bendixen, G., Egeberg, J. & Poulsen, J.E. (1971). Antipancreatic cellular hypersensitivity in diabetes mellitus. *Diabetes*, **20**, 424–7.

Nishimoto, H., Kikutani, H., Yamamura, K. & Kishimoto, T. (1987). Prevention of auto-immune insulitis by expression of I-E molecules in NOD mice. *Nature*, **328**, 432–4.

Notkins, A.L. (1977). Virus induced diabetes mellitus. Brief review. *Archives of Virology*, **54**, 1–17.

Oldstone, M.B.A. (1988). Prevention of type I diabetes in nonobese diabetic mice by virus infection. *Science*, **239**, 500–2.

Oldstone, M.B.A. (1990). Viruses as therapeutic agents. I. Treatment of non-obese insulin-dependent diabetes mice with virus prevents insulin-dependent diabetes mellitus while maintaining general immune competence. *Journal of Experimental Medicine*, **171**, 2077–89.

Oliveira, D.B.G. & Peters, D.K. (1990). The immunogenetic basis of autoimmunity. *Autoimmunity*, **5**, 293–306.

Onodera, T., Toniolo, A., Ray, U.R., Bennett Jenson, A., Knazek, R.A. & Notkins, A.L. (1981). Virus-induced diabetes mellitus. XX. Polyendocrinopathy and autoimmunity. *Journal of Experimental Medicine*, **153**, 1457–73.

Onodera, T., Ray, U.R., Melez, K.A., Suzuki, H., Toniolo, A. & Notkins, A.L. (1982). Virus-induced diabetes mellitus: autoimmunity and polyendocrine disease prevented by immunosuppression. *Nature*, **297**, 66–8.

Oschilewski, U., Kiesel, U. & Kolb, H. (1985). Administration of silica prevents diabetes in BB-rats. *Diabetes*, **34**, 197–9.

Owerbach, D., Lernmark, Å., Platz, P., Ryder, L.P., Rask, L., Peterson, P.A. & Ludvigsson, J. (1983). HLA-D region β-chain DNA endonuclease fragments differ between HLA-DR identical healthy and insulin-dependent diabetic individuals. *Nature*, **303**, 815–17.

Pak, C.Y., Eun, H.-M., McArthur, R.G. & Yoon, J.-W. (1988). Association of cytomegalo-virus infection with autoimmune type 1 diabetes. *Lancet*, **ii**, 1–4.

Palmer, J.P., Asplin, C.M., Clemons, P., Lyen, K., Tatpati, O., Raghu, P.K. & Paquette, T.L. (1983). Insulin antibodies in insulin-dependent diabetics before insulin treatment. *Science*, **222**, 1337–9.

Peig, M., Gomis, R., Ercilla, G., Casamitjana, R., Bottazzo, G.F. & Pujol-Borrell, R. (1989). Correlation between residual β-cell function and islet cell antibodies in newly diagnosed type I diabetes. Follow-up study. *Diabetes*, **38**, 1396–401.

Plamondon, C., Kottis, V., Brideau, C., Métroz-Dayer, M.-D. & Poussier, P. (1990). Abnormal thymocyte maturation in spontaneously diabetic BB rats involves the deletion of CD4⁻8⁺ cells. *Journal of Immunology*, **144**, 923–8.

Platz, P., Jakobsen, B.K., Morling, N., Ryder, L.P., Svejgaard, A., Thomsen, M., Christy, M., Kromann, H., Benn, J., Nerup, J., Green, A. & Hauge, M. (1981). HLA-D and DR antigens in genetic analysis of insulin-dependent diabetes mellitus. *Diabetologia*, **21**, 108–15.

Prochazka, M., Leiter, E.H., Serreze, D.V. & Coleman, D.L. (1987). Three recessive loci required for insulin-dependent diabetes in non-obese diabetic mice. *Science*, **237**, 286–9.

Prud'homme, G.J., Fuks, A., Colle, E. & Guttmann, R.D. (1984). Isolation of T-lymphocyte lines with specificity for islet cell antigens from spontaneously diabetic (insulin-dependent) rats. *Diabetes*, **33**, 801–3.

Pujol-Borrell, R., Todd, I., Doshi, M., Bottazzo, G.F., Sutton, R., Gray, D., Adolf, G.R. & Feldmann, M. (1987). HLA class II induction in human islet cells by interferon-γ plus tumour necrosis factor or lymphotoxin. *Nature*, **326**, 304–6.

Pukel, C., Baquerizo, H. & Rabinovitch, A. (1988). Destruction of rat islet cell monolayers by cytokines. Synergistic interactions of interferon-γ tumor necrosis factor, lymphotoxin and interleukin 1. *Diabetes*, **37**, 133–6.

Rabinovitch, A., Sumoski, W., Rajotte, R.V. & Warnock, G.L. (1990). Cytotoxic effects of cytokines on human pancreatic islet cells in monolayer culture. *Journal of Clinical Endocrinology and Metabolism*, **71**, 152–6.

Raum, D., Awdeh, Z., Yunis, E., Alper, C.A. & Gabbay, K.H. (1984). Extended major histocompatibility complex haplotypes in type I diabetes mellitus. *Journal of Clinical Investigation*, **74**, 449–54.

Rayfield, E.J., Kelly, K.J. & Yoon, J.-W. (1986). Rubella virus-induced diabetes in the hamster. *Diabetes*, **35**, 1278–81.

Reddy, S., Bibby, N.J. & Elliott, R.B. (1988). Ontogeny of islet cell antibodies, insulin autoantibodies and insulitis in the non-obese diabetic mouse. *Diabetologia*, **31**, 322–8.

Reich, E.P., Sherwin, R.S., Kanagawa, O. & Janeway, C.A. (1989). An explanation for the protective effect of the MHC class II I-E molecule in murine diabetes. *Nature*, **341**, 326–8.

Reijonen, H., Silvennoinen-Kassinen, S., Ilonen, J. & Knip, M. (1990). Lack of association of T cell receptor beta-chain constant region polymorphism with insulin-dependent diabetes mellitus in Finland. *Clinical and Experimental Immunology*, **81**, 396–9.

Rochet, N., Sadoul, J.L., Ferrua, B., Kubar, J., Tanti, J.F., Bougneres, P., Vialettes, B., Van Obberghen, E., Le Marchand-Brustel, Y. & Freychet, P. (1990). Autoantibodies to the insulin receptor are infrequent findings in type I (insulin-dependent) diabetes mellitus of recent onset. *Diabetologia*, **33**, 411–16.

Roep, B.O., Arden, S.D., De Vries, R.R.P. & Hutton, J.C. (1990). T-cell clones from type-1 diabetes patient respond to insulin secretory granule proteins. *Nature*, **345**, 632–4.

Roman, L.M., Simons, L.F., Hammer, R.E., Sambrook, J.F. & Gething, M.H. (1990). The expression of influenza virus haemagglutinin in the pancreatic β cells of transgenic mice results in autoimmune diabetes. *Cell*, **61**, 383–96.

Rossini, A.A., Williams, R.M., Mordes, J.P., Appel, M.C. & Like, A.A. (1979). Spontaneous diabetes in the gnotobiotic BB/W rat. *Diabetes*, **28**, 1031–2.

Rossini, A.A., Faustman, D., Woda, B.A., Like, A.A., Szymanski, I. & Mordes, J.P. (1984). Lymphocyte transfusions prevent diabetes in the Bio-Breeding/Worcester rat. *Journal of Clinical Investigation*, **74**, 39–46.

Rotter, J.I., Anderson, C.E., Rubin, R., Congleton, J.E., Terasaki, P.I. & Rimoin, D.L. (1983). HLA genotypic study of insulin-dependent diabetes. The excess of DR3/DR4 heterozygotes allows rejection of the recessive hypothesis. *Diabetes*, **32**, 169–74.

Sarvetnick, N., Liggitt, D., Pitts, S.L., Hansen, S.E. & Stewart, T.A. (1988). Insulin-dependent diabetes mellitus induced in transgenic mice by ectopic expression of class II MHC and interferon-gamma. *Cell*, **52**, 773–82.

Scott, F.W., Mongeau, R., Kardish, M., Hatinka, G., Trick, K.D. & Wojcinski, Z. (1985). Diet can prevent diabetes in the BB rat. *Diabetes*, **34**, 1059–62.

Sheehy, M.J., Scharf, S.J., Rowe, J.R., Neme de Gimenez, M.H., Meske, L.M., Erlich, H.A. & Nepom, B.S. (1989). A diabetes-susceptible HLA haplotype is best defined by a combination of HLA-DR and -DQ alleles. *Journal of Clinical Investigation*, **83**, 830–5.

Signore, A., Pozzilli, P., Gale, E.A.M., Andreani, D. & Beverley, P.C.L. (1989). The natural history of lymphocyte subsets infiltrating the pancreas of NOD mice. *Diabetologia*, **32**, 282–9.

Singal, D.P. & Blajchman, M.A. (1973). Histocompatibility (HL-A) antigens, lymphocyto-toxic antibodies and tissue antibodies in patients with diabetes mellitus. *Diabetes*, **22**, 429–32.

Spinas, G.A., Mandrup-Poulsen, T., Mølvig, J., Baek, L., Bendtzen, K., Dinarello, C.A. & Nerup, J. (1986). Low concentrations of interleukin-1 stimulate and high concentrations inhibit insulin release from isolated rat islets of Langerhans. *Acta Endocrinologica*, **113**, 551–8.

Srikanta, S., Ganda, O.P., Rabizadeh, A., Soeldner, J.S. & Eisenbarth, G. (1985). First-degree relatives of patients with type 1 diabetes mellitus. Islet-cell antibodies and abnormal insulin secretion. *New England Journal of Medicine*, **313**, 461–4.

Stiller, C.R., Dupré, J., Gent, M., Jenner, M.R., Keown, P.A., Laupacis, A., Martell, R., Rodger, N.W. & Graffenried, B.V. (1984). Effects of cyclosporine immunosuppression in insulin-dependent diabetes mellitus of recent onset. *Science*, **223**, 1362–7.

Sumoski, W., Baquerizo, H. & Rabinovitch, A. (1989). Oxygen free radical scavengers protect rat islet cells from damage by cytokines. *Diabetologia*, **32**, 792–6.

Sutherland, D.E.R. (1990). Pancreas transplantation or insulin? *Lancet*, **336**, 110.

Tait, B.D., Propert, D.N., Harrison, L., Mandel, T. & Martin, F.I.R. (1986). Interaction between HLA antigens and immunoglobulin (Gm) allotypes in susceptibility to type I diabetes. *Tissue Antigens*, **27**, 249–55.

Tarn, A.C., Smith, C.P., Spencer, K.M., Bottazzo, G.F. & Gale, E.A.M. (1987). Type I (insulin-dependent) diabetes: a disease of slow clinical onset? *British Medical Journal*, **294**, 342–5.

Taylor, S.I., Barbetti, F., Accili, D., Roth, J. & Gorden, P. (1989). Syndromes of autoimmu-nity and hypoglycaemia. Autoantibodies directed against insulin and its receptor. *Endocrin-ology and Metabolism Clinics of North America*, **18**, 123–43.

Thomsen, M., Mølvig, J., Zerbib, A, de Preval, C., Abbal, M., Dugoujon, J.M., Ohayon, E., Svejgaard, A., Cambon-Thomsen, A. & Nerup, J. (1988). The susceptibility to insulin-dependent diabetes mellitus is associated with C4 allotypes independently of the association with HLA-DQ alleles in HLA-DR3/4 heterozygotes. *Immunogenetics*, **28**, 320–7.

Thomson, G., Robinson, W.P., Kuhner, M.K., Joe, S., MacDonald, M.J., Gottschall, J.L., Barbosa, J., Rich, S.S., Bertrams, J., Baur, M.P., Partanen, J., Tait, B.D., Schober, E.,

Mayr, W.R., Ludvigsson, J., Lindblom, B., Farid, N.R., Thompson, C. & Deschamps, I. (1988). Genetic heterogeneity, modes of inheritance, and risk estimates for a joint study of Caucasians with insulin-dependent diabetes mellitus. *American Journal of Human Genetics*, **43**, 799–816.

Tiwari, J.L. & Terasaki, P.I. (1985). Juvenile diabetes mellitus. In *HLA and Disease Associations*, pp. 185–212., Berlin: Springer-Verlag.

Todd, J.A., Bell, J.I. & McDevitt, H.O. (1987). HLA-DQβ gene contributes to susceptibility and resistance to insulin-dependent diabetes mellitus. *Nature*, **329**, 599–604.

Todd, J.A., Mijovic, C., Fletcher, J., Jenkins, D., Bradwell, A.R. & Barnett, A.H. (1989). Identification of susceptibility loci for insulin-dependent diabetes mellitus by trans-racial gene mapping. *Nature*, **338**, 587–9.

Todd, J.A., Fukui, Y., Kitigawa, T. & Sasazuki, T. (1990). The A3 allele of the HLA-DQA1 locus is associated with susceptibility to type 1 diabetes in Japanese. *Proceedings of the National Academy of Science, USA*, **87**, 1094–8.

Topliss, D., How, J., Lewis, M., Row, V.V. & Volpé, R. (1983). Evidence for cell-mediated immunity and specific suppressor T lymphocyte dysfunction in Graves' disease and diabetes mellitus. *Journal of Clinical Endocrinology and Metabolism*, **57**, 700–5.

Tuomilehto-Wolf, E., Tuomilehto, J., Cepaitis, Z., Lounamaa, R. & DIME Study Group (1989). New susceptibility haplotype for type 1 diabetes. *Lancet*, **ii**, 299–302.

Uchigata, Y., Yao, K., Takayama-Hasumi, S. & Hirata, Y. (1989). Human monoclonal IgG1 insulin autoantibody from insulin autoimmune syndrome directed at determinant at asparagine site on insulin B-chain. *Diabetes*, **38**, 663–6.

Vague, P., Vialettes, B., Lassmann-Vague, V. & Vallo, J.J. (1987). Nicotinamide may extend remission phase in insulin-dependent diabetes. *Lancet*, **i**, 619–20.

Van De Winkel, M., Smets, G., Gepts, W. & Pipeleers, D. (1982). Islet cell surface antibodies from insulin-dependent diabetics bind specifically to pancreatic β cells. *Journal of Clinical Investigation*, **70**, 41–9.

Van Rees, E.P., Voorbij, H.A.M. & Dijkstra, C.D. (1988). Neonatal development of lymphoid organs and specific immune responses *in situ* in diabetes-prone BB rats. *Immunology*, **65**, 465–72.

Walker, R., Cooke, A., Bone, A.J., Dean, B.M:, Van Der Meide, P. & Baird, J.D. (1986). Induction of class II MHC antigens in vitro on pancreatic β cells isolated from BB/E rats. *Diabetologia*, **29**, 749–51.

Walker, R., Bone, A.J., Cooke, A. & Baird, J. (1988). Distinct macrophage subpopulations in the pancreas of prediabetic BB/E rats. Possible role for macrophages in pathogenesis of IDDM. *Diabetes*, **37**, 1301–4.

Warram, J.H., Krolewski, A.S. & Kahn, C.R. (1988). Determinants of IDDM and perinatal mortality in children of diabetic mothers. *Diabetes*, **37**, 1328–34.

Wassmuth, R. & Lernmark, Å. (1989). The genetics of susceptibility to diabetes. *Clininical Immunology and Immunopathology*, **53**, 358–99.

Webb, S.R., Loria, R.M., Madge, G.E. & Kirbrick, S. (1976). Susceptibility of mice to group B Coxsackie virus is influenced by the diabetic gene. *Journal of Experimental Medicine*, **143**, 1239–48.

WHO-HLA Nomenclature Committee (1988). Nomenclature for factors of the HLA system. *Vox Saguinis*, **55**, 119–26.

Wicker, L.S., Miller, B.J. & Mullen, Y. (1986). Transfer of autoimmune diabetes mellitus with splenocytes from nonobese diabetic (NOD) mice. *Diabetes*, **35**, 855–60.

Wicker, L.S., Miller, B.J., Coker, L.Z., McNally, S.E., Scott, S., Mullen, Y. & Appel, M.C. (1987). Genetic control of diabetes and insulitis in the nonobese diabetic (NOD) mouse. *Journal of Experimental Medicine*, **165**, 1639–54.

Wicker, L.S., Miller, B.J., Fischer, P.A., Pressey, A. & Peterson, L.B. (1989). Genetic control of diabetes and insulitis in the non-obese diabetic mouse. Pedigree analysis of a diabetic H-2nod/b heterozygote. *Journal of Immunology*, **142**, 781–4.

Wilkin, T.J. (1990). Insulin autoantibodies as markers for type I diabetes. *Endocrine Reviews*, **11**, 92–104.

Wilkin, T., Armitage, M., Casey, C., Pyke, D.A., Hoskins, P.J., Rodier, M., Diaz, J.-L. & Leslie, R.D.G. (1985). Value of insulin autoantibodies as serum markers for insulin-dependent diabetes mellitus. *Lancet*, **i**, 480–2.

Wilson, C.A., Jacobs, C., Baker, P., Baskin, D.G., Dower, S., Lernmark, Å., Toivola, B., Vertrees, S. & Wilson, D. (1990). IL-1β modulation of spontaneous autoimmune diabetes and thyroiditis in the BB rat. *Journal of Immunology*, **144**, 3784–8.

Winter, W.E., Shimpo, K., Obata, M., Yamada, K. & Luchetta, R. (1990). Immunogenetic analysis of β-cell autoimmunity in NOD mice. Relationship of insulitis to T-lymphocyte-receptor β nod and Aβ nod genes. *Diabetes*, **39**, 975–82.

Woda, B.A. & Biron, C.A. (1986). Natural killer cell number and function in the spontaneously diabetic BB/W rat. *Journal of Immunology*, **137**, 1860–6.

Wolf, E., Spencer, K.M. & Cudworth, A.G. (1983). The genetic susceptibility to type I (insulin-dependent) diabetes: analysis of the HLA-DR association. *Diabetologia*, **24**, 224–30.

Yale, J.-F., Grose, M. & Marliss, E.B. (1985). Time course of the lymphopenia in BB rats. Relation to the onset of diabetes. *Diabetes*, **34**, 955–9.

Yamada, K., Nonaka, K., Hanafusa, T., Miyazaki, A., Toyoshima, H. & Tarui, S. (1982). Preventitive and therapeutic effects of large-dose nicotinamide injections on diabetes associated with insulitis. An observation in non obese diabetic (NOD) mice. *Diabetes*, **31**, 749–53.

Yamagata, K., Nakajima, H., Hanafusa, T., Noguchi, T., Miyazaki, A., Miyagawa, J., Sada, M., Amemiya, H., Tanaka, T., Kono, N. & Tarui, S. (1989). Aspartic acid at position 57 of DQβ chain does not protect against type I (insulin-dependent) diabetes mellitus in Japanese subjects. *Diabetologia*, **32**, 762–4.

Yoon, J.-W., Austin, M., Onodera, T. & Notkins, A.L. (1979). Virus-induced diabetes mellitus. Isolation of a virus from the pancreas of a child with diabetic ketoacidosis. *New England Journal of Medicine*, **300**, 1173–9.

Young, L.H.Y., Peterson, L.B., Wicker, L.S., Persechini, P.M. & Young, J.D. (1989). *In vivo* expression of perforin by CD8+ lymphocytes in autoimmune disease. Studies on spontaneous and adoptively transferred diabetes in non-obese diabetic mice. *Journal of Immunology*, **143**, 3994–9.

Ziegler, A.G., Ziegler, R., Vardi, P., Jackson, R.A., Soeldner, J.S. & Eisenbarth, G.S. (1989). Life-table analysis of progression to diabetes of anti-insulin autoantibody-positive relatives of individuals with type 1 diabetes. *Diabetes*, **38**, 1320–5.

Ziegler, A.G., Herskowitz, R.D., Jackson, R.A., Soeldner, J.S. & Eisenbarth, G.S. (1990). Predicting type I diabetes. *Diabetic Care*, **13**, 762–75.

Zielasek, J., Burkart, V., Naylor, P., Goldstein, A., Kiesel, U. & Kolb, H. (1990). Interleukin-2-dependent control of disease development in spontaneously diabetic BB rats. *Immunology*, **69**, 209–14.

Adrenal autoimmunity

Autoimmune Addison's disease

Addison (1855) originally described 11 cases of aetiologically diverse adrenal failure and, for many years subsequently, tuberculosis was the main cause of this disorder. However, it is now apparent that autoimmune adrenalitis is by far the commonest form of Addison's disease, being responsible in 79% of 329 British patients (Irvine & Barnes, 1975). The average age of onset is 30–35 years. The prevalence is between 30 and 60 per million, with a female to male ratio of 2.5:1, but when diagnosed in the first two decades of life, the sex ratio is almost equal.

Determining that autoimmunity underlies the disease is important, to avoid missing the diagnosis of adrenal destruction caused by tumour, infection or infiltration. There are also recent reports of Addison's disease occurring as a result of venous thrombosis in the primary antiphospholipid syndrome, marked by the presence of lupus anticoagulants or cardiolipin antibodies in the absence of defined systemic lupus erythematosus (Asherson & Hughes, 1989). In many patients with conventional autoimmune adrenal failure, the disorder is accompanied by other endocrinopathies, which helps in making this diagnosis: polyendocrine autoimmunity is considered separately in Chapter 8. In contrast to tuberculous adrenal failure, the glands are not calcified on plain abdominal radiography and are small or undetectable by computerised tomography at the time of diagnosis (Vita *et al.*, 1985). The adrenal histology is of cortical atrophy and disruption, with variable amounts of lymphocytic infiltration (including germinal centre formation) and fibrosis. The medulla is preserved but often contains lymphocytes (Irvine, Stewart & Scarth, 1967; Petri & Nerup, 1971). Focal accumulations of lymphocytes occur in around 2% of ostensibly normal adrenals at post-mortem (Petri & Nerup, 1971).

Experimental autoimmune adrenalitis

Immunisation of animals with adrenal gland extracts in complete Freund's adjuvant results in specific adrenalitis with formation of autoantibodies which may cross-react with ovary (Colover & Glynn, 1958; Barnett, Dumonde & Glynn, 1963). The disease is transferable with lymph node-derived cells (Levine & Wenk, 1968). As well as infiltration of other endocrine tissues, T cell depletion in certain strains of mice also results in adrenalitis and the production of adrenocortical autoantibodies, although combined thymectomy and cyclosporin A treatment is necessary (Sakaguchi & Sakaguchi, 1989). Murine cytomegalovirus infection of BALB/c mice induces adrenalitis and antibody formation (Bartholomaeus et al., 1988). However, the specificity of this response is poor, with adrenal antibodies reacting with both the cortex and the medulla and a wide range of other organs being involved.

Immunogenetics and environmental factors

HLA-B8 was the first MHC antigen to be associated with Addison's disease, the relative risk being 8.3 (Thomsen et al., 1975) and an association between the presence of adrenocortical autoantibodies and B8 was also noted. However, subsequent studies have shown that the primary association is with HLA-DR3 in linkage disequilibrium with HLA-B8. In a study of 34 patients with Addison's disease in the USA, which excluded those with type 1 polyendocrine autoimmunity, the relative risk was 12.1 for DR3 with an aetiological fraction of 0.7 (Maclaren & Riley, 1986). DR4 also conferred susceptibility with a relative risk of 8.9 and when DR3 and DR4 were present together, the relative risk was 46.8. This is reminiscent of the findings in type 1 diabetes mellitus, but the results remained significant when those Addison's patients with concurrent diabetes were excluded. However, in 34 European patients, only DR3 was significantly associated with the disease, the relative risk being 3.4 and the association was stronger in those patients with adrenal antibodies and associated endocrinopathies (Latinne et al., 1987). In 33 UK patients we have studied by analysis of restriction fragment polymorphisms, DR3 alone was significantly associated, with a relative risk of 3.6 and an aetiological fraction of 0.45 (Weetman et al., unpublished data). Only two patients had diabetes, and there was no association of DR4 with particular alleles of the DQB1 locus in the other subjects. No environmental factors are known to operate in Addison's disease.

T cell responses

A high percentage of circulating T cells in recently diagnosed patients express Ia or class II MHC molecules, in common with many other autoimmune disorders (Rabinowe *et al.*, 1984). Peripheral blood T cells also appear to be sensitised to adrenal mitochondrial antigens in autoimmune adrenalitis. Using a MIF assay, eight of 11 men and six of 19 women (46% of total) gave positive responses, whereas the test was negative in all seven patients with Addison's disease caused by tuberculosis (Nerup & Bendixen, 1969). There was no correlation between this cellular immune response and the presence of adrenal antibodies. Surprisingly, a similar antigen preparation was unable to induce blastogenesis in T cells from patients with autoimmune Addison's disease (Nerup, Anderson & Bendixen, 1970).

Studies on the infiltrating lymphocytes have not been performed. A minority of normal adrenal zona reticularis cells express Ia whereas in autoimmune Addison's disease all the remaining cortical cells, irrespective of type, are strongly Ia^+ (Jackson *et al.*, 1988). However, a similar appearance was found in tuberculous glands associated with areas of inflammation. These features in normal and non-autoimmune adrenal tissue indicate that Ia^+ cortical cells are most unlikely to stimulate T cells and lead to an autoimmune response.

B cell responses

The earliest description of adrenal autoantibodies documented positive complement fixation tests using adrenal extracts in two of 10 Addison's patients (Anderson *et al.*, 1957). Soon afterwards, indirect immunofluorescence assays were used to show that 51% of 71 patients with idiopathic Addison's disease had adrenal antibodies, only two-thirds of which were detected by the complement fixation assay (Blizzard & Kyle, 1963). The reactivity was organ-specific, with antigenic reactivity in both microsomal and mitochondrial fractions of adrenal homogenate. Twelve years later, a review of 511 published cases showed that the proportion of patients with adrenal antibodies by immunofluorescence remained at 58% (Irvine & Barnes, 1975). Although 8% of 154 tuberculous Addison's patients also had adrenal antibodies, those positive were found in the earliest studies. The antibodies disappear in 17% of cases within five years of diagnosis and may persist for at least 20 years in some patients (Sotsiou, Bottazzo & Doniach, 1980).

Patients with various other autoimmune disorders have been assessed for the presence of adrenal antibodies and only in idiopathic hypoparathyroidism was a high prevalence (30% of 20 subjects) noted (Irvine & Barnes, 1975), presumably related to the incipient occurrence of a polyendocrine autoimmunity syndrome. In a subsequent study of 628 autoimmune endocrine patients, (excluding Addison's disease but of unspecified nature), the prevalence of adrenal antibodies was 7% (Sotsiou *et al.*, 1980). Of 518 patients with autoimmune thyroid disease, 5.2% had adrenal antibodies by immunofluorescence, as did 3.1% of 130 patients with myasthenia gravis; none of 268 controls were positive (Scherbaum & Berg, 1982). Thirty of these non-Addisonian patients with antibodies were followed for up to three and a half years. Three had impaired adrenal reserve and two developed adrenal insufficiency, suggesting that autoimmune Addison's disease, like thyroiditis, may have a subclinical form reflecting the slow evolution of the condition. A rather lower prevalence of adrenal antibodies was detected by complement fixation, positive tests being found in 1.6% of 250 patients with thyroid autoimmunity, 1.2% of 251 diabetic patients and 14% of 14 patients with hypoparathyroidism (Betterle et al., 1983). Within 1–31 months four of these (two diabetic and both the hypoparathyroid subjects) developed Addison's disease. These studies suggest that adrenal antibodies are a marker for susceptibility to develop adrenal failure.

The antigens identified by immunofluorescence are located particularly in the innermost cells of the cortex and are not species-specific, being found in canine, bovine, porcine, simian, feline and guinea pig adrenals (Blizzard & Kyle, 1963; Anderson et al., 1968; Irvine, Chan & Scarth, 1969). Mouse and rat adrenals do not contain antigens reactive with human sera (Nerup, 1974). Because there is considerable autofluorescence and interindividual variation in the glands used as substrate, attempts have been made to improve the assay of adrenal autoantibodies and to define the exact antigens recognised. Human adrenal cell suspensions and monolayer cultures express surface autoantigens and, although these can be recognised by Addison's sera, bound antibody does not fix complement (Khoury et al., 1981). The immunofluorescence results using cells were no different to those with tissue sections in sensitivity for antibodies. An ELISA has been described which is more sensitive and reproducible than previous techniques, 79% of idiopathic Addison's patients giving positive results (Stechemesser et al., 1985). A solid-phase radioimmunoassay using adrenal microsomes from patients with Cushing's disease was also more sensitive than immunofluorescence for low antibody titres (Kosowicz, Gryczynska & Bottazzo, 1986).

In a preliminary immunoprecipitation study, autoimmune Addison's sera reacted with a 38 kd adrenal microsome component (Banga et al., 1985). However, others have shown that 57% of 23 Addison's sera recognise a 55 kd protein which was specific for adrenal tissue and this reactivity correlated closely with the results of immunofluorescence (Furmaniak et al., 1988). By Western blotting, a wider range of specific reactivity was noted: of 15 patients tested, antibodies reacting against adrenal antigens of 75, 60 or 55 kd were found in six patients (Weetman et al., unpublished data). To determine the intracellular localisation of antigen, antibody binding to enzymatically defined subcellular fractions of adrenal homogenate was monitored by fluorescence spectromicroscopy. Autoantigens were defined in both the microsomes and the plasma membrane, but not the mitochondria (Bright & Singh, 1990). The exact nature of the autoantigens and indeed whether they are multiple, a presumption made on the basis of heterogeneous patterns of immunofluorescent staining (Khoury et al., 1981; Chapter 6), remains to be elucidated.

However, one distinct cell surface autoantigen may be the adrenocorticotrophic hormone (ACTH) receptor. Based on the fact that, occasionally, autoimmune hypothyroidism may be the result of TSH receptor-blocking antibodies, serum from a patient with Addison's disease and type 1 polyglandular syndrome was tested for ACTH receptor-blocking antibodies (Kendall-Taylor et al., 1988). A crude IgG preparation was found to inhibit ACTH-stimulated cortisol synthesis by dispersed guinea pig adrenal cells, but the site of immunoglobulin action was not determined. An unusual feature of this patient was the absence of increased pigmentation typical of Addison's disease, which is compatible with the putative antibodies also blocking the effect of ACTH on melanocytes. A subsequent study used both this assay and one of ACTH-stimulated adrenal DNA synthesis (estimated by the cytochemical bioassay) to assess ACTH-blocking antibodies in 25 patients with idiopathic Addison's disease, not in association with type 1 polyendocrine autoimmunity (Wulffraat et al., 1989). IgG preparations from 92% of these patients blocked ACTH stimulation of adrenal cells, whereas IgG from 10 controls was inactive. However, two of nine patients with miscellaneous adrenal disorders, not conventionally thought of as autoimmune, were positive for this blocking activity. Clearly these results are very exciting, but much further study is required to identify the epitope recognised (which need not be the ACTH receptor itself), the mode of action of these antibodies and the reasons why ACTH is still able to stimulate melanocytes in these patients.

Effector mechanisms

There is little firm evidence to support any particular mode of tissue injury in Addison's disease. The ACTH-blocking antibodies just described represent one possible cause of gland dysfunction. Complement fixation and ADCC mediated by cell surface adrenal antibodies are also possible, although neither have been shown in vitro (Khoury et al., 1981). A priori it would seem that the adrenal lymphocytic infiltrate must also contribute to gland destruction by cell-mediated cytotoxicity or lymphokine release, but this is purely speculative. The pathophysiological role of leucocyte-derived ACTH and other potential modulators of adrenal cell function remains to be defined (Buckingham, 1987).

Treatment

Patients require lifelong replacement with glucocorticoids and mineralocorticoids, usually given as hydrocortisone and fludrocortisone. No immunomodulatory treatment has been tried or is warranted; one might expect that the steroid deficiency and replacement itself could have an immunological effect.

Cushing's syndrome

The primary pigmented and nodular form of Cushing's syndrome is a very rare cause of hypercortisolism. It may be sporadic or familial, the latter sometimes being part of a multisystem tumour syndrome, termed the Carney complex. Patients with both familial types of the disorder have been described in whom serum immunoglobulins stimulated guinea pig adrenal segments to produce cortisol and synthesise DNA (determined by the Feulgen reaction). These antibodies were also found in five of 11 first degree relatives with normal adrenal function (Van Berkhout *et al.*, 1986; 1989; Young *et al.*, 1989). A perivascular lymphocytic infiltrate composed mainly of CD4$^+$ T cells was also observed in the nodular adrenal glands. It is therefore possible that these unusual patients may have antibodies which mimic the action of ACTH on the adrenal cell receptor, although this requires more comprehensive study. A local effect of the lymphocytic infiltrate is also conceivable: for instance, IL-6 can stimulate steroid production by adrenal cells *in vitro* (Salas *et al.*, 1990).

Adrenal medullary autoantibodies

No syndrome of adrenal medullary dysfunction has been ascribed to autoimmunity but specific complement-fixing antibodies against cells in the medulla have been reported in 16% of 107 newly diagnosed diabetics, in whom they correlated with the presence of islet cell antibodies (Scherbaum *et al.*, 1988). Medullary antibodies were not found in other autoimmune conditions, except three of 103 Addison's patients and there was no apparent effect on circulating basal adrenaline and noradrenaline levels, so that their pathophysiological significance is unclear. Another study found that a third of diabetics and their first degree relatives who had islet cell antibodies were also positive for adrenal medullary antibodies (Brown *et al.*, 1988). The authors speculated that medullary autoimmunity may account for the impaired adrenaline response to hypoglycaemia in some diabetics, but this clearly needs formal assessment. Adrenal fibrosis, apparently without lymphocytic infiltration, has been described in long-standing diabetes: whether this too is part of some autoimmune process is unknown (Brown *et al.*, 1989).

Summary

The autoimmune basis for the majority of cases of idiopathic Addison's disease is firmly established. This is now the commonest cause of the disorder and is strongly associated with HLA-DR3. Autoimmune adrenalitis can be reproduced in animals and these models suggest that defective T cell-dependent immunoregulation may be as aetiologically important in this as in other endocrinopathies. However, there have been few studies of T cell function *in vitro* in man. In contrast, there is an extensive literature on adrenal autoantibodies, but the nature of the autoantigens recognised by Addison's sera and the role of autoantibodies in mediating tissue injury are unclear. In at least 20% of patients, circulating adrenal antibodies cannot be found: some of these cases may not be autoimmune, while in others alternative effector mechanisms may operate. There has been recent interest in the possibility that autoantibodies may block the action of ACTH in Addison's disease and the reverse phenomenon, namely stimulation of ACTH-dependent functions by immunoglobulins, has also been described in a very rare form of Cushing's syndrome. Whether these phenomena are mediated by ACTH receptor antibodies is so far unknown.

References

Addison, T. (1855). On the constitutional and local effects of disease of the suprarenal capsules. In *A Collection of the Published Writings of the Late Thomas Addison MD, Physician at Guy's Hospital, London*. New Sydenham Society, London (1868).

Anderson, J.R., Goudie, R.B., Gray, K.G. & Timbury, G.C. (1957). Auto-antibodies in Addison's disease. *Lancet*, **i**, 1123–4.

Anderson, J.R., Goudie, R.B., Gray, K. G. & Stuart-Smith, D.A. (1968). Immunological features of idiopathic Addison's disease: an antibody to cells producing steroid hormones. *Clinical and Experimental Immunology*, **3**, 107–17.

Asherson, R.A. & Hughes, G.R.V. (1989). Addison's disease and primary antiphospholipid syndrome. *Lancet*, **ii**, 874.

Banga, J.P., Pryce, G., Hammond, L. & Roitt, I.M. (1985). Structural features of the autoantigens involved in thyroid autoimmune disease: the thyroid microsomal/microvillar antigen. *Molecular Immunology*, **22**, 629–42.

Barnett, E.V., Dumonde, D.C. & Glynn, L.E. (1963). Induction of autoimmunity to adrenal gland. *Immunology*, **6**, 382–402.

Bartholomaeus, W.N., O'Donoghue, H., Foti, D., Lawson, C.M., Shellam, G. R. & Reed, W.D. (1988). Multiple autoantibodies following cytomegalovirus infection: virus distribution and specificity of autoantibodies. *Immunology*, **64**, 397–405.

Betterle, C., Zanette, F., Zanchetta, R., Pedini, B., Trevisan, A., Mantero, F. & Rigon, F. (1983). Complement-fixing adrenal autoantibodies aş a marker for predicting onset of idiopathic Addison's disease. *Lancet*, **i**, 1238–41.

Blizzard, R.M. & Kyle, M. (1963). Studies of the adrenal antigens and antibodies in Addison's disease. *Journal of Clinical Investigation*, **42**, 1653–60.

Bright, G.M. & Singh, I. (1990). Adrenal autoantibodies bind to adrenal subcellular fractions enriched in cytochrome-c reductase and 5'-nucleotidase. *Journal of Clinical Endocrinology and Metabolism*, **70**, 95–9.

Brown, F.M., Kamalesh, M., Adri, M.N.S. & Rabinowe, S.L. (1988). Anti-adrenal medullary antibodies in IDDM subjects and subjects at high risk of developing IDDM. *Diabetes Care*, **11**, 30–3.

Brown, F.M., Zuckerman, M., Longway, S. & Rabinowe, S.L. (1989). Adrenal medullary fibrosis in IDDM of long duration. *Diabetes Care*, **12**, 494–7.

Buckingham, J.C. (1987). A role for leucocytes in the control of adrenal steroidogenesis? *Journal of Endocrinology*, **114**, 1–2.

Colover, J. & Glynn, L.E. (1958). Experimental iso-immune adrenalitis. *Immunology*, **1**, 172–8.

Furmaniak, J., Talbot, D., Reinwein, D., Benker, G., Creagh, F.M. & Rees Smith, B. (1988). Immunoprecipitation of human adrenal microsomal antigen. *FEBS Letters*, **231**, 25–8.

Irvine, W.J., Stewart, A.G. & Scarth, L. (1967). A clinical and immunological study of adrenocortical insufficiency (Addison's disease). *Clinical and Experimental Immunology*, **2**, 31–70.

Irvine, W.J., Chan, M.M.W. & Scarth, L. (1969). The further characterization of auto-antibodies reactive with extra-adrenal steroid-producing cells in patients with adrenal disorders. *Clinical and Experimental Immunology*, **4**, 489–503.

Irvine, W.J. & Barnes, E.W. (1975). Addison's disease, ovarian failure and hypopara-thyroidism. *Clinics in Endocrinology and Metabolism*, **4**, 379–434.

Jackson, R., McNicol, A.M., Farquharson, M. & Foulis, A.K. (1988). Class II MHC expression in normal adrenal cortex and cortical cells in autoimmune Addison's disease. *Journal of Pathology*, **155**, 113–20.

Kendall-Taylor, P., Lambert, A., Mitchell, R. & Robertson, W.R. (1988). Antibody that blocks stimulation of cortisol secretion by adrenocorticotrophic hormone in Addison's disease. *British Medical Journal*, **296**, 1489–91.

Khoury, E.L., Hammond, L., Bottazzo, G.F. & Doniach, D. (1981). Surface-reactive antibodies to human adrenal cells in Addison's disease. *Clinical and Experimental Immunology*, **45**, 48–55.

Kosowicz, J., Gryczynska, M. & Bottazzo, G.F. (1986). A radioimmunoassay for the detection of adrenal autoantibodies. *Clinical and Experimental Immunology*, **63**, 671–9.

Latinne, D., Vandeput, Y., De Bruyere, M., Bottazzo, F., Sokal, G. & Crabbe, J. (1987). Addison's disease: immunological aspects. *Tissue Antigens*, **30**, 23–4.

Levine, S. & Wenk, E.J. (1968). The production and passive transfer of allergic adrenalitis. *American Journal of Pathology*, **52**, 41–53.

Maclaren, N.K. & Riley, W.J. (1986). Inherited susceptibility to autoimmune Addison's disease is linked to human leukocyte antigens -DR3 and/or DR4, except when associated with type I autoimmune polyglandular syndrome. *Journal of Clinical Endocrinology and Metabolism*, **62**, 455–9.

Nerup, J. (1974). Addison's disease – serological studies. *Acta Endocrinologica*, **76**, 142–58.

Nerup, J. & Bendixen, G. (1969). Anti-adrenal cellular hypersensitivity in Addison's disease. II. Correlation with clinical and serological findings. *Clinical and Experimental Immunology*, **5**, 341–53.

Nerup, J., Anderson, V. & Bendixen, G. (1970). Antiadrenal cellular hypersensitivity in Addison's disease. IV In vivo and in vitro investigations of the mitochondrial fraction. *Clinical and Experimental Immunology*, **6**, 733–9.

Petri, M. & Nerup, J. (1971). Addison's adrenalitis. *Acta Pathologica et Microbiologica Scandinavica*, **79**, 381–8.

Rabinowe, S.L., Jackson, R.A., Dluhy, R.G. & Williams, G.H. (1984). Ia-positive T lymphocytes in recently diagnosed idiopathic Addison's disease. *American Journal of Medicine*, **77**, 597–601.

Sakaguchi, S. & Sakaguchi, N. (1989). Organ-specific autoimmune disease induced in mice by elimination of T cell subsets. V. Neonatal administration of cyclosporin A causes auto-immune disease. *Journal of Immunology*, **142**, 471–80.

Salas, M.A., Evans, S.W., Levell, M.J. & Whicher, J.T. (1990). Interleukin-6 and ACTH act synergistically to stimulate the release of corticosterone from adrenal gland cells. *Clinical and Experimental Immunology*, **79**, 470–3.

Scherbaum, W.A. & Berg, P.A. (1982). Development of adrenocortical failure in non-Addisonian patients with antibodies to adrenal cortex. *Clinical Endocrinology*, **16**, 345–52.

Scherbaum, W.A., Mogel, H., Boehm, B.O., Hedderich, U., Gluck, M., Schernthaner, G., Bottazzo, G.F. & Pfeiffer, E.F. (1988). Autoantibodies to adrenal medullary and thyroid calcitonin cells in type I diabetes mellitus – a prospective study. *Journal of Autoimmunity*, **1**, 219–30.

Sotsiou, F., Bottazzo, G.F. & Doniach, D. (1980). Immunofluorescence studies on autoantibodies to steroid-producing cells, and to germline cells in endocrine diseases and infertility. *Clinical and Experimental Immunology*, **39**, 97–111.

Stechemesser, E., Scherbaum, W.A., Grossmann, T. & Berg, P.A. (1985). An ELISA method for the detection of autoantibodies to adrenal cortex. *Journal of Immunological Methods*, **80**, 67–76.

Thomsen, M., Platz, P., Ortved Anderson, O., Christy, M., Lyngsoe, J., Nerup, J., Rasmussen, K., Ryder, L.P., Staub-Nielsen, L. & Svejgaard, A. (1975). MLC typing in juvenile diabetes mellitus and idiopathic Addison's disease. *Transplantation Reviews*, **22**, 125–47.

Van Berkhout, F.T., Croughs, R.J.M., Kater, L., Schuurman, H.J., Gruelig Meyling, F.J.H., Kooyman, C.D., Van Der Gaag, R.D., Jolink, D. & Drexhage, H.A. (1986). Familial Cushing's syndrome due to nodular adrenocortical dysplasia. A putative receptor-antibody disease? *Clinical Endocrinology*, **24**, 299–310.

Van Berkhout, F.T., Croughs, R.J.M., Wulffraat, N.M. & Drexhage, H.A. (1989). Familial Cushing's syndrome due to nodular adrenocortical dysplasia is an inherited disease of immunological origin. *Clinical Endocrinology*, **31**, 185–91.

Vita, J.A., Silverberg, S.J., Goland, R.S., Austin, J.H.M. & Knowlton, A.I. (1985). Clinical clues to the cause of Addison's disease. *American Journal of Medicine*, **78**, 461–6.

Wulffraat, N.M., Drexhage, H.A., Bottazzo, G.F., Wiersinga, W.M., Jeucken, P. & Van der Gaag, R. (1989). Immunoglobulins of patients with idiopathic Addison's disease block the *in vitro* action of adrenocorticotropin. *Journal of Clinical Endocrinology and Metabolism*, **69**, 231–8.

Young, W.F., Carney, J.A., Musa, B.U., Wulffraat, N.M., Lens, J.W. & Drexhage, H.A. (1989). Familial Cushing's syndrome due to primary pigmented nodular adrenocortical disease. *New England Journal of Medicine*, **321**, 1659–64.

–6–

Gonadal autoimmunity

Autoimmune oophoritis

This presents as premature ovarian failure resulting in oestrogen deficiency, although there is some variation between studies in defining the age at which a menopause is premature. In a review of records from the Mayo Clinic, the incidence of a natural menopause in women less than 40 years old was 1% (Coulam, Adamson & Annegers, 1986). It is uncertain how many of these cases have an autoimmune aetiology. The first hint that autoimmunity could cause ovarian failure came from observations that this disorder preceded the onset of Addison's disease by 8–14 years in four women, while three men with adrenal failure were noted to have testicular atrophy (Turkington & Lebovitz, 1967). This association has been amply confirmed by others: in one large series of 157 women with idiopathic Addison's disease, 6% had oligomenorrhoea and 24% amenorrhoea (Irvine & Barnes, 1975). However, Addison's disease is far less prevalent than premature ovarian failure and several studies have sought to establish an autoimmune aetiology in some of these patients without adrenal disease.

After excluding chromosome disorders, 17α-hydroxylase deficiency and galactosaemia, another non-autoimmune and genetically determined subset of women exists with (probable) autosomal dominant inheritance of ovarian failure (Coulam, Stringfellow & Hoefnagel, 1983; Mattison *et al.*, 1984). For the remainder, no clearly accepted criteria of autoimmune oophoritis exist to define its prevalence. The occurrence of ovarian autoantibodies is considered in detail below. Several groups have used the coincidence of other autoimmune disorders besides Addison's disease as a marker for ovarian autoimmunity and certainly these conditions have an increased prevalence in patients with premature ovarian failure (Table 6.1). Abnormalities in non-specific tests of immune function, including the presence of circulating immune complexes and low NK cell activity, have been documented in about a third of patients with unexplained premature ovarian failure (Pekonen *et al.*, 1986).

Table 6.1. *Prevalence of non-adrenal autoimmune disease in women with premature ovarian failure[a]*

Study	Number of patients	Percentage with autoimmune disease	Type of disease
Rebar, Erickson & Yen (1982)	26	12%	Autoimmune thyroid disease ($n = 3$)
Alper & Garner (1985)	33	39%[b]	Autoimmune thyroid disease ($n = 11$), Addison's disease ($n = 1$), vitiligo ($n = 1$)
Aiman & Smentek (1985)	35	9%[c]	Type 1 diabetes ($n = 1$), SLE + Graves' disease ($n = 1$), Crohn's disease ($n = 1$)
Pekonen et al. (1986)	18	11%[d]	SLE ($n = 1$), polyendocrine autoimmunity ($n = 1$)
Miyake, Sato & Takeuchi (1987)	20	10%[e]	Hashimoto's thyroiditis ($n = 1$), myasthenia gravis ($n = 1$)

[a] Patients not preselected for the coincident presence of Addison's disease.
[b] One patient with Addison's disease: 36% excluding this subject.
[c] A further three patients (9%) had thyroid antibodies.
[d] A further four patients (22%) had thyroid or nuclear antibodies.
[e] A further 12 patients (60%) had thyroid, gastric parietal cell or nuclear antibodies; adrenal antibodies were undetectable.

The established histological appearance of the ovary in autoimmune oophoritis is a lymphocytic and plasma cell infiltrate associated with the endocrine hilar cells, the theca interna of growing follicles (but not the primordial follicles) and the corpora lutea (Irvine & Barnes, 1975; Gloor & Hurlimann, 1984). However, ovarian biopsy is not always obtained in women with premature ovarian failure. When the ovaries are examined more than half of such women have no evidence of lymphocytic infiltration (Aiman & Smentek, 1985), but the absence of a lymphocytic oophoritis cannot be regarded as conclusive evidence against an autoimmune aetiology, as this could equally be due to the duration of disease or the operation of some other process such as blocking autoantibodies. It seems possible that around 20% of women with premature ovarian failure but without Addison's disease may have an autoimmune cause for this disorder (Coulam et al., 1983), although much more work is required to establish this firmly.

Experimental autoimmune oophoritis

Immunisation of rats with ovarian extract and complete Freund's adjuvant leads to the production of antiovarian antibodies and oophoritis (Jankovic *et al.*, 1973). However, the histology is unlike that seen in women with autoimmune ovarian failure, as the secondary follicles and corpora lutea are spared while the primordial follicles and interfollicular tissue bear the brunt of lymphocytic infiltration. Neonatal thymectomy in certain strains of mice results in oophoritis (with a similar appearance to the human disease) and the formation of anti-oocyte antibodies (Nishizuka & Sakakura, 1971; Taguchi *et al.*, 1980; Miyake *et al.*, 1988). The end result is a fibrotic ovarian remnant. Antibodies against ovarian steroid cells, which are present in women with autoimmune ovarian failure, are infrequent or of low titre. The disease can be transferred to normal newborn or athymic nude mice with Lyt-1 (helper) but not Lyt-2,3 (cytotoxic/suppressor) T cells (Sakaguchi, Takahashi & Nishizuka, 1982a). Surprisingly, there was no requirement for MHC compatibility between donor and recipient in these transfer experiments. The Lyt-1^+ population also contained cells capable of suppressing disease induction, as the transfer of Lyt-1^+ cells from normal adult female mice two weeks after thymectomy prevented the development of oophoritis (Sakaguchi *et al.*, 1982b). Direct elimination of the Lyt-1^+ population from normal adult mice also resulted in multiple autoimmune diseases, including oophoritis in 50% of the animals, as shown by transfer of Lyt-1-depleted spleen cells from untreated BALB/c heterozygous nude (nu/+) mice to nude (nu/nu) littermates (Sakaguchi *et al.*, 1985). These results resemble those obtained in similar experimental models of autoimmune thyroiditis (indeed thyroiditis also occurred in 10–20% of the recipient nude mice) and they support a central role for T cells both as effectors and, under normal circumstances, suppressors of autoimmune oophoritis.

Immunogenetics and environmental factors

As indicated in the introduction, patients are often diagnosed because there is an accompanying autoimmune endocrinopathy, which prevents the delineation of any separate immunogenetic susceptibility to the ovarian component. However, in one study, 19 patients with premature ovarian failure, who had no detectable ovarian antibodies and only one of whom had another endocrine disease, were tested for HLA associations (Walfish *et al.*, 1983). Seven (37%) were Bw35-positive, although the significance of this did not survive correction. HLA-DR3 was present in 11 (53%), compared to 23% of controls, a significant association with a relative risk of 4.34. There was little overlap between these two antigens, suggesting that there may be two subgroups of ovarian failure in this population, those with HLA-DR3 being likely to have an autoimmune aetiology.

There are no known environmental factors which precipitate autoimmune oophoritis. Smoking is associated with an increased risk of premature ovarian failure, but this has not been further delineated regarding the aetiology of the ovarian disorder. *In vitro* fertilisation results in the formation of ovarian autoantibodies, which increase during successive attempts (Moncayo, Moncayo & Dapunt, 1990; Gobert *et al.*, 1990). This does not appear to be due to the primary pathology causing the infertility, but may reflect autoimmunisation with ovarian antigens released by repeated microtrauma.

T cell responses

In contrast to the strong evidence adduced for T cell mediation of experimental autoimmune oophoritis, there have been few attempts to define a similar role for T cells in the human disorder. In one biopsied patient who also had Addison's disease, there was a mixed lymphocytic infiltrate around maturing or atretic follicles, but T cells predominated and these were largely CD4$^+$ (Sedmak, Hart & Tubbs, 1987). Only a few NK cells were seen, but a lot of macrophages were present in the granulosa cell layers. There are conflicting data on circulating T cells subsets, presumably reflecting aetiology, heterogeneity and duration of disease. In a group of 20 women with premature ovarian failure (14 of whom had a variety of autoantibodies), circulating Ia$^+$ T cells were increased and the CD4:CD8 T cell ratio was elevated compared to controls (Miyake, Sato & Takeuchi, 1987). CD4$^+$ T cells were increased but CD8$^+$ T cells remained normal in another group of patients with premature ovarian failure, an abnormality associated with reduced MIF responses to non-specific microbial antigens (Mignot *et al.*, 1989). However, others have found the CD4:CD8 ratio to be normal (Rabinowe *et al.*, 1989), or low and dependent on circulating oestrogen concentrations (Ho *et al.*, 1988). In agreement with a previous study, circulating numbers of Ia$^+$ T cells were abnormally high in eight of 23 women with premature ovarian failure, five of whom had no associated endocrinopathy (Rabinowe *et al.*, 1989). Although non-specific, this increase in activated T cells at least is suggestive of an autoimmune component operating in these patients. Sensitisation of circulating T cells to ovarian antigens is poorly documented; in one study, T cells from three (17%) of 18 women produced MIF in response to ovarian antigens (Pekonen *et al.*, 1986).

B cell responses

As in Addison's disease, considerable attention has been paid to the humoral autoimmune response. This began with the description of antibodies found in a man with Addison's disease which reacted by indirect immunofluorescence with ovarian theca interna and corpus luteum, testicular Leydig cells, hilar cells of both organs and placental trophoblast, as well as with adrenal cortex (Anderson et al., 1968). These were termed steroid cell antibodies and their presence was subsequently detected in 26% of 182 women and 4% of 76 men with Addison's disease (Irvine & Barnes, 1975). In this series, steroid cell antibodies were not found in 329 controls or 140 women with unexplained amenorrhoea and were only detected very rarely in other autoimmune conditions. However, their presence strongly correlated with primary or secondary amenorrhoea in the Addisonian patients. It was also apparent from the variety of immunofluorescent staining patterns that several steroid cell antigens were recognised, all of which appeared to be present in the adrenal cortex but with differing distributions in the testis, ovary and placenta.

The dictum that steroid cell antibodies are only found in adrenal antibody-positive sera was supported by others (Ruehsen et al., 1972; Sotsiou, Bottazzo & Doniach, 1980), although two patients were found out of the 302 tested in which this did not apply. As well as the previously noted strong association with ovarian failure, more than half of the sera from Addisonian patients with thyroiditis, type 1 diabetes or pernicious anaemia had steroid cell antibodies compared to only 22% of Addisonian patients without another endocrinopathy. (All of these patients with Addison's disease were selected for the presence of adrenal antibodies.) Many of the women with steroid cell antibodies also had antibodies which reacted with ova (Sotsiou et al., 1980). An even larger series, which analysed 325 controls, 505 diabetics, 37 patients with adrenal antibodies and 15 with unexplained primary ovarian failure, tested for steroid cell antibodies by immunofluorescence on human testis and only 12 positive sera were found, which all came from patients with adrenal antibodies (Elder, Maclaren & Riley, 1981). As before, these antibodies also reacted with the theca interna and granulosa layers of ovarian follicles and, while powdered adrenal could absorb out all of the gonadal reactivity, adrenal reactivity was not absorbed out by gonadal antigens. Thus, steroid cell antibodies appeared to be a subset of adrenal antibodies, the remainder being adrenal-specific.

However, this dogma has been challenged by alternative tests for ovarian antibodies. By radioimmunoassay, sera from all but one of 15 patients with premature ovarian failure bound more strongly to ovarian antigens than premenopausal control sera (Coulam & Ryan, 1979). By immunofluorescence and immunohistochemistry, 52% of 27 patients with premature menopause had ovarian antibodies, predominantly against granulosa cells and oocytes, compared to 29% of 17 patients with other autoimmune disorders and none of 24 menstruating controls (Damewood et al., 1986). Significantly, none of the 27 women with ovarian failure had any other autoimmune disorder (Damewood, 1987). Patients with endometriosis have also been screened for ovarian antibodies, because secondary infertility is common in this disorder. In 13 such patients (12 with normal menses), serum antibody binding to human ovarian antigens was measured by immunofluorescence and haemagglutination assays and was significantly higher than controls (Mathur *et al.*, 1982).

An ELISA using antigenic extracts of bovine corpora lutea has confirmed the presence of ovarian antibodies in about half of the endometriosis patients tested and also documented their occurrence in 84% of 19 patients with SLE, although it was not reported whether there was any association with disturbed gonadal function (Moncayo *et al.*, 1989; Moncayo-Naveda *et al.*, 1989). The antigens recognised in these two studies appear to be the unoccupied luteinising hormone (LH) receptor and the LH receptor–hormone complex. An alternative ELISA, using human ovarian homogenate as a source of antigen, detected antibodies in 46% of 24 patients with idiopathic premature ovarian failure and 33% of nine patients in whom the disorder was associated with another autoimmune disease (Luborsky *et al.*, 1990). Separate antibodies against oocytes were also detected by ELISA in a proportion of these women, as well as in some without ovarian autoimmunity, but antibodies against LH were rare (6%) and none were detected against follicle stimulating hormone (FSH).

The findings of Moncayo *et al.* (1989) suggest the existence of gonadotrophin receptor-blocking antibodies as a cause of ovarian failure, although these have previously been sought without success (Austin, Coulam & Ryan, 1979). Such a possibility clearly requires further exploration, particularly with functional assays. Two patients with myasthenia gravis and amenorrhoea have been described with antibodies which inhibited FSH binding to testicular receptors and suppressed two FSH-stimulated functions, cAMP production and androgen-binding protein release from seminiferous tubules *in vitro* (Chiauzzi *et al.*, 1982; Escobar *et al.*, 1982). Both of these patients had evidence of the gonadotrophin-resistant ovary syndrome, especially the presence of morphologically normal but immature ovarian follicles in the face of high circulating gonadotrophin levels. These features certainly fit with the concept of a receptor-blocking antibody as the cause. However, the resistant ovary syndrome accounted for premature ovarian failure in only 11% of women in one series studied by ovarian biopsy (Aiman & Smentek, 1985), so even if caused by receptor antibodies in a proportion of cases, this is probably a rare form of gonadal autoimmunity. Further studies are obviously needed.

Effector mechanisms

Practically nothing is known about the pathogenesis of ovarian failure but, as in other autoimmune endocrinopathies, several effector processes are likely to operate in combination. Antibodies from nine of 23 Addisonian patients with clinical evidence of gonadal failure were cytotoxic to cultured human granulosa cells in the presence of complement and also inhibited progesterone production *in vitro* (McNatty *et al.*, 1975). Cell-mediated immune mechanisms seem likely to be involved, as judged by the histological appearances and the absence of ovarian antibodies in many patients. Finally, lymphokines may also be important: TNF inhibits gonadotrophin-stimulated steroidogenesis by murine granulosa cells (Adashi *et al.*, 1990).

Treatment

There are now many case reports of conception occurring after premature ovarian failure. Of 246 patients in one review, 5.9% had subsequent pregnancies, but of course the frequency of autoimmune oophoritis was not clearly established in these patients (Alper & Garner, 1985). Nonetheless, certain women with a definite autoimmune aetiology for this disorder do resume menstruation and steroids have been advocated as immunosuppressive treatment if pregnancy is wanted (Table 6.2). In the remaining women, oestrogen and progesterone replacement and careful follow-up are necessary as some of these patients may develop other autoimmune disorders.

Autoimmune orchitis

Experimental autoimmune orchitis can be induced readily in rats or mice by thymectomy or immunisation with testicular antigens plus adjuvant and several spontaneous models exist, but in all cases the immune response is against sperm antigens (Tung, 1987; Yokochi *et al.*, 1990). Although the original description of steroid cell antibodies was in a clinically normal man with Addison's disease (Anderson *et al.*, 1968), this is a rare phenomenon, such antibodies being found in just three of 79 Addisonian men subsequently (Irvine & Barnes, 1975). Only one of these, a 15 year old, had any evidence of clinical disease, with left testicular atrophy and gynaecomastia, which could equally have had a non-autoimmune basis. Five men with Addison's disease were described as having primary hypogonadism in a review of polyendocrine autoimmunity, but the basis for this diagnosis and further details were not given (Turkington & Lebovitz, 1967; Neufeld, Maclaren & Blizzard, 1981). Patients with steroid cell antibodies do not have sperm antibodies, which contrasts with the frequency of antibodies against ova in such women (Sotsiou *et al.*, 1980). While it seems likely that testicular endocrine function may be impaired by autoimmune orchitis, particularly in conjunction with Addison's disease, there is no detailed study of Leydig cell function or histological appearance in such patients.

Table 6.2. *Recovery of ovarian function in women with autoimmune oophoritis*

Case Report	Biopsy	Ovarian antibodies	Other endocrinopathy	Treatment	Outcome
Coulam et al. (1981)	Oophoritis	+	None	Steroids	Transient menses
Finer et al. (1985)	ND[a]	+	Thyroiditis + Addison's disease	Replacement steroids[c]	Menses + conception
Rabinowe et al. (1986)	Oophoritis	+	Thyroiditis	Steroids	Menses[b]
Tan et al. (1986)	No oophoritis or ova	+	Thyroiditis + Addison's disease	Nil	Spontaneously resumed menses
Cowchok et al. (1988)	ND	ND (adrenal ab+)	Addison's disease	Replacement steroids[c]	Menses + conception
Taylor et al. (1989)	ND	+	Addison's disease	Nil	Spontaneously resumed menses and conceived
Luborsky et al. (1990)	ND	+[d]	Graves' disease + type 1 diabetes	Steroids	Menses + conception
		+[d]	None	Steroids	Menses + conception

[a]ND = not done.
[b]Elevated circulating Ia⁻ T cells decreased after treatment.
[c]Physiological replacement for Addison's disease rather than therapeutic doses of steroids temporally related to resumption of menstruation.
[d]Antibody levels fell with steroid treatment.

Summary

There are close parallels between autoimmune adrenalitis and oophoritis; not only do these conditions frequently coexist and share autoantigens, but also their investigation has centred around a role for T cells in animals and for autoantibodies in the human counterpart. However, a particular problem with interpreting studies on autoimmune oophoritis is its distinction from other causes of premature ovarian failure, in turn highlighting the need for a specific and sensitive diagnostic test. At least one subset of patients can be identified with coincident Addison's disease, in whom the ovarian failure is associated with circulating antibodies against both steroid cells and ova. *In vitro* evidence indicates that these autoantibodies may be pathogenic, although the histological appearances are at least compatible with a role for cell-mediated tissue injury, by extrapolation from experimental models and other endocrinopathies. In a second subset, antibodies which block the gonadotrophin receptor may be responsible for ovarian failure. Although firm evidence for this is available in only two patients, recent work suggests a more important role for such antibodies. There remains a group of patients who have ovarian antibodies detectable by immunofluorescence, ELISA or radioimmunoassay in the absence of Addison's disease. The nature of their disorder is unclear. Since autoimmune premature ovarian failure may be reversed by steroids (Table 6.2), it will be particularly important to delineate further the immunological features of the disease in this subgroup. Auto-immune orchitis is a far less distinct entity and evidence for endocrine dysfunction as a result of this is sparse, being largely confined to observations on men with Addison's disease. However, unlike the ovary in which both steroid cells and ova give rise to autoantibodies, the main testicular autoantigens appear to be spermatic, presumably the result of difference in the anatomical location of endocrine and germ cell elements.

References

Adashi, E.Y., Resnick, C.E., Packman, J.N., Hurwitz, A. & Payne, D.W. (1990). Cytokine-mediated regulation of ovarian function: tumor necrosis factor-α inhibits gonadotropin-supported progesterone accumulation by differentiating and luteinized murine granulosa cells. *American Journal of Obstetrics and Gynaecology*, **162**, 889–99.

Aiman, J. & Smentek, C. (1985). Premature ovarian failure. *Obstetrics and Gynaecology*, **66**, 9–14.

Alper, M.M. & Garner, P.R. (1985). Premature ovarian failure: its relationship to auto-immune disease. *Obstetrics and Gynaecology*, **66**, 27–30.

Anderson, J.R., Goudie, R.B., Gray, K. & Stuart-Smith, D.A. (1968). Immunological features of idiopathic Addison's disease: an antibody to cells producing steroid hormones. *Clinical and Experimental Immunology*, **3**, 107–17.

Austin, G.E., Coulam, C.B. & Ryan, R.J. (1979). A search for antibodies to luteinizing hormone receptors in premature ovarian failure. *Mayo Clinic Proceedings*, **54**, 394–400.

Chiauzzi, V., Cigorraga, S., Escobar, M.E., Rivarola, M.A. & Charreau, E.H. (1982). Inhibition of follicle-stimulating hormone receptor binding by circulating immunoglobulins. *Journal of Clinical Endocrinology and Metabolism*, **54**, 1221–8.

Coulam, C.B. & Ryan, R.J. (1979). Premature menopause. I. Etiology. *Americal Journal of Obstetrics and Gynaecology*, **133**, 639–43.

Coulam, C.B., Kempers, R.D. & Randall, R.V. (1981). Premature ovarian failure: evidence for the autoimmune mechanism. *Fertility and Sterility*, **36**, 238–40.

Coulam, C.B., Stringfellow, S. & Hoefnagel, D. (1983). Evidence for a genetic factor in the etiology of premature ovarian failure. *Fertility and Sterility*, **40**, 693–5.

Coulam, C.B., Adamson, S.C. & Annegers, J.F. (1986). Incidence of premature ovarian failure. *Obstetrics and Gynaecology*, **67**, 604–6.

Cowchok, F.S., McCabe, J.L. & Montgomery, B.B. (1988). Pregnancy after corticosteroid administration in premature ovarian failure (polyglandular endocrinopathy syndrome). *American Journal of Obstetrics and Gynaecology*, **158**, 118–19.

Damewood, M.D. (1987). Circulating antiovarian antibodies in premature ovarian failure. *Obstetrics and Gynaecology*, **70**, 144.

Damewood, M.D., Zacur, H.A., Hoffman, G.J. & Rock, J.A. (1986). Circulating antiovarian antibodies in premature ovarian failure. *Obstetrics and Gynaecology*, **68**, 850–4.

Elder, M., Maclaren, N. & Riley, W. (1981). Gonadal autoantibodies in patients with hypogonadism and/or Addison's disease. *Journal of Clinical Endocrinology and Metabolism*, **52**, 1137–42.

Escobar, M.E., Cigorraga, S.B., Chiauzzi, V.A., Charreau, E.H. & Rivarola, M.A. (1982). Development of the gonadotrophic resistant ovary syndrome in myasthenia gravis: suggestion of similar autoimmune mechanisms. *Acta Endocrinologica*, **99**, 431–6.

Finer, N., Fogelman, I. & Bottazzo, G.F. (1985). Pregnancy in a woman with premature ovarian failure. *Postgraduate Medical Journal*, **61**, 1079–80.

Gloor, E. & Hurlimann, J. (1984). Autoimmune oophoritis. *American Journal of Clinical Pathology*, **81**, 105–9.

Gobert, B., Barabarino-Monnier, P., Guillet-Rosso, F., Bene, M.C. & Faure, G.C. (1990). Ovary antibodies after IVF. *Lancet*, **335**, 723.

Ho, P.C., Tang, G.W.K., Fu, K.H., Fau, M.C. & Lawton, J.W.M. (1988). Immunologic studies in patients with premature ovarian failure. *Obstetrics and Gynaecology*, **71**, 622–6.

Irvine, W.J. & Barnes, E.W. (1975). Addison's disease, ovarian failure and hypoparathyroidism. *Clinics in Endocrinology and Metabolism*, **4**, 379–434.

Jankovic, B.D., Markovic, B.M., Petrovic, S. & Isakovic, K. (1973). Experimental autoimmune oophoritis in the rat. *European Journal of Immunology*, **3**, 375–7.

Luborsky, J.L., Visintin, L., Boyers, S., Asari, T., Caldwell, B. & DeCherney, A. (1990). Ovarian antibodies detected by immobilized antigen immunoassay in patients with premature ovarian failure. *Journal of Clinical Endocrinology and Metabolism*, **70**, 69–75.

McNatty, K.P., Short, R.V., Barnes, E.W. & Irvine, W.J. (1975). The cytotoxic effect of serum from patients with Addison's disease and autoimmune ovarian failure on human granulosa cells in culture. *Clinical and Experimental Immunology*, **22**, 378–84.

Mathur, S., Peress, M.R., Williamson, H.O., Youmans, C.D., Maney, S.A., Garvin, A.J., Rust, P.F. & Fudenberg, H.H. (1982). Autoimmunity to endometrium and ovary in endometriosis. *Clinical and Experimental Immunology*, **50**, 259–66.

Mattison, D.R., Evans, M.I., Schwimmer, W.B., White, B.J., Jensen, B. & Schulman, J.D. (1984). Familial premature ovarian failure. *American Journal of Human Genetics*, **36**, 1341–8.

Mignot, M.H., Drexhage, H.A., Kleingeld, M., Van de Plassche-Boers, E.M., Ramanath Rao, B. & Schoemaker, J. (1989). Premature ovarian failure. II: Considerations of cellular immunity defects. *European Journal of Obstetrics & Gynaecology and Reproductive Biology*, **30**, 67–72.

Miyake, T., Sato, Y. & Takeuchi, S. (1987). Implications of circulating autoantibodies and peripheral blood lymphocytes for the genesis of premature ovarian failure. *Journal of Reproductive Immunology*, **12**, 163–71.

Miyake, T., Taguchi, O., Ikeda, H., Sato, Y., Takeuchi, S. & Nishizuka, Y. (1988). Acute oocyte loss in experimental autoimmune oophoritis as a possible model of premature ovarian failure. *Americal Journal of Obstetrics and Gynaecology*, **158**, 186–92.

Moncayo, H., Moncayo, R., Benz, R., Wolf, A. & Lauritzen, C. (1989). Ovarian failure and autoimmunity. Detection of autoantibodies directed against both the unoccupied luteinizing hormone/human chorionic gonadotropin receptor and the hormone–receptor complex of bovine corpus luteum. *Journal of Clinical Investigation*, **84**, 1857–65.

Moncayo, R., Moncayo, H. & Dapunt, O. (1990). Immunological risks of IVF. *Lancet*, **335**, 180.

Moncayo-Naveda, H., Moncayo, R., Benz, R., Wolf, A. & Lauritzen, C. (1989). Organ-specific antibodies against ovary in patients with systemic lupus erythematosus. *American Journal of Obstetrics and Gynaecology*, **160**, 1227–9.

Neufeld, M., Maclaren, N.K. & Blizzard, R.M. (1981). Two types of autoimmune Addison's disease associated with different polyglandular autoimmune (PGA) syndromes. *Medicine*, **60**, 355–62.

Nishizuka, Y. & Sakakura, T. (1971). Ovarian dysgenesis induced by neonatal thymectomy in the mouse. *Endocrinology*, **89**, 886–93.

Pekonen, F., Siegberg, R., Makinen, T., Miettinen, A. & Yli-Korkala, O. (1986). Immunological disturbances in patients with premature ovarian failure. *Clinical Endocrinology*, **25**, 1–6.

Rabinowe, S.L., Berger, M.J., Welch, W.R. & Dluhy, R.G. (1986). Lymphocyte dysfunction in autoimmune oophoritis. Resumption of menses with corticosteroids. *American Journal of Medicine*, **81**, 347–50.

Rabinowe, S.L., George, K.L., Ravnikar, V.A., Dluhy, R.G. & Dib, S.A. (1989). Premature menopause: monoclonal antibody defined T lymphocyte abnormalities and antiovarian antibodies. *Fertility and Sterility*, **51**, 450–4.

Rebar, R.W., Erickson, G.F. & Yen, S.S.C. (1982). Idiopathic premature ovarian failure: clinical and endocrine characteristics. *Fertility and Sterility*, **37**, 35–41.

Ruehsen, M.M., Blizzard, R.M., Garcia-Bunuel, R. & Jones, G.S. (1972). Autoimmunity and ovarian failure. *American Journal of Obstetrics and Gynaecology*, **112**, 693–703.

Sakaguchi, S., Takahashi, T. & Nishizuka, Y. (1982a). Study on cellular events in post-thymectomy autoimmune oophoritis in mice. I. Requirement of Lyt-1 effector cells for oocytes damage after adoptive transfer. *Journal of Experimental Medicine*, **156**, 1565–76.

Sakaguchi, S., Takahashi, T. & Nishizuka, Y. (1982b). Study on cellular events in post-thymectomy autoimmune oophoritis in mice. II. Requirement of Lyt-1 cells in normal female mice for the prevention of oophoritis. *Journal of Experimental Medicine*, **156**, 1577–86.

Sakaguchi, S., Fukuma, K., Kuribayashi, K. & Masuda, T. (1985). Organ-specific autoimmune diseases induced in mice by elimination of T cell subset. I. Evidence for the active participation of T cells in natural self-tolerance; deficit of a T cell subset as a possible cause of autoimmune disease. *Journal of Experimental Medicine*, **161**, 72–87.

Sedmak, D.D., Hart, W.R. & Tubbs, R.R. (1987). Autoimmune oophoritis: a histopathological study of involved ovaries with immunological characterization of the mononuclear cell infiltrate. *International Journal of Gynaecological Pathology*, **6**, 73–81.

Sotsiou, F., Bottazzo, G.F. & Doniach, D. (1980). Immunofluorescence studies on autoantibodies to steroid-producing cells, and to germline cells in endocrine disease and infertility. *Clinical and Experimental Immunology*, **39**, 97–111.

Taguchi, O., Nishizuka, Y., Sakakura, T. & Kojima, A. (1980). Autoimmune oophoritis in thymectomized mice: detection of circulating antibodies against oocytes. *Clinical and Experimental Immunology*, **40**, 540–53.

Tan, S.L., Hague, W.M., Becker, F. & Jacobs, H.S. (1986). Autoimmune premature ovarian failure with polyendocrinopathy and spontaneous recovery of ovarian follicular activity. *Fertility and Sterility*, **45**, 421–4.

Taylor, R., Smith, N.M., Angus, B., Horne, C.H.W. & Dunlop, W. (1989). Return of fertility after twelve years of autoimmune ovarian failure. *Clinical Endocrinology*, **31**, 305–8.

Tung, K. (1987). Immunologic basis of male infertility. *Laboratory Investigation*, **57**, 1–4.

Turkington, R.W. & Lebovitz, H.E. (1967). Extra-adrenal endocrine deficiencies in Addison's disease. *American Journal of Medicine*, **43**, 499–507.

Walfish, P.G., Gottesman, I.S., Shewchuk, A.B., Bain, J., Hawe, B.S. & Farid, N.R. (1983). Association of premature ovarian failure with HLA antigens. *Tissue Antigens*, **21**, 168–9.

Yokochi, T., Ikeda, H., Inone, Y., Kimura, Y., Ito, H., Fujii, Y. & Kato, N. (1990). Characterization of autoantigens relevant to experimental autoimmune orchitis (EAO) in mice immunized with syngeneic testis homogenate and Klebsiella 03 lipopolysaccharide. *American Journal of Reproductive Immunology*, **22**, 42–8.

Pituitary autoimmunity

The anatomical site of the pituitary has made study of autoimmune hypophysitis difficult. It is possible that pituitary autoimmunity could be more important than previously suspected in a variety of pituitary disorders, although the dramatic condition of lymphocytic hypophysitis seems to be rare.

Experimental autoimmune hypophysitis

The first inkling of the importance of neonatal tolerance to autoantigens was in fact provided by observations on pituitary autoimmunity. Triplett (1962) removed the pituitary glands from frog embryos, maintained their viability by transplantation into other tadpoles and found that the glands were rejected when reimplanted into the adult donor. This was correctly interpreted as showing the requirement for self recognition by the developing immune system in order to prevent autoimmunity. Autoantibodies to uncharacterised pituitary antigens were elicited by immunisation of rabbits with homologous and heterologous pituitary extract in adjuvant; although these could fix complement, no pathological lesions in the pituitary were detected (Beutner, Djanian & Witebsky, 1964). However, immunisation of Lewis strain rats with homogenised pituitary tissue, emulsified in completed Freund's adjuvant, produced a severe focal and diffuse lymphocytic infiltrate in the pituitary two to three weeks later (Levine, 1967). In addition, pituitary cells appeared to be undergoing lysis in the areas of infiltration. These changes were confined almost exclusively to the anterior pituitary, rather than the posterior and intermediate lobes and there was little evidence of lesions elsewhere. It is particularly interesting, in relation to the human counterpart, that the severity of the disease appeared to be worse in animals postpartum.

As discussed in Chapter 4, there is impressive evidence for a viral aetiology in certain types of experimental autoimmune diabetes mellitus. In one such model, reovirus type 1 infection in mice results in hyperglycaemia and lymphocytic infiltration of the islets of Langerhans and about half the infected mice show retarded growth (Onodera *et al.*, 1981). The anterior lobe of the pituitary in these animals contains a mononuclear cell infiltrate and viral antigens are also localised in this area, particularly in the growth hormone-producing cells. Growth hormone levels are lower in the runted mice and antibodies against the pituitary are detectable by immunofluorescence; these react specifically with somatotrophs. Antibodies to other endocrine tissues (apart from islet cells) are not found in these animals. The pituitary dysfunction appears to be the result of autoreactivity rather than a direct effect of the reovirus since immunosuppressive agents reverse the disease without affecting viral titres (Onodera *et al.*, 1982).

Other viral infections, including Japanese encephalitis virus, lymphocytic choriomeningitis, measles, rabies and vaccinia, can trigger the formation of anterior pituitary autoantibodies in mice, often as part of a generalised response against endocrine tissues (Srinivasappa *et al.*, 1986). These antibodies are thought to arise by molecular mimicry, the B cell response against particular viral sequences or configurations resulting by chance in the formation of anti-self antibodies. However, it is likely that many of these pituitary antibodies are of low affinity and so far there is no good evidence, apart from the reovirus model, that they have a pathogenic role resulting in pituitary dysfunction.

Pituitary autoimmunity in man

There are two forms of human pituitary autoimmunity, marked by the presence of lymphocytic hypophysitis or antibodies against the pituitary, which only occasionally appear to overlap.

Lymphocytic hypophysitis

The first patient described with histologically proven autoimmune hypophysitis was a 22 year old woman who died 14 months postpartum and shortly after appendicectomy, as a result of previously unsuspected hypopituitarism (Goudie & Pinkerton, 1962). At autopsy there was typical Hashimoto's thyroiditis and a lymphocytic infiltrate in the anterior pituitary, which was half normal size. The pituitary contained no fibrosis but the glandular elements were reduced and the acidophils were less granular than normal. The patient had had amenorrhoea for the preceding 6 months.

This single case highlights the typical features of autoimmune hypophysitis revealed by subsequent reports, namely the association with other autoimmune endocrinopathies, the onset of symptoms during the postpartum period and the difficulty in making the diagnosis, as witnessed by the frequently fatal nature of the condition. The disease appears rare, given the number of patients reported (Table 7.1). However, in view of the severity of symptoms with which the majority of known patients have presented, usually the result either of a mass compressing the optic chiasm or of hypopituitarism, it would not be surprising if milder forms of the condition are more common than recognised so far. This is particularly so for women in the postpartum period. If the autoimmune response against the pituitary mirrors that against the thyroid, then transient forms of hypophysitis might be expected, although it must be said that several patients have developed symptoms in the last trimester, possibly because the pituitary normally enlarges during pregnancy. This association with pregnancy also begs the question as to whether any cases of Sheehan's syndrome (hypopituitarism resulting from ischaemic pituitary necrosis, usually ascribed to blood loss and hypotension around the time of delivery) are in fact the result of pituitary autoimmunity.

Only two men with autoimmune hypophysitis have so far been reported and in one nulliparous woman the disorder presented at 74 years old (Table 7.1). Little is known of the immunogenetics of the disorder. One patient tested was found to be HLA-DR1,5 (Guay et al., 1987) and in two others the class I, II and III genes were shared, DR types being 4, 7 and 4, 13 (Pestell, Best & Alford, 1990). The pituitary enlargement can be confined to the sella or may give rise to parasellar or suprasellar extension. Hyperprolactinaemia has been reported in several patients, sometimes sufficient to result in galactorrhoea (Quencer, 1980; Asa et al., 1981; Portocarrero et al., 1981; Cebelin et al., 1981; Mazzone, Kelly & Ensinck, 1983). This is presumably the result of stalk compression, preventing the normal dopaminergic inhibition of prolactin secretion. In two cases, selective ACTH deficiency was associated with hypophysitis (Richtsmeier et al., 1980; Jensen et al., 1986) and this will be discussed in detail below. Complete recovery of pituitary function has been recorded in one patient within a year of transphenoidal biopsy (McGrail et al., 1987).

In the other patients, the pituitary appears to have failed generally, accompanied by a diffuse and follicular lymphocytic infiltrate which usually occupies 10–20% of the gland. This was characterised in one study as being a mixture of $CD4^+$ and $CD8^+$ T cells, with B cells present in well-defined follicles (Jensen et al., 1986). There may be a minor degree of lymphocytic infiltration even in apparently normal pituitary tissue and as many as 43% of glands show this at routine post-mortem (Shanklin, 1951). However, in the patients reported with hypophysitis, the infiltrate is much more extensive than this. It remains unclear whether the frequent presence of lymphocytes in the normal pituitary has any pathological significance. In none of the cases in Table 7.1 were granulomata observed. This is an important diagnostic point since the obscure entity of intrasellar giant-cell granuloma can mimic the presentation of lymphocytic hypophysitis, but the histological appearance includes giant cells as well as a lymphocytic infiltrate (Del Pozo *et al.*, 1980). Confusing the distinction are reports of granulomatous hypophysitis in women who also had lymphocytic adrenalitis and/or thyroiditis; (Kler & Norgaard, 1969; Ludmerer & Kissane, 1984), so that some of these cases may have an autoimmune aetiology.

Pituitary autoantibodies

Circulating pituitary antibodies have been sought in only six cases of lymphocytic hypophysitis. By indirect immunofluorescence using normal human pituitary tissue sections, these could not be detected in five patients (Asa *et al.*, 1981; Jensen *et al.*, 1986; Guay *et al.*, 1987; Pestell *et al.*, 1990). A low titre of antibodies staining all anterior pituitary cell types was found in the sixth patient, but direct immunofluorescence failed to reveal any immunoglobulin bound to the pituitary cells of the diseased gland (Mayfield *et al.*, 1980).

In contrast to this rather poor detection rate in patients with florid lymphocytic hypophysitis, pituitary antibodies were reported in as many as 18% of healthy women one week postpartum, although the same patients were negative for these antibodies before delivery; a single patient with Sheehan's syndrome also had high levels of these antibodies (Engelberth & Jezkova, 1965). This study measured antibodies by a complement consumption assay and does not appear to have been followed up, although I have been unable to detect any significant antibody binding to human pituitary membranes by ELISA in sequential sera from 50 women with postpartum thyroiditis (Weetman, unpublished data). Immunofluorescence techniques have been used in all other studies on pituitary antibodies; these methods generally have proved difficult to perform and to quantitate accurately.

Autoantibodies to the surface and cytoplasm of prolactin-secreting cells were found by indirect double immunofluorescence on pituitary sections in 6.6% of 287 patients with a variety of autoimmune disorders, particularly in those with hypoparathyroidism associated with polyendocrine autoimmunity (Bottazzo *et al.*, 1975). There were no clinical features to suggest pituitary dysfunction in patients with these antibodies, although subsequently two hypopituitary patients were found to have antibodies binding to lactotrophs (Bottazzo & Doniach, 1978). The quality of the pituitary used to provide sections for this assay seems critical, reactivity being clearest using specimens obtained at hypophysectomy for breast cancer. Another methodological problem is the non-specific binding of immunoglobulins to ACTH-secreting cells, thought to be mediated by Fc receptors on the cell surface (Pouplard *et al.*, 1976).

Table 7.1. *Summary of clinical details in patients with autoimmune hypophysitis*

Authors	Sex	Age	Presentation	Other autoimmune disorders
Goudie & Pinkerton (1962)	F	22	Fatal hypopituitarism; 14 mo postpartum	Hashimoto's thyroiditis
Hume & Roberts (1967)	F	74	Fatal hypopituitarism	Pernicious anaemia; focal thyroiditis
Egloff, Fischbacher & von Groumoens (1969)	F	29	Fatal hypopituitarism; 1 year postpartum	None
Lack (1975)	F	42	Fatal hypopituitarism	Parathyroid lymphocytic infiltrate
Gleason, Stebbins & Shanahan (1978)	F	49	Fatal hypopituitarism	None
Mayfield et al. (1980)	F	23	Hypopituitarism; 7 mo postpartum	None
Quencer (1980)	F	25	Galactorrhoea; 5 mo postpartum	None (increased serum IgG)
Richtsmeier et al. (1980)	F	31	Fatal selective ACTH deficiency; 1 mo postpartum	Lymphocytic thyroiditis
Asa et al. (1981)	F	28	Visual failure; pregnant at 6 mo	None
	F	29	Hypopituitarism; 6 mo postpartum	None

Reference	Sex	Age	Presentation	Associated conditions
Cebelin et al. (1981)	F	22	Galactorrhoea; 14 mo postpartum	None
Portocarrero et al. (1981)	F	25	Headache; 5 mo postpartum	None
Baskin et al. (1982)	F	33	Visual failure; pregnant at 8 mo	None
	F	28	Visual failure; 1 mo postpartum	None
Hungerford et al. (1982)	F	27	Visual failure + hypopituitarism; 1 mo postpartum	None
Mazzone, Kelly & Ensinck (1983)	F	37	Hypopituitarism; 2 mo postpartum	Pernicious anaemia
Sobrinho-Simoes et al. (1985)	F	24	Fatal hypopituitarism; 26 mo postpartum	Lymphocytic thyroiditis and adrenalitis
Jensen et al. (1986)	F	32	Selective ACTH deficiency; 3 mo postpartum	Possible transient thyroiditis
Guay et al. (1987)	M	52	Hypopituitarism	Positive anti-nuclear antibodies
Meichner et al. (1987)	F	24	Visual failure; 2 wk post-partum	Positive smooth muscle antibodies
McGrail et al. (1987)	F	27	Visual failure; 1 wk post-partum	None
Pestell et al. (1990)	F	22	Visual failure; 27 wk gestation	None
	M	61	Hypopituitarism	Positive anti-parietal cell antibodies

Guinea pig pituitary seems to be a suitable alternative substrate and antibodies binding to this material have been found in 44% of 54 patients with a variety of idiopathic and acquired pituitary hormone deficiencies, compared to 4.7% of 42 controls and 7.8% of 51 patients with autoimmune endocrinopathies (Pouplard, 1982). These antibodies were IgG, fixed complement and, in some patients, bound to particular types of anterior pituitary cells that correlated with the type of hormone deficiency. In addition, two children have been described with growth retardation in whom antibodies against somatotrophs were detected by indirect double immunofluorescence (Bottazzo & Doniach, 1978; Bottazzo et al., 1980). One had Turner's syndrome, in which the prevalence of thyroid autoimmunity is increased and the mother of the other child had thyroiditis and Addison's disease. Pituitary antibodies, detected using transformed rodent cell lines secreting ACTH or prolactin, were found in 78% of selected patients with primary empty sella syndrome (Komatsu et al., 1988).

Several other patient populations have been tested for pituitary antibodies. Of 52 children with cryptorchidism, 48% were positive for antibodies against gonadotrophs and these were also found in five of 12 mothers who had affected children, indicating possible transplacental transfer as a pathogenic mechanism for this congenital problem (Pouplard-Barthelaix et al., 1984). Using rat and porcine pituitary, antibody binding to lactotrophs and/or somatotrophs was found in sera from 14 of 22 patients with untreated Graves' disease (Hansen et al., 1989). In type 1 diabetes mellitus, 16.6% of patients with recent onset disease were positive for pituitary antibodies, in contrast to only 2% with long-standing diabetes (Mirakian et al., 1982). However, the antibodies in the diabetic patients were generally of low titre and stained a wide variety of pituitary cells. These results were confirmed in another study using rat rather than human tissue, with 22% of diabetic patients positive (Sugiura et al., 1986). In the same report, 10 of 21 patients with isolated ACTH deficiency were found initially to have pituitary antibodies, although in eight the reactivity was absorbed out by rat liver acetone powder, suggesting a non-specific reactivity.

Isolated ACTH deficiency is rare but, when reported, has frequently been associated with other autoimmune endocrinopathies such as type 1 diabetes mellitus (Giustina et al., 1988), Graves' disease (Stephens et al., 1985) and polyglandular autoimmunity (Kojima, Nejima & Ogata, 1982). There are also two cases previously mentioned in which ACTH deficiency was associated with lymphocytic hypophysitis (Richtsmeier et al., 1980; Jensen et al., 1986). In a recently studied patient, corticotroph antibodies were detected which reacted specifically with the secretory granules but not with ACTH or its precursors (Sauter et al., 1990). Corticotroph destruction could result from complement fixation or be ADCC-mediated by these antibodies; alternatively the antibodies could affect processing or secretion of ACTH.

However, no actual effector mechanism has yet been proven in this or any other form of pituitary autoimmunity.

Hormone secretion by the posterior lobe of the pituitary depends on hormone transported from the hypothalamus; using sections of human hypothalamus in indirect double immunofluorescence assays, antibodies against vasopressin-producing cells were detected in 11 of 30 patients with idiopathic diabetes insipidus, seven of whom also had other forms of endocrine autoimmunity (Scherbaum & Bottazzo, 1983). One patient, a 74 year old man with a four month history of diabetes insipidus, has been described who had a predominantly T cell lymphocytic infiltration of the infundibulum, stalk and posterior lobe of the pituitary with loss of vasopressin-containing neurones (Kojima et al., 1989). Antibodies were not assayed but the case does suggest that autoimmune processes may be involved in some patients with this condition.

Summary

There is good experimental and clinical evidence for pituitary autoimmunity. This seems particularly likely to occur during or after pregnancy, which may relate to the increased size and vascularity of the gland at this time. Lymphocytic hypophysitis usually presents as a pituitary mass causing generalised hypopituitarism or chiasmal compression and treatment is directed at relieving the mass effect and anterior pituitary hormone replacement. There is no obvious way of making the diagnosis except at surgery. In particular, pituitary antibodies have only been detected in one of four patients examined. This contrasts with the frequent occurrence of such antibodies in a wide variety of other conditions, often in association with more conventional autoimmune endocrinopathies. By analogy with experimental models, one wonders if some of these antibodies may be the result of viral infections. In diabetes mellitus and Graves' disease they seem to have little pathological effect. Therefore it is difficult to assert that pituitary antibodies have an aetiological role in other conditions such as cryptorchidism, short stature and diabetes insipidus, their presence as a secondary phenomenon being an equally likely possibility. Isolated ACTH deficiency may be an exception, particularly since there is a known association with lymphocytic hypophysitis. Further studies of pituitary antibodies are required, aimed at developing robust, homologous assays for population studies, identifying the autoantigens recognised and analysing possible pathophysiological effects. If these antibodies do act as markers for lymphocytic hypophysitis, it may then be possible to estimate the real prevalence of this disorder.

References

Asa, S.L., Bilbao, J.M., Kovacs, K., Josse, R.G. & Kreines, K. (1981). Lymphocytic hypophysitis of pregnancy resulting in hypopituitarism: a distinct clinicopathologic entity. *Annals of Internal Medicine*, **95**, 166–71.

Baskin, D.S., Townsend, J.J. & Wilson, C.B. (1982). Lymphocytic adenohypophysitis of pregnancy simulating a pituitary adenoma: a distinct pathological entity. Report of two cases. *Journal of Neurosurgery*, **56**, 148–53.

Beutner, E.H., Djanian, A. & Witebsky, E. (1964). Serological studies on rabbit antibodies to the anterior pituitary. *Immunology*, **7**, 172–81.

Bottazzo, G.F., Pouplard, A., Florin-Christensen, A. & Doniach, D. (1975). Autoantibodies to prolactin-secreting cells of human pituitary. *Lancet*, **ii**, 97–101.

Bottazzo, G.F. & Doniach, D. (1978). Pituitary autoimmunity: a review. *Journal of the Royal Society of Medicine*, **71**, 433–6.

Bottazzo, G.F., McIntosh, C., Stanford, W. & Preece, M. (1980). Growth hormone cell antibodies and partial growth hormone deficiency in a girl with Turner's syndrome. *Clinical Endocrinology*, **12**, 1–9.

Cebelin, M.S., Velasco, M.E., De Las Mulas, J.M. & Druet, R.L. (1981). Galactorrhea associated with lymphocytic adenohypophysitis. Case report. *British Journal of Obstetrics and Gynaecology*, **88**, 675–80.

Del Pozo, J.M., Roda, J.E., Montoya, J.G., Iglesias, J.R. & Hurtado, A. (1980). Intrasellar granuloma. Case report. *Journal of Neurosurgery*, **53**, 717–19.

Egloff, B., Fischbacher, W. & von Groumoens, E. (1969). Lymphomatose hypophysitis mit hypophysenin-suffizieng. *Schweizerische Medizinische Wochenschrift*, **99**, 1499–502.

Engelberth, O. & Jezkova, Z. (1965). Autoantibodies in Sheehan's syndrome. *Lancet*, **i**, 1075.

Giustina, A., Candrina, R., Cimino, A. & Romanelli, G. (1988). Development of isolated ACTH deficiency in a man with type I diabetes mellitus. *Journal of Endocrinological Investigation*, **11**, 373–7.

Gleason, T.H., Stebbins, P.L. & Shanahan, M.F. (1978). Lymphoid hypophysitis in a patient with hypoglycemic episodes. *Archives of Pathology and Laboratory Medicine*, **102**, 46–8.

Goudie, R.B. & Pinkerton, P.H. (1962). Anterior hypophysitis and Hashimoto's disease in a young woman. *Journal of Pathology and Bacteriology*, **83**, 584–5.

Guay, A.T., Agnello, V., Tronic, B.C., Gresham, D.G. & Freidberg, S.R. (1987). Lymphocytic hypophysitis in a man. *Journal of Clinical Endocrinology and Metabolism*, **64**, 631–4.

Hansen, B.L., Hedgedus, L., Hansen, G.N., Hagen, C., Hansen, J.M. & Hoier-Madsen, M. (1989). Pituitary-cell autoantibody diversity in sera from patients with untreated Graves' disease. *Autoimmunity*, **5**, 49–57.

Hume, R. & Roberts, G.H. (1967). Hypophysitis and hypopituitarism: report of a case. *British Medical Journal*, **2**, 548–50.

Hungerford, G.D., Biggs, P.J., Levine, J.H., Shelley, B.E., Perot, P.L. & Chambers, J.K. (1982). Lymphoid adenohypophysitis with radiologic and clinical findings resembling a pituitary tumour. *American Journal of Neuroradiology*, **3**, 444–6.

Jensen, M.D., Handwerger, B.S., Scheithauer, B.W., Carpenter, P.C., Mirakian, R. & Banks, P.M. (1986). Lymphocytic hypophysitis with isolated corticotropin deficiency. *Annals of Internal Medicine*, **105**, 200–3.

Kler, W. & Norgaard, J.O. (1969). Granulomatous hypophysitis and thyroiditis with lymphocytic adrenalitis. *Acta Pathologica et Microbiologica Scandanavica*, **76**, 229–38.

Kojima, I., Nejima, I. & Ogata, E. (1982). Isolated adrenocorticotropin deficiency associated with polyglandular failure. *Journal of Clinical Endocrinology and Metabolism*, **54**, 182–6.

Kojima, H., Nojima, T., Nagashima, K., Kudo, M. & Ishikura, M. (1989). Diabetes insipidus caused by lymphocytic infundibulo-neurohypophysitis. *Archives of Pathology and Laboratory Medicine*, **113**, 1399–401.

Komatsu, M., Kondo, T., Yamauchi, K., Yokokawa, N., Ichikawa, K., Ishihara, M., Aizawa, T., Yamada, T., Imai, Y., Tanaka, K., Taniguchi, K., Watanabe, T. & Takahashi, Y. (1988). Antipituitary antibodies in patients with the primary empty sella syndrome. *Journal of Clinical Endocrinology and Metabolism*, **67**, 633–8.

Lack, E. (1975). Lymphoid 'hypophysitis' with end organ insufficiency. *Archives of Pathology*, **99**, 215–19.

Levine, S. (1967). Allergic adenohypophysitis: new experimental disease of the pituitary gland. *Science*, **158**, 1190–1.

Ludmerer, K.M., & Kissane, J.M. (1984). Primary hypothyroidism and hypopituitarism in a young woman. *American Journal of Medicine*, **77**, 319–30.

Mayfield, R.K., Levine, J.H., Gordon, L., Powers, J., Galbraith, R.M. & Rawe, S.E. (1980). Lymphoid adenohypophysitis presenting as a pituitary tumour. *American Journal of Medicine*, **69**, 619–23.

Mazzone, T., Kelly, W. & Ensinck, J. (1983). Lymphocytic hypophysitis associated with antiparietal cell antibodies and vitamin B12 deficiency. *Archives of Internal Medicine*, **143**, 1794–5.

McGrail, K.M., Beyerl, B.D., Black, P.M., Klibanski, A. & Zervas, N.T. (1987). Lymphocytic adenohypophysitis of pregnancy with complete recovery. *Neurosurgery*, **20**, 791–3.

Meichner, R., Riggio, S., Manz, H.J. & Earll, J.M. (1987). Lymphocytic hypophysitis causing pituitary mass. *Neurology*, **37**, 158–61.

Mirakian, R., Cudworth, A.G., Bottazzo, G.F. Richardson, C.A. & Doniach, D. (1982). Autoimmunity to anterior pituitary cells and the pathogenesis of insulin-dependent diabetes mellitus. *Lancet*, **i**, 755–8.

Onodera, T., Toniolo, A., Ray, U.R., Jenson, A.B., Knazek, R.A. & Notkins, A.L. (1981). Virus-induced diabetes mellitus. XX. Polyendocrinopathy and autoimmunity. *Journal of Experimental Medicine*, **153**, 1457–73.

Onodera, T., Ray, U.R., Melez, K.A., Suzuki, H., Toniolo, A. & Notkins, A.L. (1982). Virus-induced diabetes mellitus: autoimmunity and polyendocrine disease prevented by immunosuppression. *Nature*, **297**, 66–9.

Pestell, R.G., Best, J.D. & Alford, F.P. (1990). Lymphocytic hypophysitis. The clinical spectrum of the disorder and evidence for an autoimmune pathogenesis. *Clinical Endocrinology*, **33**, 457–66.

Portocarrero, C.J., Robinson, A.G., Taylor, A.L. & Klein, I. (1981). Lymphoid hypophysitis. An unusual cause of hyperprolactinemia and enlarged sella turcica. *Journal of the American Medical Association*, **246**, 1811–12.

Pouplard, A. (1982). Pituitary autoimmunity. *Hormone Research*, **16**, 289–97

Pouplard, A., Bottazzo, G.F., Doniach, D. & Roitt, I.M. (1976). Binding of human immunoglobulins to pituitary ACTH cells. *Nature*, **261**, 142–4.

Pouplard-Barthelaix, A., Lepinard, V., Luxembourger, L., Rohmer, V., Berthelot, J. & Bigorgne, J.C. (1984). Circulating pituitary autoantibodies against cells secreting luteinising and follicle stimulating hormones in children with cryptorchidism. *Lancet*, **ii**, 631–2.

Quencer, R.M. (1980). Lymphocytic adenohypophysitis: autoimmune disorder of the pituitary gland. *American Journal of Neuroradiology*, **1**, 343–5.

Richtsmeier, A.J., Henry, R.A., Bloodworth, J.M.B. & Ehrlich, E.N. (1980). Lymphoid hypophysitis with selective adrenocorticotropic hormone deficiency. *Archives of Internal Medicine*, **140**, 1243–5.

Sauter, N.P., Toni, R., McLaughlin, C.D., Dyess, E.M., Kritzman, J. & Lechan, R.M. (1990). Isolated adrenocorticotropin deficiency associated with an autoantibody to a corticotroph antigen that is not adrenocorticotropin or other proopiomelanocortin-derived peptides. *Journal of Clinical Endocrinology and Metabolism*, **70**, 1391–7.

Scherbaum, W.A. & Bottazzo, G.F. (1983). Autoantibodies to vasopressin cells in idiopathic diabetes insipidus: evidence for an autoimmune variant. *Lancet*, **i**, 897–901.

Shanklin, W.M. (1951). Lymphocytes and lymphoid tissue in the human pituitary. *Anatomical Record*, **111**, 177–91.

Sobrinho-Simoes, M., Brandao, A., Paiva, M.E., Vilela, B., Fernandes, E. & Carneiro-Chaves, F. (1985). Lymphoid hypophysitis in a patient with lymphoid thyroiditis, lymphoid adrenalitis, and idiopathic retroperitoneal fibrosis. *Archives of Pathology and Laboratory Medicine*, **109**, 230–3.

Srinivasappa, J., Saegusa, J., Prabhakar, B.S., Gentry, M.K., Buchmeier, M.J., Wiktor, T.J., Koprowski, H., Oldstone, M.B.A. & Notkins, A.L. (1986). Molecular mimicry: frequency of reactivity of monoclonal antiviral antibodies with normal tissues. *Journal of Virology*, **57**, 397–401.

Stephens, W.P., Goddard, K.J., Laing, I. & Adams, J.E. (1985). Isolated adrenocorticotrophin deficiency and empty sella associated with hypothyroidism. *Clinical Endocrinology*, **22**, 771–6.

Sugiura, M., Hashimoto, A., Shizawa, M., Tsukada, M., Maruyama, S., Ishido, T., Kasahara, T. & Hirata, Y. (1986). Heterogeneity of anterior pituitary cell antibodies detected in insulin-dependent diabetes mellitus and adrenocorticotropic hormone deficiency. *Diabetes Research*, **3**, 111–14.

Triplett, E. (1962). On the mechanism of immunologic self recognition. *Journal of Immunology*, **89**, 505–10.

Note added in proof

Three further women with lymphocytic hypophysitis have been described with visual failure or hypopituitarism presenting within 6 months of delivery; none had concurrent autoimmune disorders. (Cosman, F., Post, K.D., Haub, D.A. & Wardlow, S.L. (1989). Lymphocytic hypophysitis. Report of 3 new cases and review of the literature. *Medicine*, **68**, 240–56.)

–8–

Polyendocrine autoimmunity

In the preceding chapters, frequent reference has been made to the concurrence of autoimmune endocrine diseases and the two main polyendocrine syndromes are considered in this section. The Type 1 syndrome comprises patients who have at least two of the triad of Addison's disease, hypoparathyroidism and chronic mucocutaneous candidiasis, whereas the term Type 2 syndrome was originally proposed to replace the eponymous Schmidt's syndrome, in which Addison's disease is associated with thyroid disease and/or type 1 diabetes (Neufeld, Maclaren & Blizzard, 1981). The Type 3 syndrome covered patients with thyroiditis plus any other endocrinopathy excluding Addison's disease, but these patients are now usually included in the Type 2 group. In addition, two unusual clusters of autoimmune disorders with endocrine importance exist: the POEMS syndrome and Type B insulin resistance.

Experimental polyendocrine autoimmunity

Immunisation with antigens from one endocrine organ only results in an autoimmune response against the target gland. Similarly, neonatal thymectomy in appropriate strains of mice usually produces only a single autoimmune disorder, but reconstitution of athymic nude mice with normal, Lyt-1-depleted spleen cells induces oophoritis in 50% of the recipients, with coincident gastritis or thyroiditis in a small proportion of these (Sakaguchi *et al.*, 1985). These three disorders, plus adrenalitis and insulitis, were also seen in various combinations in mice given cyclosporin A from birth and thymectomised on day 7 (Sakaguchi & Sakaguchi, 1989). Such results obviously suggest that polyendocrine autoimmunity results from a more profound T cell disturbance (intolerance or suppression) than that required for single organ disease in the same immunogenetically susceptible strain.

Spontaneous endocrine autoimmunity may involve several glands. The OS chicken develops antibodies to adrenal and gastric antigens but clinical disease does not result (Khoury *et al.*, 1982). Diabetic BB rats frequently have coincident thyroiditis and antibodies to gastric mucosa have been

Table 8.1. *Components of the type 1 polyendocrine autoimmunity syndrome[a]*

	Neufeld *et al.* (1981) ($n = 71$)	Ahonen *et al.* (1988) ($n = 45$)
Major components		
Addison's disease	100%[b]	78%
Hypoparathyroidism	76%	84%
Chronic mucocutaneous candidiasis	73%	100%
Minor components		
Ovarian failure	17%	58%[c]
Alopecia	32%	35%
Vitiligo	8%	28%
Diabetes mellitus	4%	13%
Pernicious anaemia	13%	13%

[a] Other features include keratopathy and hypoplasia of dental enamel and nails.
[b] Patients were selected for study because they had Addison's disease.
[c] Of women.

found in some animals, but adrenal, gonadal and pituitary autoantibodies have not been detected (Yale & Marliss, 1984). Thyroiditis and salivary gland lymphocytic infiltration (resembling Sjögren's syndrome) occur in a small proportion of diabetic NOD mice but there is no evidence of adrenalitis or hypophysitis (Pontesilli *et al.*, 1987). Viruses can also produce a polyendocrinopathy in mice but the pattern of disease is not typical of the human syndromes, particularly as the autoantibodies are against hormones or cross-react with several target organs (Onodera *et al.*, 1981; Haspel *et al.*, 1983).

Type 1 polyendocrine autoimmunity

This is a rare syndrome, usually recognised in childhood by the coincidence of chronic mucocutaneous candidiasis and hypoparathyroidism (peak age of onset at 5 years), followed 5–10 years later by Addison's disease (Neufeld *et al.*, 1981; Eisenbarth & Jackson, 1981). Other autoimmune disorders occur in these patients (Table 8.1). The inheritance appears to be autosomal recessive and is not linked to HLA genes (Wirfalt, 1981; Eisenbarth & Jackson, 1981; Maclaren & Riley, 1986). One problem in these studies is incomplete penetrance; family members may show only one or two components of the syndrome at the time of analysis yet develop other features subsequently. In one group of 34 families with members rather older than previously reported, there appeared to be an association of hypoparathyroidism and diabetes with HLA-A28, but the absence of any DR association was confirmed (Ahonen *et al.*, 1988). Linkage of disease to genes in the HLA region was excluded by sib-pair analysis, and it is therefore possible that HLA-A28 (and other genes) may modify the expression of the syndrome initiated by a gene whose location is currently unknown.

There are very few reports of the histology of parathyroid tissue in autoimmune hypoparathyroidism, although hyperplastic parathyroiditis, resembling Hashimoto's thyroiditis, has been found at routine post-mortem (Irvine & Barnes, 1975; Boyce, Doherty & Mortimer, 1982). In three patients with chronic mucocutaneous candidiasis (one each with concurrent diabetes or Addison's disease), there was general cutaneous anergy by skin testing with multiple antigens including *Candida*, yet *in vitro* the T cells from these individuals proliferated in response to *Candida* (Chilgren *et al.*, 1969). This suggests that some defect in T cell effector function is responsible for the candidiasis component of the syndrome. Non-specific abnormalities of circulating suppressor T cell function, defined by measuring the proliferative response to concanavalin A, have been demonstrated in two patients and a clinically normal sibling (Arulanantham, Dwyer & Genel, 1979).

Antibodies to adrenal and parathyroid tissue have been detected by indirect immunofluorescence in type 1 syndrome patients (Blizzard, Chee & Davies, 1966; Ahonen, Miettinen & Perheentupa, 1987), although those against the parathyroid have proved difficult to detect in other studies (Irvine & Barnes, 1975). Adrenal antibodies were associated with steroidal cell antibodies in more than 90% of patients, in contrast to the frequent occurrence of adrenal antibodies alone in other forms of Addison's disease (Chapter 5). These antibodies preceded and closely correlated with the development of adrenal and ovarian failure in patients followed sequentially (Ahonen *et al.*, 1987).

Antibodies which lysed bovine parathyroid cells in the presence of complement were detected in seven patients with autoimmune hypoparathyroidism, comprising four individuals with additional mucocutaneous candidiasis with or without Addison's disease and three related individuals (mother and twins) with isolated hypoparathyroidism (Brandi *et al.*, 1986). These antibodies appeared to cross-react with adrenal tissue. Subsequent studies with sera from six of these patients (excluding the mother of the twins) identified an IgM antibody which reacted with bovine endothelium by immunofluorescence (Fattorossi *et al.*, 1988). There was only variable and weak reactivity of these sera with human parathyroid tissue. It was postulated that the endothelial antigen was transferred to parathyroid cells *in vitro* to account for the previous results.

Isolated autoimmune hypoparathyroidism is a rare entity that has received little attention: most patients with this condition have an associated

Table 8.2. *Components of the type 2 polyendocrine autoimmunity syndrome*

	Frequency in patients with Addison's disease plus the type 2 syndrome[a]
Addison's disease	100%
Autoimmune thyroid disease	69%
Type 1 diabetes mellitus	52%
Gonadal failure	4%
Vitiligo	5%
Alopecia	1%
Pernicious anaemia	<1%
Myasthenia gravis	ND[b]
Coeliac disease	ND
Autoimmune hypophysitis	ND

[a]Data from Neufeld *et al.* (1981), who analysed reports of 224 patients with Addison's disease plus another endocrinopathy; results would be different if thyroid disease or diabetes were chosen as the index disorder.
[b]Not determined; these disorders are probably associated with the type 2 syndrome.

endocrinopathy and usually present at an early age. However, it is possible that remitting forms of the disease exist, making identification difficult. In eight of 23 patients with idiopathic hypoparathyroidism, serum antibodies were detected which reacted by immunofluorescence with dispersed human parathyroid cells or parathyroid sections (Posillico *et al.*, 1986). Two of these patients also had adrenal antibodies. The sera from three subjects (two men: age range 56–76) inhibited parathyroid hormone secretion by parathyroid cells *in vitro*. In one subject the antibodies and clinical course fluctuated. Thus parathyroid autoantibodies may have a primary role in the pathogenesis of sporadic and polyendocrinopathy-associated hypoparathyroidism by causing cytotoxicity and by inhibiting gland function.

Type 2 polyendocrine autoimmunity

The occurrence of two or more of the endocrinopathies detailed in Table 8.2 constitutes evidence for this syndrome in a patient. Family members usually differ in their individual spectra of endocrinopathies and associated disorders. In keeping with the sporadic diseases, the mean age of onset is usually around the fourth decade except for diabetes. Vitiligo, alopecia and pernicious anaemia are also frequently found, as well as other less common autoimmune disorders (Neufeld *et al.*, 1981). Early reports do not mention autoimmune hypophysitis as part of the type 2 syndrome. However, as discussed in Chapter 7, several patients with lymphocytic hypophysitis or isolated ACTH deficiency presumed to be caused by autoimmunity have other endocrinopathies, which suggests that this is truly a feature of the syndrome, albeit rare. In addition, two men with Addison's disease (one of whom also had primary myxoedema) have been reported with isolated gonadotroph failure, which was postulated to be the result of autoimmune hypophysitis (Barkan, Kelch & Marshall, 1985).

There seems nothing to distinguish the autoimmune responses against the target organs in this syndrome from those occurring in the common sporadic forms. However, the HLA-B8, -DR3 haplotype is more frequent in these patients than in those with the individual components of the syndrome, with a relative risk of up to 48 (Eisenbarth & Jackson, 1981; Maclaren & Riley, 1986). Ascertainment bias, sex differences and incomplete penetrance affect studies on the mode of inheritance, but the high prevalence of disease in parents and evidence from a proportion of families suggest a dominant pattern. It seems likely that the various components of the syndrome are modified by other genes, such as those linked to HLA-DR2 and -DR4 in diabetes and pernicious anaemia respectively (Chapter 4; Ungar et al., 1981). In addition, non-MHC genes and environmental factors probably affect disease expression.

Other HLA-DR3-associated autoimmune diseases are not conventionally regarded as part of the type 2 syndrome, including SLE, Sjögren's syndrome, dermatitis herpetiformis and chronic active hepatitis, but thyroid autoimmunity is more frequent in these disorders (Doniach et al., 1966; Ayala et al., 1979; Weetman & Walport, 1987; Weetman et al., 1988). It is likely that these clusters are due to the increased chance of concurrence with possession of DR3 haplotypes. Autoimmune thyroid disease and type 1 diabetes are common and only a small proportion of these patients will have the polyendocrine syndrome. In a survey of 1779 patients with type 1 diabetes mellitus, 5.7% had autoimmune thyroid disease, 0.45% pernicious anaemia and only 0.11% Addison's disease (Nabarro et al., 1979). However, for patients with Addison's disease, the prevalence of associated premature ovarian failure is 20–25%, thyroid disease 15–20% and type 1 diabetes 8–20% (Eisenbarth & Jackson, 1981). Therefore all patients with Addison's disease should be followed up to detect the occurrence of the type 2 polyendocrine syndrome, whereas this is not indicated in patients with thyroid autoimmunity or diabetes.

There appear to be further polyendocrine syndromes, which are variants of the type 1 and type 2 forms and two recent examples illustrate this. The first is the association of hyperthyroidism and hypoparathyroidism in four separate patients, one with Down's syndrome in addition (Blumberg & AvRuskin, 1987). Secondly, five Persian Jews have been described with primary hypoparathyroidism and hypogonadism; two had Addison's disease, and one each had type 1 diabetes mellitus and hypothyroidism (Shapiro *et al.*, 1987). There appeared to be an association with HLA-DR5.

Type B insulin resistance syndrome

This syndrome is produced by autoantibodies against the insulin receptor and usually causes extremely insulin-resistant diabetes and acanthosis nigricans (Flier *et al.*, 1975). It is very rare (less than 50 cases reported) but in such patients other autoimmune phenomena are frequent. It is more prevalent in women, who have ovarian hyperandrogenism in addition to diabetes, and most cases have been among Blacks. Occasional patients have mild glucose intolerance or hypoglycaemia, presumably caused by antibodies with receptor-stimulating activity (Flier *et al.*, 1978; Taylor *et al.*, 1982, 1989). However, the typical picture is of symptomatic diabetes, mild or absent ketoacidosis, endogenous hyperinsulinaemia and the requirement for massive doses of insulin (over 100 000 units/day in some cases) to control the blood glucose.

Antibodies from these patients are polyclonal, recognise the insulin receptor and impair insulin binding *in vitro* (Flier *et al.*, 1976). A wide range of functional effects are observed on cultured adipocytes and lymphocytes, such antibodies often having transient insulin-like activity followed by the induction of insulin resistance which is probably due to both receptor degradation and an action on post receptor events (Khan *et al.*, 1977; Taylor & Marcus-Samuels, 1984). One patient has been described with atypical antibodies which did not inhibit insulin binding *in vitro* but could be detected by immunoprecipitation of affinity-labelled receptors (Bloise *et al.*, 1989). This means that at least two separate assays are required to exclude completely the presence of insulin receptor autoantibodies.

The other autoimmune features of the syndrome are shown in Table 8.3 (Tsokos *et al.*, 1985). Spontaneous remission has been observed in a few patients; in others, diabetes has proved resistant over years, even to heroic doses of insulin (Flier *et al.*, 1978). Treatment with steroids or plasma exchange has been tried but it is difficult to evaluate the effects of these, given the fluctuation naturally seen in this condition (Flier *et al.*, 1978; Muggeo *et al.*, 1979).

POEMS syndrome

The acronym stands for polyneuropathy, organomegaly (splenomegaly and lymphadenopathy), endocrinopathy, M-proteins (monoclonal gammopathy

Table 8.3. *Autoimmune features in 14 patients with type B insulin resistance syndrome (Tsokos et al., 1985)*

Non-specific abnormalities	Prevalence
Leukopenia	86%
Antinuclear antibodies	86%
Raised erythrocyte sedimentation rate	79%
Raised circulating total IgG	79%
Hypocomplementaemia	29%
Specific disorders[a]	
Systemic lupus erythematosus	36%
Alopecia	36%
Vitiligo	14%
Autoimmune haemolytic anaemia	14%

[a]Sjögrens syndrome, systemic sclerosis and other connective tissue disorders have also been associated.

which is lambda light chain-restricted) and skin changes (hyperpigmentation and thickening; Bardwick *et al.*, 1980). The endocrine disorders include insulin-dependent diabetes mellitus in 50% of cases and gonadal failure in 70%; hypothyroidism, hyperprolactinaemia and adrenal failure are less frequent. Conventional autoantibodies against endocrine organs are not detectable and the aetiology of the syndrome is unknown, but it is possible that some unusual plasma cell product may be the cause.

Summary

Type 2 polyendocrine autoimmunity is reasonably common and seems related to a dominant gene, possibly in linkage disequilibrium with genes on the HLA-B8, -DR3 haplotype. Results in animal models suggest that an extreme form of disordered T cell immunoregulation may be involved. Other genes and environmental factors may modify the expression of the syndrome in individual family members. The Type 1 syndrome is much less common, being inherited as an autosomal recessive disorder; the gene responsible is undefined. However, these patients develop autoimmune adrenal and ovarian failure, associated with autoantibody production which resembles the sporadic forms of these conditions. Could the unknown, non-MHC gene have a role in some conventional cases of Addison's disease? Type B insulin resistance and the POEMS syndrome are extremely rare disorders and the nature of the abnormal immune responses in both remains to be defined.

References

Ahonen, P., Miettinen, A. & Perheentupa, J. (1987). Adrenal and steroidal cell antibodies in patients with autoimmune polyglandular disease type 1 and risk of adrenocortical and ovarian failure. *Journal of Clinical Endocrinology and Metabolism*, **64**, 494–500.

Ahonen, P., Koskimies, S., Lokki, M.-L., Tiilikainen, A. & Perheentupa, J. (1988). The expression of autoimmune polyglandular disease type 1 appears associated with several HLA-A antigens but not with HLA-DR. *Journal of Clinical Endocrinology and Metabolism*, **66**, 1151–7.

Arulanantham, K., Dwyer, J.M. & Genel, M. (1979). Evidence for defective immunoregulation in the syndrome of familial candidiasis endocrinopathy. *New England Journal of Medicine*, **300**, 164–8.

Ayala, A., Canales, E.S., Karchmer, S., Alarcon, D. & Zarate, A. (1979). Premature ovarian failure and hypothyroidism associated with sicca syndrome. *Obstetrics and Gynaecology*, **53** (Suppl. 3), 98S–101S.

Bardwick, P.A., Zvaifler, N.J., Gill, G.N., Newman, D., Greenway, G.D. & Resnick, D.L. (1980). Plasma cell dyscrasia with polyneuropathy, organomegaly, endocrinopathy, M protein, and skin changes: the POEMS Syndrome. *Medicine*, **59**, 311–22.

Barkan, A.L., Kelch, R.P. & Marshall, J.C. (1985). Isolated gonadotroph failure in the polyglandular autoimmune syndrome. *New England Journal of Medicine*, **312**, 1535–40.

Blizzard, R.M., Chee, D. & Davis, W. (1966). The incidence of parathyroid and other antibodies in the sera of patients with idiopathic hypoparathyroidism. *Clinical and Experimental Immunology*, **1**, 119–28.

Bloise, W., Wajchenberg, B.L., Moncada, V.Y., Marcus-Samuels, B. & Taylor, S.I. (1989). Atypical antiinsulin receptor antibodies in a patient with type B insulin resistance and scleroderma. *Journal of Clinical Endocrinology and Metabolism*, **68**, 227–31.

Blumberg, D. & AvRuskin, T. (1987). Down's syndrome, autoimmune hyperthyroidism, and hypoparathyroidism: a unique triad. *American Journal of Diseases of Childhood*, **141**, 1149.

Boyce, B.E., Doherty, V.R. & Mortimer, G. (1982). Hyperplastic parathyroiditis – a new autoimmune disease? *Journal of Clinical Pathology*, **35**, 812–14.

Brandi, M.-L., Aurbach, G.D., Fattorossi, A., Quarto, R., Marx, S.J. & Fitzpatrick, L.A. (1986). Antibodies cytotoxic to bovine parathyroid cells in autoimmune hypoparathyroidism. *Proceedings of the National Academy of Sciences, USA*. **83**, 8366–9.

Childgren, R.A., Meuwissen, H.J., Quie, P.G., Good, R.A. & Hong, R. (1969). The cellular immune defect in chronic mucocutaneous candidiasis. *Lancet*, **i**, 1286–8.

Doniach, D., Roitt, I.M., Walker, J.G. & Sherlock, S. (1966). Tissue antibodies in primary biliary cirrhosis, active chronic (lupoid) hepatitis, cryptogenic cirrhosis and other liver diseases and their clinical implications. *Clinical and Experimental Immunology*, **1**, 237–62.

Eisenbarth, G.S. & Jackson, R.A. (1981). Immunogenetics of polyglandular failure and related diseases. In *HLA in Endocrine and Metabolic Disorders*, ed. N.R. Farid, pp. 235–64. New York: Academic Press.

Fattorossi, A., Aurbach, G.D., Sakaguchi, K., Cama, A., Marx, S.J., Streeten, E.A., Fitzpatrick, L.A. & Brandi, M.L. (1988). Anti-endothelial cell antibodies: detection and characterization in sera from patients with autoimmune hypoparathyroidism. *Proceedings of the National Academy of Sciences, USA*, **85**, 4015–19.

Flier, J.S., Kahn, C.R., Roth, J. & Bar, R.S. (1975). Antibodies that impair insulin receptor binding in an unusual diabetic syndrome with severe insulin resistance. *Science*, **190**, 63–5.

Flier, J.S., Kahn, R.C., Jarrett, D.B. & Roth, J. (1976). Characterization of antibodies to the insulin receptor. A cause of insulin-resistant diabetes in man. *Journal of Clinical Investigation*, **58**, 1442–9.

Flier, J.S., Bar, R.S., Muggeo, M., Khan, C.R., Roth, J. & Gorden, P. (1978). The evolving clinical course of patients with insulin receptor autoantibodies: spontaneous remission or receptor proliferation with hypoglycaemia. *Journal of Clinical Endocrinology and Metabolism*, **47**, 985–95.

Haspel, M.V., Onodera, T., Prabhakar, B.S., Horita, M., Suzuki, H. & Notkins, A.L. (1983). Virus-induced autoimmunity: monoclonal antibodies that react with endocrine tissues. *Science*, **220**, 304–6.

Irvine, W.J. & Barnes, E.W. (1975). Addison's disease, ovarian failure and hypoparathyroidism. *Clinics in Endocrinology and Metabolism*, **4**, 379–434.

Khan, C.R., Baird, K., Flier, J.S. & Jarrett, D.B. (1977). Effects of autoantibodies to the insulin receptor on isolated adipocytes. *Journal of Clinical Investigation*, **60**, 1094–106.

Khoury, E.L., Bottazzo, G.F., Pontes de Carvalho, L.C., Wick, G. & Roitt, I.M. (1982). Predisposition to organ-specific autoimmunity in obese strain (OS) chickens: reactivity to thyroid, gastric, adrenal and pancreatic cytoplasmic antigens. *Clinical and Experimental Immunology*, **49**, 273–82.

Maclaren, N.K. & Riley, W.J. (1986). Inherited susceptibility to autoimmune Addison's disease is linked to human leukocyte antigens-DR3 and/or DR4, except when associated with type 1 autoimmune polyglandular syndrome. *Journal of Clinical Endocrinology and Metabolism*, **62**, 455–9.

Muggeo, M., Flier, J.S., Abrams, R.A., Harrison, L.C., Diesseroth, A.B. & Khan, C.R. (1979). Treatment by plasma exchange of a patient with autoantibodies to the insulin receptor. *New England Journal of Medicine*, **300**, 477–80.

Nabarro, J.D.N., Mustaffa, B.E., Morris, D.V., Walport, M.J. & Kurtz, A.B. (1979). Insulin deficient diabetes: contrasts with other endocrine deficiencies. *Diabetologia*, **16**, 5–12.

Neufeld, M., Maclaren, N.K. & Blizzard, R.M. (1981). Two types of autoimmune Addison's disease associated with different polyglandular autoimmune (PGA) syndromes. *Medicine*, **60**, 355–62.

Onodera, T., Toniolo, A., Ray, U.R., Bennett-Johnson, A., Knazek, R.A. & Notkins, A.L. (1981). Virus-induced diabetes mellitus. XX. Polyendocrinopathy and autoimmunity. *Journal of Experimental Medicine*, **153**, 1457–73.

Pontesilli, O., Carotenuto, P., Gazda, L.S., Pratt, P.F. & Prowse, S.J. (1987). Circulating lymphocyte populations and autoantibodies in non-obese (NOD) mice: a longitudinal study. *Clinical and Experimental Immunology*, **70**, 84–93.

Posillico, J.T., Wortsman, J., Srikanta, S., Eisenbarth, G.S., Mallette, L.W. & Brown E.M. (1986). Parathyroid cell surface autoantibodies that inhibit parathyroid hormone secretion from dispersed human parathyroid cells. *Journal of Bone and Mineral Research*, **1**, 475–83.

Sakaguchi, S., Fukuma, K., Kuribayashi, K. & Masuda, T. (1985). Organ-specific autoimmune diseases induced in mice by elimination of T cell subset. *Journal of Experimental Medicine*, **161**, 72–87.

Sakaguchi, S. & Sakaguchi, N. (1989). Organ-specific autoimmune disease induced in mice by elimination of T cell subsets. *Journal of Immunology*, **142**, 471–80.

Shapiro, M.S., Zamir, R., Weiss, E., Radnay, J. & Shenkman, L. (1987). The polyglandular deficiency syndrome: a new variant in Persian Jews. *Journal of Endocrinological Investigation*, **10**, 1–7.

Taylor, S.I., Grunberger, G., Marcus-Samuels, B., Underhill, L.H., Dons, R.F., Ryan, J., Roddam, R.F., Rupe, C.F. & Gorden, P. (1982). Hypoglycaemia associated with antibodies to the insulin receptor. *New England Journal of Medicine*, **307**, 1422–446.

Taylor, S.I. & Marcus-Samuels, B. (1984). Anti-receptor antibodies mimic the effect of insulin to down-regulate insulin receptors in cultured human lymphoblastoid (IM-9) cells. *Journal of Clinical Endocrinology and Metabolism*, **58**, 182–6.

Taylor, S.I., Barbetti, F., Accili, D., Roth, J. & Gorden, P. (1989). Syndromes of autoimmunity and hypoglycaemia: autoantibodies directed against insulin and its receptor. *Endocrine and Metabolic Clinics of North America*, **18**, 123–43.

Tsokos, G.C., Gorden, P., Antonovych, T., Wilson, C.B. & Balow, J.E. (1985). Lupus nephritis and other autoimmune features in patients with diabetes mellitus due to autoantibody to insulin receptors. *Annals of Internal Medicine*, **102**, 176–81.

Ungar, B., Mathews, J.D., Tait, B.D. & Cowling, D.C. (1981). HLA-DR patterns in pernicious anaemia. *British Medical Journal*, **282**, 768–70.

Weetman, A.P. & Walport, M.J. (1987). The association of autoimmune thyroiditis with systemic lupus erythematosus. *British Journal of Rheumatology*, **26**, 359–61.

Weetman, A.P., Burrin, J.M., MacKay, D., Leonard, J.N., Griffiths, C.E.M. & Fry, L. (1988). The prevalence of thyroid autoantibodies in dermatitis herpetiformis. *British Journal of Dermatology*, **118**, 377–83.

Wirfalt, A. (1981). Genetic heterogeneity in autoimmune polyglandular failure. *Acta Medica Scandinavica*, **210**, 7–13.

Yale, J.F. & Marliss, E.B. (1984). Altered immunity and diabetes in the BB rat. *Clinical and Experimental Immunology*, **57**, 1–11.

Index